Milestones in Drug Therapy

Series Editors

Michael J. Parnham, Fraunhofer IME & Goethe University Frankfurt, Germany
Jacques Bruinvels, Bilthoven, The Netherlands

Series Editors

J.C. Buckingham, Imperial College School of Medicine, London, UK
R.J. Flower, The William Harvey Research Institute, London, UK
A.G. Herman, Universiteit Antwerpen, Antwerp, Belgium
P. Skolnick, National Institute on Drug Abuse, Bethesda, MD, USA

For further volumes:
http://www.springer.com/series/4991

Philipp Y. Maximov • Russell E. McDaniel •
V. Craig Jordan

Tamoxifen

Pioneering Medicine in Breast Cancer

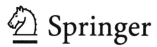 Springer

Philipp Y. Maximov
Russell E. McDaniel
V. Craig Jordan
Lombardi Comprehensive Cancer Center
Georgetown University Medical Center
Washington, DC
USA

ISBN 978-3-0348-0663-3   ISBN 978-3-0348-0664-0 (eBook)
DOI 10.1007/978-3-0348-0664-0
Springer Basel Heidelberg New York Dordrecht London

Library of Congress Control Number: 2013941548

Printed on acid-free paper

Springer is part of Springer Science+Business Media (www.springer.com)

Thanks to all the "Tamoxifen Teams" who translated ideas into lives saved over the past 35 years

With the indispensable assistance of Fadeke Agboke, Puspanjali Bhatta, and Amy Botello

Foreword

I joined the Clinical Research Department of ICI Americas (ICI) in Wilmington, Delaware, in 1973, after competing in the World Championships for Rowing in Moscow, Russia, as a member of the first US women's rowing team. I mention this competition because as I was part of a team who was pioneering the international competition of women's crew, I was among the team at ICI who was pioneering the support and development of "targeted therapies," the first being tamoxifen. The operative word here is *team*. Having previously worked at the National Cancer Institute supporting the Breast Cancer Task Force, I was considered the most qualified individual at the time in the newly formed ICI to plan and organize the clinical investigation of the antiestrogen ICI46,474 in the United States!

I remember asking my director how long it takes to have a drug approved. He told me about 8 years; as a competitor, and not understanding all the aspects of pharmaceutical drug development, I said to myself, "We will do it *four years*." As it is known, the Food and Drug Administration (FDA) approved the labeling for tamoxifen on December 31, 1977, just 4 years and 5 months from the day I was hired. Thinking back over those early years, I recall a number of my colleagues as dedicated individuals who understood the importance of developing tamoxifen— Beverly Bach, Fran Ehrlich, David Sofi, and Bruce Decker—working in clinical research, regulatory affairs, market research, and marketing. Eventually, dozens of staff were all on the mission as a *team* to make tamoxifen available as quickly as possible to those patients who were most likely to benefit.

As you will read throughout this book, the early clinical development of tamoxifen was driven by clinical investigators and scientists in the United States, Canada, and Europe, who devoted their lives to the treatment of patients with breast cancer, such as Pierre Band, Harvey Lerner, and Lucien Israel. In fact, it was Harvey Lerner who demonstrated to Stuart Pharmaceuticals the urgency of continuing to develop this agent when the financial forecast was not compelling.

As you will read, the story of ICI46,474 began with its discovery in the fertility control program at ICI Pharmaceuticals, Alderley Park, Cheshire. It was an excellent morning-after pill in rats, but in fact stimulated ovulation in subfertile women. Although marketed in the United Kingdom for the induction of ovulation, the agent's main focus in the United States was to treat breast cancer. A few small clinical studies of ICI46,474 conducted in Europe had reported modest activity in metastatic breast cancer (Cole et al. *British Journal of Cancer*, 1971;25:270–275 and Ward *British Medical Journal*, 1973;5844:13–14).

In the early 1970s, US clinical trial cooperative groups were focusing on the use of combination cytotoxic chemotherapy with the goal of curing breast cancer. Endocrine therapy was largely viewed as palliative; so there was little possibility that this antiestrogen would make much of an impact in the treatment of metastatic breast cancer or provide reasonable financial returns for investment in clinical studies. Then, in 1973, I met Craig Jordan, one of the few people in the world with a background in, and understanding of, the pharmacology of nonsteroidal antiestrogens. I arranged with my management to provide Craig with an unrestricted research grant at the Worcester Foundation and visited him to discuss the progress as he reinvented the strategic therapeutic use of ICI46,474 to become the drug tamoxifen that we know today. Craig's laboratory studies supported the exclusive use of tamoxifen to treat estrogen receptor (ER)-positive tumors. We used his results, prior to their publication, in our "investigators brochure."

I suggested that Craig become our scientific advisor for tamoxifen and arranged for him to meet the senior leadership of the Eastern Cooperative Oncology Group (ECOG): Doug Tormey, head of the ECOG Breast Committee, and Paul Carbone, chairman of ECOG. ICI Americas continued supporting his research, and in the laboratory, Craig discovered the strategy used today, that of long-term adjuvant tamoxifen therapy specifically targeting ER-positive breast tumors.

Looking at "the good, the bad, and the ugly" of tamoxifen, Craig's laboratory raised the question of whether the agent would increase the incidence of endometrial cancer. It did. This led to the recruitment of gynecologists to the breast cancer patient's care team, an extremely valuable advance at the end of the 1980s, as tamoxifen was about to be tested as a chemopreventive agent in high-risk women.

On a personal note, Craig and I had numerous adventures over the years, coincident with various clinical trial meetings. Here, I relate a story that demonstrates his philosophy of honoring commitment. In 1979, Craig was to be the opening speaker at the tamoxifen meeting in Sorrento, Italy. He was working in Bern, Switzerland, and was scheduled to fly down on an Alitalia flight from Zurich to Naples on the evening before his talk. Craig had to leave Zurich on the last flight that evening, as he had a site visit at the Ludwig Institute for Cancer Research in Bern earlier in the day. Then disaster struck. I learned that Alitalia was to go on strike that evening and urged him to leave Bern at lunch time, if there was to be any hope of his presenting at the meeting. Craig declared, "But I have a room full of site visitors from America—not possible," followed by, "Don't worry, I will be there." After my call, Craig immediately contacted his technician Brigitte Haldemann to drive him through the night over the 730 miles to Sorrento. With an hour to spare and after a shower, he presented his talk.

To this day, tamoxifen remains in the news. The Adjuvant Tamoxifen Longer Against Shorter (ATLAS) trial shows that 10 years of adjuvant tamoxifen is superior to 5 years of tamoxifen (Davies C et al., *Lancet*, 2012; epub 12/12/

2012). The therapeutic strategy is again being tested successfully, but the benefit in decreasing mortality occurs in the second decade after stopping longer-duration tamoxifen. This phenomenon (Wolf D, and Jordan VC, *Recent Results in Cancer Research*, 1993;127:23–33) led to the new biology of estrogen-induced apoptosis.

What happened to chemoprevention? Tamoxifen became the first agent to be approved by the Food and Drug Administration for reduction of breast cancer incidence in high-risk premenopausal and postmenopausal women. In January 2013, the National Institute for Health and Clinical Excellence (NICE) recommended tamoxifen be made available through the National Health Service in the United Kingdom for the chemoprevention of breast cancer.

This book tells the humanistic story of the development of tamoxifen. It is a tribute of gratitude to the tens of thousands of women and men who participated in clinical trials throughout the development of tamoxifen, which is now a therapeutic agent for the prevention as well as the treatment of minimal through advanced stages of breast cancer, depending on the patient's hormonal receptor status. It is also an acknowledgment of hundreds of clinical oncology health teams working to advance our understanding of the biology of breast cancer as well as thousands of clinicians caring for those with breast cancer.

I am amazed and so grateful that so many millions of lives have been extended and many more have benefited from the research and therapeutic strategies retold in this book. I am personally grateful to have played a role, minimal as it was and is, in the development of tamoxifen.

West Conshohocken, PA, USA

Lois Trench-Hines
Founder and Chief Executive Officer
Meniscus Limited

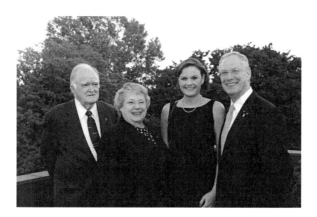

Pictured from *left* to *right*, George Hines, Lois Trench-Hines, Alexandra Jordan-Noel, and V. Craig Jordan. Photographed at a celebration at the Swiss Ambassador's Residence in Washington, DC, to celebrate the award of the St. Gallen Prize for Outstanding Accomplishments in the Adjuvant Treatment of Breast Cancer in 2011

Preface

The story of tamoxifen is unique. This pioneering medicine was not conceived as part of a major development plan in the pharmaceutical industry to create a blockbuster, but rather tamoxifen (ICI46,474) was an orphan product that had failed its first indication as a "morning-after pill." Breast cancer was a consideration, but the company terminated clinical development of the medicine in 1972. The resurrection of the medicine then occurred and, after a period of dismissal by the clinical community in the mid-1970s, successes went from strength to strength.

The success of the product depended upon individuals being in the right place at the right time and a "gentleman's agreement" between industry (ICI Pharmaceuticals Division now AstraZeneca) and academia (Worcester Foundation and the Leeds University) to create a new strategy for the treatment and prevention of breast cancer. The gestation period for that strategy was the whole of the 1970s [1–4]. The principles conceived of targeting the tumor estrogen receptor (ER) and using long-term adjuvant endocrine therapy translated effectively to clinical trials that demonstrated dramatic and lasting reduction in mortality [5]. It is estimated that the hundreds of thousands, perhaps millions, of women are alive today because of the successful translation of research conducted in the 1970s.

Additionally, laboratory research on the prevention of mammary carcinogenesis [2, 3] in animals would translate to successful clinical trials [6–8] with tamoxifen being the first medicine to be approved by the Food and Drug Administration (FDA) for the reduction of the incidence of breast cancer in pre- and postmenopausal women at high risk. Tamoxifen was the first medicine to be approved to reduce the risk for any cancer.

Without the economic success of tamoxifen, there would have been no incentive to develop the aromatase inhibitors for the adjuvant treatment of ER-positive breast cancer in postmenopausal women. Without the study of the "good, the bad, and the ugly" of the tamoxifen, there would be no selective ER modulators (SERMs). The chance finding that tamoxifen and also a failed breast cancer drug keoxifene (to be renamed 5 or 6 years later as raloxifene) would maintain bone density in ovariectomized rats [9] opened the door to the suggestion that

Important clues have been garnered about the effects of tamoxifen on bone and lipids so it is possible that derivatives could find targeted applications to retard osteoporosis or athero-sclerosis. The ubiquitous application of novel compounds to prevent diseases associated with the progressive changes after menopause may, as a side effect, significantly retard the development of breast cancer. [10]

Today, raloxifene is approved by the FDA for the prevention and treatment of osteoporosis in postmenopausal women and for the prevention of breast cancer in high-risk postmenopausal women [11]. However, tamoxifen became the pioneering SERM that switched on or switched off estrogen target sites around a woman's body. This new drug group also led to the idea of now being able to treat diseases via any member of the nuclear hormone receptor superfamily. Specificity would be enhanced and side effects reduced.

This monograph documents the milestones achieved during the curious twists and turns in the development of tamoxifen over the past 40 years. The story starts with the systemic synthesis of nonsteroidal estrogens that through serendipity suddenly gave us the nonsteroidal antiestrogens. The discovery by Leonard Lerner in the 1950s of MER25 (or ethamoxytriphetol) and subsequently clomiphene [10] and the finding that they were antifertility agents in rats [10] aroused the interest of the pharmaceutical industry to develop "morning-after pills." Nonsteroidal antiestrogens, however, were excellent contraceptives in rats but actually induced ovulation in subfertile women. Interest in nonsteroidal antiestrogens waned.

Cancer treatment was a consideration because of the known link between estrogen and the growth of some metastatic breast cancers. However, again there was no real enthusiasm from the pharmaceutical industry. Tamoxifen, after an unlikely start in the 1960s, advanced alone during the 1970s to become the "gold standard" for the antihormone treatment and prevention of breast cancer for the next 20 years. Despite all the "ups and downs" of the story, tamoxifen remains a cheap and effective lifesaving drug around the world. Indeed, the concept first described by our studies in the 1970s that "longer was better" as the treatment strategy for adjuvant therapy with tamoxifen for patients with ER-positive breast cancer continues to go from strength to strength in clinical trial. Ten years of adjuvant therapy is now known to be superior to 5 years of adjuvant therapy, but the profound decrease in mortality occurs during the decade after stopping tamoxifen at 10 years [12]. Again, there is a prediction we made in the 1990s that tamoxifen causes the evolution of drug resistance in the undetected micrometastases that exposes a vulnerability to estrogen-induced apoptosis in the tumor cells [13].

Lois Trench-Hanes generously accepted my invitation to contribute our Fore-word. She was there at the beginning of tamoxifen in the United States and was the one who recruited me, on Arthur Walpole's recommendation, to advance the science and to support clinical development. We had many adventures over the years but her attitude of "get the job done" was essential to the start of this milestone. She was a force to be reckoned with, that through her willingness to see the project succeed for her company by establishing the correct clinical contacts not only propelled tamoxifen forward but helped my career development. She and her husband George are lifelong friends and Lois is a godmother to my youngest daughter Alexandra (see pictures in Lois's Foreword).

This monograph has been put together by my Tamoxifen Team (VCJ) at the Lombardi Comprehensive Cancer Center at Georgetown University, Washington, DC. It is intended to illustrate and document the real journey traveled by this milestone in medicine.

V. Craig Jordan

Russell E. McDaniel

Philipp Y. Maximov

References

1. Jordan VC, Koerner S (1975) Tamoxifen (ICI 46,474) and the human carcinoma 8S oestrogen receptor. Eur J Cancer 11:205–206
2. Jordan VC (1976) Effect of tamoxifen (ICI 46,474) on initiation and growth of DMBA-induced rat mammary carcinomata. Eur J Cancer 12:419–424
3. Jordan VC, Allen KE (1980) Evaluation of the antitumour activity of the non-steroidal antioestrogen monohydroxytamoxifen in the DMBA-induced rat mammary carcinoma model. Eur J Cancer 16:239–251
4. Jordan VC (2008) Tamoxifen: catalyst for the change to targeted therapy. Eur J Cancer 44:30–38
5. Davies C, Godwin J, Gray R et al (2011) Relevance of breast cancer hormone receptors and other factors to the efficacy of adjuvant tamoxifen: patient-level meta-analysis of randomised trials. Lancet 378:771–784
6. Fisher B, Costantino JP, Wickerham DL et al (1998) Tamoxifen for prevention of breast cancer: report of the National Surgical Adjuvant Breast and Bowel Project P-1 Study. J Natl Cancer Inst 90:1371–1388
7. Fisher B, Costantino JP, Wickerham DL et al (2005) Tamoxifen for the prevention of breast cancer: current status of the National Surgical Adjuvant Breast and Bowel Project P-1 study. J Natl Cancer Inst 97:1652–1662
8. Powles TJ, Ashley S, Tidy A, Smith IE, Dowsett M (2007) Twenty-year follow-up of the Royal Marsden randomized, double-blinded tamoxifen breast cancer prevention trial. J Natl Cancer Inst 99:283–290
9. Jordan VC, Phelps E, Lindgren JU (1987) Effects of anti-estrogens on bone in castrated and intact female rats. Breast Cancer Res Treat 10:31–35
10. Lerner LJ, Jordan VC (1990) Development of antiestrogens and their use in breast cancer: eighth Cain memorial award lecture. Cancer Res 50:4177–4189
11. Vogel VG, Costantino JP, Wickerham DL et al (2006) Effects of tamoxifen vs raloxifene on the risk of developing invasive breast cancer and other disease outcomes: the NSABP Study of Tamoxifen and Raloxifene (STAR) P-2 trial. JAMA 295:2727–2741

12. Davies C, Pan H, Godwin J et al (2013) Long-term effects of continuing adjuvant tamoxifen to 10 years versus stopping at 5 years after diagnosis of oestrogen receptor-positive breast cancer: ATLAS, a randomised trial. Lancet 381:805–816
13. Wolf DM, Jordan VC (1993) A laboratory model to explain the survival advantage observed in patients taking adjuvant tamoxifen therapy. Recent Results Cancer Res 127:23–33

Acknowledgments

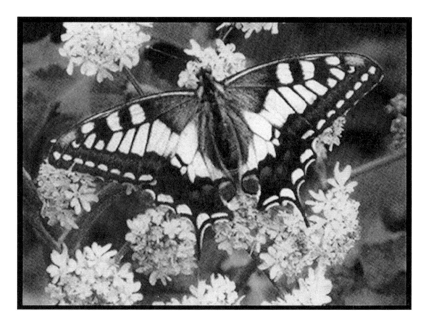

"We are in it for life"™
Tamoxifen Team Georgetown University

Dr. Jordan wishes to thank all of his "Tamoxifen Teams," who for the past four decades have converted ideas into lives saved. He also wishes to thank the Department of Defense Breast Program under award number W81XWH-06-1-0590 Center of Excellence; subcontract under the SU2C (AACR) grant number SU2C-AACR-DT0409; the Susan G Komen for the Cure Foundation under award number SAC100009; and the Lombardi Comprehensive Cancer Center Support Grant (CCSG) Core Grant NIH P30 CA051008 for his current research funding. The views and opinions of the author(s) do not reflect those of the US Army or the Department of Defense.

Contents

About the Authors

V. Craig Jordan, OBE, Ph.D., D.Sc., FMedSci, member of the National Academy of Sciences, is known as the "father of tamoxifen." He was educated in England, obtaining his Ph.D. in Pharmacology (1973) studying a group of failed anti-fertility agents called nonsteroidal antiestrogens. There was no interest in drug development until then, but his work in academia blossomed into tamoxifen. Over a 40-year career, he researched all aspects of antiestrogens and then SERMs using structure-function relationships to investigate molecular mechanisms, developed new models, studied metabolism, developed the first realistic models of SERM resistance in vivo, and 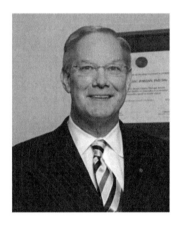 translated all of his concepts into clinical trials. He was there for the birth of tamoxifen as he is credited for reinventing a "failed morning-after contraceptive" to become the "gold standard" for the treatment of breast cancer. During his work, Jordan has held professorships at University of Wisconsin (1985–1993), Northwestern University (1993–2004) (also the Diana Princess of Wales Professor), the Fox Chase Cancer Center (2004–2009) (also the Alfred Knudson Professor), and currently Georgetown Lombardi Cancer Center where he is the scientific director. He has contributed more than 600 scientific articles with more than 23,000 citations. His work on SERMs has been recognized with the ACS Medal of Honor, the BMS Award, the Kettering Prize, the Karnofsky Award (ASCO), the Landon Award (AACR), and the St. Gallen Prize. He is a member of the National Academy of Sciences, Fellow of the Academy of Medical Sciences (UK), Fellow of the AACR Academy, one of the 90 honorary fellows of the Royal Society of Medicine worldwide, and he received the Order of the British Empire (OBE) for services to International Breast Cancer Research from Her Majesty Queen Elizabeth II in 2002. The chapters described in this book are all written by Dr. Jordan as he contributed personally to every aspect of tamoxifen application in therapeutics and all aspects of tamoxifen's pharmacology. He discovered SERMs and the new biology of estrogen-induced apoptosis. Each chapter is a personal journey with a few decades of discovery that forever changed women's health.

Philipp Y. Maximov, M.D., Ph.D., graduated from the Russian National Research Medical University named after N. I. Pirogov (RNRMU) in Moscow, Russia, specializing in medical biochemistry in 2006, and completed his postgraduate program in 2010, receiving the Candidate of Medical Sciences degree (equivalent to Ph.D. in the USA) in medical biochemistry and molecular biology with a thesis titled "Structure-functional relationship of triphenylethylene estrogens and the estrogen receptor alpha in human breast cancer cells" under the mentorship of Dr. V. Craig Jordan, OBE, Ph.D., D.Sc. Dr. Maximov during his last year of medical school was chosen to be one of the top students in his class to represent his university in an exchange program between Fox Chase Cancer Center (FCCC) in Philadelphia, PA.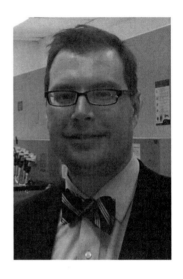
From 2005 to 2010, Dr. Maximov was a graduate student at FCCC and, from 2006, was a Ph.D. student in Dr. Jordan's laboratory. After his Ph.D. thesis defense in Moscow, Dr. Maximov rejoined Dr. Jordan's lab as a Susan G. Komen for the Cure International Postdoctoral Fellow at Georgetown University in 2011. Dr. Maximov is a member of the American Association for Cancer Research (AACR) and the Overseas Fellow of Royal Society of Medicine in London, UK.

Russell E. McDaniel received his BS in Biochemistry in 2007 from Temple University in Philadelphia, PA. He served in the Peace Corps for 2 years, teaching high school chemistry in Mozambique, before joining Dr. Jordan's laboratory. At present, he is pursuing a master's degree in biotechnology at Georgetown.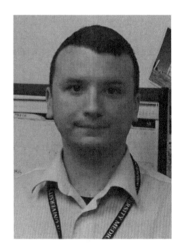

Chapter 1
Discovery and Pharmacology of Nonsteroidal Estrogens and Antiestrogens

Abstract The application of synthetic organic chemistry to establish the simplest basic structure of estrogenic compounds was a major triumph for medicinal chemistry in the 1930s. Two groups of compounds were discovered: the hydroxylated stilbenes with high potency and rapid excretion and the triphenylethylenes with high lipophilicity, metabolic activation, and a very long duration of action. A study of structure-function relationships in laboratory animals would result in the use of high-dose estrogen treatment for metastatic breast cancer in postmenopausal patients in the 1940s. The triphenylethylene-based antiestrogens would evolve into the nonsteroidal antiestrogens that in the 1960s were predicted to be potential postcoital contraceptives in women based on compelling rodent studies. This application did not succeed and enthusiasm for clinical development waned.

Introduction

It is now more than 75 years since the first compound, with known chemical structure, was shown to produce estrogenic effects in animals [1] (Fig. 1.1, compound 1). Since that time, thousands of compounds have been screened for estrogenic activity. During the past 50 years, the early events involved in the molecular mechanism of action of estrogens in their target tissues (e.g., vagina, uterus, pituitary gland, or breast), via the estrogen receptor (ER), have been described [2–4]. In this opening chapter, we will describe how the structure-function relationships of nonsteroidal estrogens set the stage for the serendipitous discoveries of nonsteroidal antiestrogens and the selective estrogen receptor modulators (SERMs). The story, with its twists and turns, is more about people and the exploitation of opportunities by individuals than a plan implicated in the drug development department of any pharmaceutical company.

P.Y. Maximov et al., *Tamoxifen*, Milestones in Drug Therapy,
DOI 10.1007/978-3-0348-0664-0_1, © Springer Basel 2013

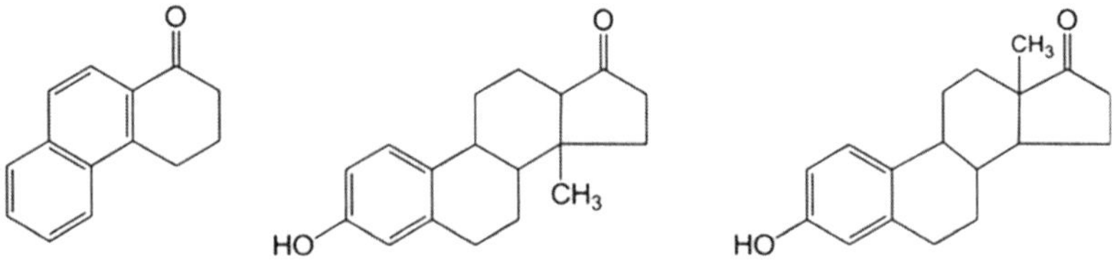

(1)   (2)   (3)

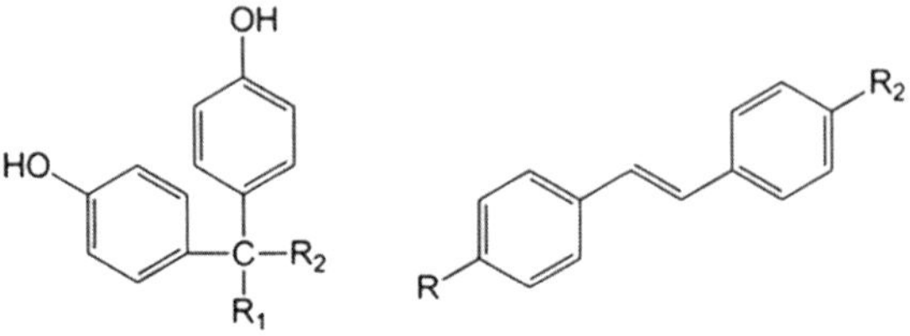

(4) $R_1=R_2=H$ (8) $R_1=R_2=H$

(5) $R_1=R_2=CH_3$ (9) $R_1=OH, R_2=H$

(6) $R_1=CH_3, R_2=C_2H_5$ (10) $R_1=R_2=OH$

(7) $R_1=CH_3, R_2=C_3H_7$

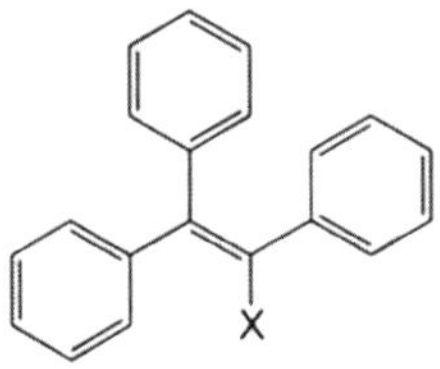

(10) X=H

(11) X=Cl

Fig. 1.1 Formulae of compounds found, in the 1930s, to have estrogenic activity in vivo. Compound 2 was believed to be the molecular structure of ketohydroxyestrin (estrone). This is now known to be incorrect and compound 3 is estrone

Testing Methods for Estrogen

To discover new knowledge about the control of fertility by hormones, animal models are required to detect target tissue-specific effects of test compounds. The Allen-Doisy test [5] depends upon the induction of vaginal cornification in castrate animals 60–80 h after the subcutaneous administration of estrogens. A colony of animals is ovariectomized and used for assays 2 weeks later. To maintain the sensitivity of the colony and retard atrophy of the uterus and vagina [6], the animals are primed with 1 μg estradiol (SC) every 6 weeks. The animals are not used for 2 weeks following either priming or experimental use. However, it is often wise to screen the animals by the vaginal smear technique to check for incomplete ovari-ectomy or test compounds with prolonged biological activity. This technique accurately identified a "principle" that Allen and Doisy called estrogen in ovarian follicular fluid [5].

Direct administration of estrogens into the vagina increases the sensitivity of the Allen-Doisy test and cornification occurs earlier since the response is not dependent upon distribution and metabolism [7, 8]. Emmens [7–10] assayed and evaluated the structural derivatives of stilbene and triphenylethylene by both intravaginal and systemic Allen-Doisy tests. This early work accurately established the relative potency of the test compounds.

Martin and Claringbold [11] developed the intravaginal assay to study the early events of estrogen stimulation by using the increase in vaginal mitoses and vaginal epithelium thickening as measures of the estrogenic response. Martin [12] further showed that the reduction of 2,3,5-triphenyltetrazolium chloride to formazan in epithelial cells of the vagina following the local application of estrogens could form the basis of a sensitive assay procedure for early estrogenic events.

The increase in uterine weight of young castrate rats was used to determine systemic estrogen and activity by Bülbring and Burn [13]. The preparation of castrate animals has been found to be an unnecessary step, and immature rats or mice are usually used [14, 15]. Estrogens induce a rapid early imbibition of water by the uterus, and this effect was used in the 6-h assay of estrogens by Astwood [16]. However, this technique cannot distinguish between full estrogens and partial agonists and also suffers from differences in the release of test compounds from the injection site which will ultimately affect the time course of the uterine response. Most assays utilize a 3-day injection technique to stimulate full uterine growth [17].

Potential estrogenic activity can be inferred for a compound by its ability to inhibit the binding of [³H]estradiol to its target tissues in vivo [18, 19]. However, many nonsteroidal antiestrogens produce the same effect [20, 21] so this effect cannot be assumed to predict biological activity. Similarly, the ability of a com-pound to inhibit the binding of [³H]estradiol to ERs in vitro suggests a potential mechanism of action via the ER but again this alone cannot predict biological activity, i.e., agonist or antagonist actions [22]. Armed with the bioassay technique in vivo, a host of compounds were screened during the 1930–1960s to find potential novel agents for clinical applications.

Structure-Activity Relationships of Estrogens

The pioneering studies by Sir Charles Dodds laid the foundation for all the subsequent research on the structure-activity relationships of nonsteroidal estrogens. The 1930s saw a remarkable expansion of knowledge that culminated in the description of the optimal structural requirements in a simple molecule to produce estrogen action. The first compound of known structure (1-keto-1,2,3,4-tertrahydrophenanthrene) (Fig. 1.1, compound 1) to be found to have estrogenic activity [1] was tested because of its structural similarity to the presumed structure of ketohydroxyestrin (Fig. 1.1, compound 2). As it turned out, the structure of the natural steroid (estrone) was incorrect (Fig. 1.1, compound 3), but this did not matter; the fact that nonsteroidal compounds can exhibit estrogenic properties was established. A phenanthrene nucleus was later found to be unnecessary for estrogenic activity [23]. Simple bisphenolic compounds are active (Fig. 1.1, compounds 4–7) and, as will be seen later in this chapter, this is a recurrent feature of many nonsteroidal estrogens. The finding that hydroxystilbenes (Fig. 1.1, compounds 8–10) possess potent estrogenic activity provided a valuable clue that stimulated a systematic investigation of analogs to optimize the potency. At this time, an interesting side issue occurred that deserves comment, as it illustrates how parallel research endeavors can eventually reach the same conclusions. Anol, a simple phenol derived from anethole (Fig. 1.2), was reported to possess extremely potent estrogenic activity with 1 μg capable of inducing estrus in all rats [24]. These results were not confirmed with different preparations of anol [25, 26], but it was found that dimerization of anol to dianol (Fig. 1.2) can occur and this impurity, which was known to have potent estrogenic [27] properties, was the compound responsible for the controversy [27]. At this time, Dodds reported [28–30] that diethyl substitution at the ethylenic bond of stilbestrol (Fig. 1.2) produces an extremely potent estrogen [31]; other substitutions produce less active compounds [28, 32]. The structural similarity between diethylstilbestrol and estradiol (the formula was established by 1938) was noted, but an attempt to mimic the rigid steroid structure by the synthesis of dihydroxyhexahydrochrysene (Fig. 1.2) resulted in a drop in estrogenic potency. Dihydroxyhexahydrochrysene is approximately 1/2,000 as potent as diethylstilbestrol [23].

There was considerable interest in the development of a long-acting synthetic estrogen because of the potential for clinical application. The duration of action of diethylstilbestrol can be increased dramatically by esterification of the phenolic groups [28]. A 10-μg dose of diethylstilbestrol dipropionate can produce estrus for more than 50 days, while the phenol at the same dose is active for only 5 days. The simple hydrocarbon triphenylethylene (Fig. 1.1, compound 11) is a weakly active estrogen [33], but 10 mg can produce vaginal cornification in mice for up to 9 weeks. Replacement of the free ethylenic hydrogen with chlorine (Fig. 1.1, compound 12) increases the potency and duration of action by subcutaneous administration [34], but when administered orally, triphenylchloroethylene has a similar duration or action as diethylstilbestrol or estradiol benzoate. In the search for orally active agents, Robson and Schonberg [35] showed that DBE (Fig. 1.2) was very effective by the oral route. The long duration of action is related to depot formation in body fat [36], but DBE did not reach clinical trial. The related compound trianisylchloroethylene (TACE) became available clinically as a long-acting estrogen (Fig. 1.2). TACE is stored in body fat for prolonged periods [37–39]. It was around the mid-1940s and early 1950s that the discovery that high-dose synthetic estrogens could cause the regression of about 30 % of metastatic breast cancers in postmenopausal women became the standard of care for the treatment of breast cancer [40, 41]. This is interesting not only because this was the

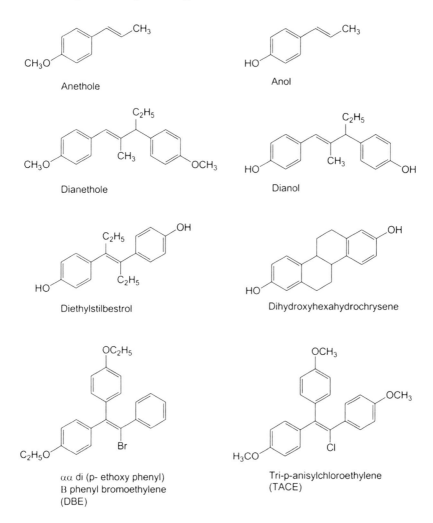

Fig. 1.2 Formulae of nonsteroidal compounds with estrogenic (or suspected) activity in vivo

first time a chemical therapy was shown to cause regression of cancer but also the compounds that Haddow used were made and provided by chemists at Imperial Chemical Industries (ICI). High-dose synthetic estrogen therapy was to remain the standard of care for the palliative treatment of breast cancer until the late 1970s early 1980s when another synthetic estrogen derivative, also produced by chemists at ICI pharmaceutical division ICI 46,474 (later to be known as tamoxifen) would revolutionize breast cancer treatment and prevention. This is the story of this book.

The first 25 years established many of the important structural features that govern the potency and duration of action of estrogens. This is a remarkable feat of structure-functional relationships without knowledge of the ER target. We will now briefly consider the evolving subcellular mechanism of estrogen action in its target tissues before describing the structure-activity relationships and pharmacological properties of the nonsteroidal antiestrogens.

Estrogen Action

The reason for the target site specificity of the estrogens remained obscure until the synthesis of tritium-labeled compounds with high specific activity. The synthesis of [^{3}H]hexestrol (reduction of diethylstilbestrol with tritium and a palladium catalyst) by Glascock working with Sir Charles Dodds [42] and the subsequent observation that there was binding of hexestrol in the uterus, vagina, mammary glands, and pituitary gland of immature female goats and sheep [43] provided the first evidence for the target tissue localization of estrogens. The subsequent applications of [^{3}H] hexestrol to determine hormone responsiveness in metastatic breast cancer was a big step in our antiestrogen story [44]. The subsequent fundamental study by Jensen and Jacobson [2] of the distribution and binding of [^{3}H]estradiol in the immature rat demonstrated that estradiol selectively binds to, and is retained by, the uterus, vagina, and pituitary gland. These systematic studies suggested there is a specific receptor for estradiol in its target tissues. The biochemical identification of an estrogen-binding protein in the immature rat uterus and the observation that [^{3}H] estradiol becomes located in the receptor nucleus of the cell provided a model to describe the initiation of estrogen-stimulated events. The early evidence for an ER system has been described [3, 4]. Simply stated, the estrogen dissociates from plasma proteins and readily diffuses into the cell. Initially it was thought that the cytoplasmic ER binds the ligand and the resulting receptor complex is activated before translocation to the nucleus. Interaction with nuclear acceptors (now referred to as promoter regions of estrogen-responsive gene) results in the activation of RNA and DNA polymerases to initiate subsequent protein synthesis and cell proliferation, respectively. There were, however, an increasing number of observations that were inconsistent with the classical two-step hypothesis. These reports have been reviewed [45]. Two innovative approaches to the question of the actual subcellular localization of unoccupied ER deserve comment. These methods, which did not require cellular disruption, settle the issue of where the unoccupied receptors resided in the cell. Therefore, if it was, in fact, cell disruption that causes the unoccupied receptor to "fall out of the nucleus" but ER complexes are "stuck" in the nucleus, this would explain the early translocation model. Indeed, a series of studies with weakly binding antiestrogens injected into the immature rat arrived at the same conclusion [46]. Monoclonal antibodies raised to the ER were used as tags for immunohistochemical studies. The antibody is linked to a peroxidase enzyme system to visualize the receptor, which appears to be located exclusively in the nuclear compartment, even in the absence of estrogen [47]. The other approach was to enucleate ER-containing GH3 rat pituitary tumor cells with cytochalasin B. Unoccupied receptors are observed in nucleoplasts rather than cytoplasts [48]. Similar studies were subsequently published using estrogen-free culture of

ER-positive MCF-7 breast cancer cells [49]. Although it was possible that these studies were generating artifactual results, the simplified model of estrogen action, i.e., unoccupied ER is a nuclear protein, is now considered to represent subcellular events in vivo.

Nonsteroidal Antiestrogens

The finding by Lerner and coworkers [50] that the compound ethamoxytriphetol (MER 25, Fig. 1.3) is an inhibitor of estrogen action provided a new tool for laboratory research and clinical investigation. It is of considerable interest that MER 25 had been synthesized as part of a cardiovascular pharmacology program and only found its way to endocrine testing at Dr. Lerner's request. Lerner had spotted that MER 25 looked like the nonsteroidal triphenylethylenes so he wanted to test it for estrogenic properties. There were none but he discovered the first nonsteroidal antiestrogen. MER 25 was subsequently found to have antifertility properties in the rat [51–53], so clinical use as an oral contraceptive seemed logical. Preliminary clinical trials with MER 25 were scientifically successful [54–56]; however, the clinical studies were discontinued because of low potency and toxic side effects. In the search for new compounds, a structural derivative of triphenylethylene, clomiphene (also called chloramiphene or MRL 41; in Fig. 1.3, the geometric isomers enclomiphene and zuclomiphene are shown. Clomiphene is a mixture of isomers) was found to be a potent antifertility agent in rats [57, 58] and it became the forerunner of many structurally similar compounds that were synthesized and tested as potential postcoital antifertility agents [59–64]. The spectrum of compounds was reviewed by Emmens [65].

Structure-Activity Relationships in the Rat

There are no published reports specifically documenting the structure-activity relationships of MER 25. Apart from one triphenylethane MRL 37, with a hydrogen substituted for MER 25's alcoholic hydroxyl [53, 66], most interest has focused on compounds related to triphenylethylene. The original antiestrogens can be classified into two major groups: substituted triphenylethylenes and bicyclic antiestrogens.

Substituted Triphenylethylenes

Early studies with clomiphene used a mixture of geometric isomers [53, 57, 58]. The *cis* and *trans* isomers were separated [67] and each has been reported to

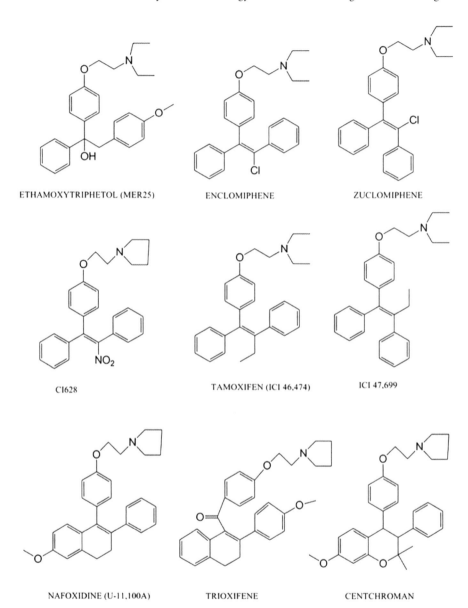

ETHAMOXYTRIPHETOL (MER25)   ENCLOMIPHENE   ZUCLOMIPHENE

C1628   TAMOXIFEN (ICI 46,474)   ICI 47,699

NAFOXIDINE (U-11,100A)   TRIOXIFENE   CENTCHROMAN

Fig. 1.3 The formulae of nonsteroidal antiestrogens mentioned in the text. Zuclomiphene and ICI 47,699 are the estrogenic geometric isomers of the antiestrogenic enclomiphene and ICI 46,474 (tamoxifen)

possess different biologic activities [68–70]; however, some controversy surrounded the designation of the isomers in relation to their observed biologic properties. They were originally mislabeled as geometric isomers! It is now clear that the *trans* isomer enclomiphene (originally named isomer B or *cis* clomiphene) has antiestrogenic properties in the rat, whereas the *cis* isomer zuclomiphene (originally named isomer A or *trans* clomiphene) is estrogenic (Fig. 1.3). Comparison of the isomers of tamoxifen and enclomiphene in the uterine weight test demonstrated only minor differences in their dose-response curves [71]. Parenthetically, in 1972, during the examination of my Ph.D. entitled "A study of the oestrogenic and anti-oestrogenic activities of some substituted triphenylethylenes and triphenylethanes," I was asked by my external examiner Dr. Arthur Walpole, head of the fertility program of ICI Pharmaceutical Division, why the biological properties of the geometric isomers of clomiphene and tamoxifen were opposite? I replied it was obviously the influence of the chlorine in clomiphene, never considering that the geometric isomers of clomiphene were misidentified. Walpole knew that!

The fundamental importance of the geometric shape of a molecule for antiestrogenic activity was realized after the report by Harper and Walpole [72] of the contrasting biological properties of the *cis* and *trans* isomers of substituted triphenylethylenes. Tamoxifen (ICI 46,474) and its *cis* isomer ICI 47,699 (Fig. 1.3) have been identified by nuclear magnetic resonance [73] and the structure of ICI 47,699 confirmed as the *cis* isomer by X-ray crystallography [74]. The simultaneous administration of tamoxifen with estradiol to immature rats prevents the increases in uterine wet weight or vaginal cornification observed with estradiol alone. In contrast, ICI 47,699 is only estrogenic in conventional tests [75]; however, very high doses have been shown to inhibit estradiol action in the uterus [71].

p-Methoxy-substituted derivatives of tamoxifen have been synthesized and tested [76] but this type of structural modification does not increase antiestrogenic activity.

CI628 (CN-55, 945–27) (Fig. 1.3) is an estrogen antagonist in the rat [77]. The isomeric mixture was used only briefly for the experimental treatment of advanced breast cancer; however, there is a considerable literature on the use of CI628 in studies with the human breast cancer ER in vitro [78]. It is an antitumor agent in the rat mammary carcinoma model [79]. There is no information on the biological properties of the separated geometric isomers; both appear to be antiestrogenic [71].

Bicyclic Antiestrogens

Scientists at the Upjohn Company, Kalamazoo, MI, focused much attention on the structure-activity relationships and properties of bicyclic (fixed ring)-based nonsteroidal antiestrogens [59–61]. Simple hydroxylated indenes [80, 81] that are superficially related to the structure of DES are potent estrogens. The structure-activity relationships of the indene nucleus have been investigated in the search for potent antifertility relationships [59] (Fig. 1.4). The 6-methoxy group is an advantage for activity but potent antifertility activity is determined by the substituted amine ethoxy side chain. Optimal activity is observed with the pyrrolidino side chain (IND 1, Fig. 1.4) and other substituted side chains (IND 2, 3, 4) have reduced

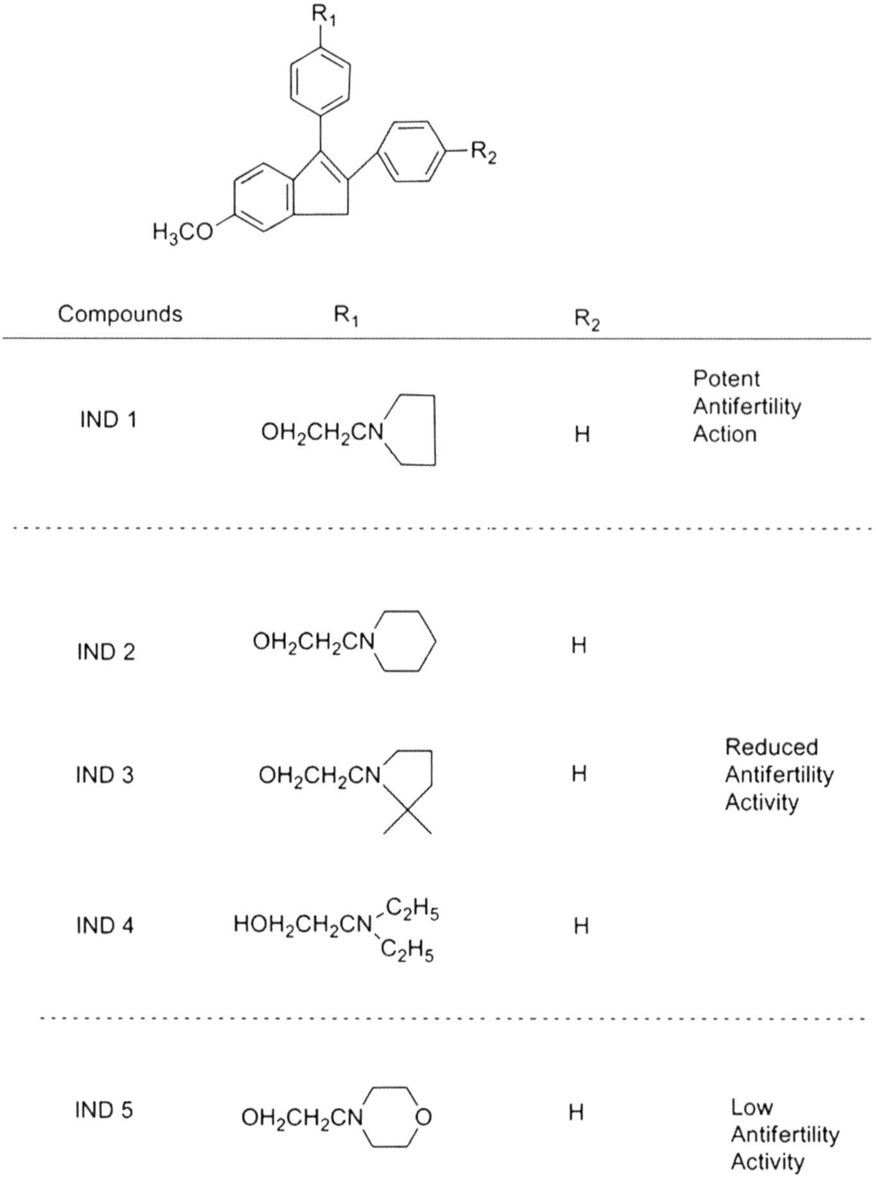

Compounds	R_1	R_2	
IND 1	OH_2CH_2CN (pyrrolidine)	H	Potent Antifertility Action
IND 2	OH_2CH_2CN (piperidine)	H	
IND 3	OH_2CH_2CN (dimethyl cyclopentane)	H	Reduced Antifertility Activity
IND 4	HOH_2CH_2CN $\overset{C_2H_5}{\underset{C_2H_5}{}}$	H	
IND 5	OH_2CH_2CN (morpholine)	H	Low Antifertility Activity

Fig. 1.4 The relative antifertility activity of substituted indenes in the rat (Data adapted from Lednicer et al. [59])

activity. A morpholino side chain (IND 5) produces a compound with approximately 1 % of the activity of IND 1 with the pyrrolidino side chain. In the same study, Lednicer and coworkers [59] showed that the 6 phenols of IND 4 had approximately 5 % of the potency of the methoxy compound. Hydroxylated derivative might be expected to have a shorter duration of action so that larger doses will be required to maintain adequate drug levels.

The 3,4-dihydronaphthalenes further exemplify the importance of the substituted side chain for optimal activity (Fig. 1.5). Nafoxidine (see Fig. 1.3 for comparison with other nonsteroidal antiestrogens) is the most potent compound of the series although the ether oxygen of the side chain can be replaced by carbon with very little loss of potency. However, decrease in the length of the side chain (NAF 1–3) (Fig. 1.5) reduces the antiestrogenic potency and in fact, removal of the side chain (NAF 6) results in the complete loss of the antagonist activity. The resulting compounds are estrogens [60, 61]. These observations led Lednicer et al. [60] to suggest that a basic group, at a given position in space, is required to obtain a molecule with estrogen antagonist activity. This point of view is further supported by the observation that dimethylation *ortho* to the aminoethoxy side chain in MER25 [82] and tamoxifen [83] reduces antiestrogen activity and receptor binding, respectively. The methyl substitutions reduce the number of positions in space that the side chain can adopt. A series of derivatives of tamoxifen with different polar side chains had been investigated [84]. The resulting biological activity related to structure is shown in Fig. 1.6. Trioxifene (available as the mesylate salt LY133314, Fig. 1.3) has been described [85] and phase I trials as a potential agent for breast cancer therapy were completed, but the drug was not developed. The unusual structural feature of trioxifene (Fig. 1.3) is the introduction of a ketone group linking the *p*-alkylaminoethoxyphenyl ring to the ethylenic bond. The structure therefore diverges from the usual triphenylethylene type. This, in the future, would turn out to be an important structural feature to create the antiestrogens with no estrogen-like actions in the uterus as raloxifene.

Centchroman (Fig. 1.3) has been studied in considerable detail in laboratory animals and women as it was investigated as a postcoital contraceptive agent [86, 87]. The structure-activity relationships of the chromans and the unsaturated chromenes have been given considerable attention. The structure with the greatest similarity to nafoxidine (3, 4-diphenylchromene) has very potent antifertility activity in rats. Substitution of hydrogen for two methyl groups at the 2 position gives a less active compound but reduction of the 3, 4 double bond restores potent antifertility activity (centchroman). It is important to note that two diastereoisomers are possible for the substituted chroman. Centchroman is the active *trans* isomer, whereas the *cis* isomer is virtually inactive [88, 89]. Like the 3, 4-dihydronaphthalenes, centchroman is antiestrogenic in the rat [90].

All the nonsteroidal antiestrogens have an alkylaminoethoxy side chain. As previously noted, moving the group further away from the double bond with the substitution of a ketone group (trioxifene) does not reduce antiestrogenic activity. Nevertheless, there seems to be a requirement for the nitrogen on the aminoethoxy side chain to be at a given position in space. A chain length of three atoms seems to be required to place the nitrogen group in the optimal position [60]. All of the studies in vivo with the structure-function relationships of antiestrogens as antifertility agents built up a strong conceptual model that the antiestrogens side chain was interacting actively with a select portion of the ER. Studies now evolved to

Fig. 1.5 The relative antiestrogenic activity of substituted 3,4-dihydronaphthalene in immature rats (Data adapted from Lednicer et al. [60, 61])

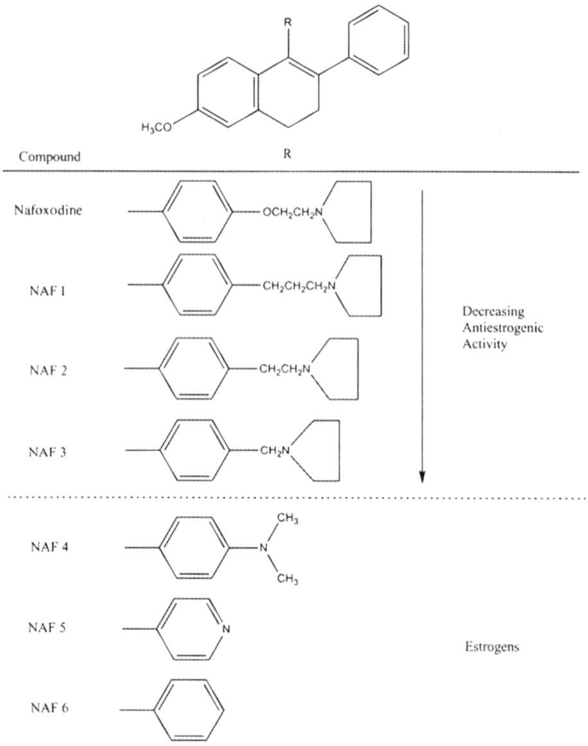

molecular mechanisms in the decades between 1970 and 2000 to predict efficacy of the ER ligand complex based on interrogation of ligand ER interactions.

The Molecular Modulation of the Estrogen Receptor by Nonsteroidal Antiestrogens

The description of the selective binding of [^{3}H]estradiol in the estrogen target tissues of the immature rat (uterus, vaginal) [2] and the subsequent isolation of the ER as an extractable protein from the rat uterus [91, 92] was not only an advance in molecular endocrinology but also an advance that would improve the therapeutics of breast cancer. The idea that by detecting the presence of the ER in a breast tumor would soon evolve from being a predictive test to decide the appropriateness of endocrine ablative surgery to become the target for antiestrogenic drugs was an important conceptual step [93]. Once it was found that the ER was extractable in the 1960s, it was possible to study and understand the binding of ligands to the ER and perhaps gain an insight into the mechanism of action of estrogens and antiestrogens. Early studies of the competitive binding of estrogens and antiestrogens with [^{3}H] estradiol for the ER in vitro [94, 95] were unable to distinguish between estrogens

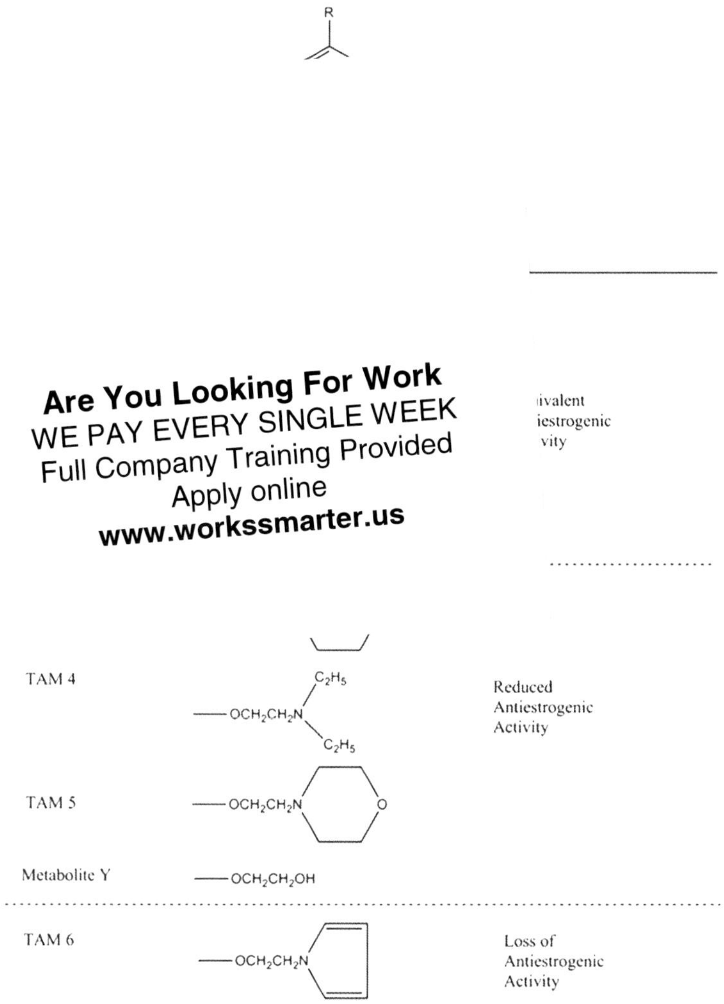

iivalent
iestrogenic
vity

TAM 4   ——OCH₂CH₂N(C₂H₅)C₂H₅   Reduced Antiestrogenic Activity

TAM 5   ——OCH₂CH₂N

Metabolite Y   ——OCH₂CH₂OH

TAM 6   ——OCH₂CH₂N   Loss of Antiestrogenic Activity

Fig 1.6 The effect of different side chains on the antiestrogenic activity of tamoxifen (Data adapted from Robertson et al. [84])

and antiestrogens biologically. All that could be concluded was that antiestrogens had low binding affinity for the ER and this, it was argued, was why such large doses were necessary to block estrogen action [94]. Also, it was concluded that the low affinity of antiestrogens for the ER was part of their mechanism of action: the ligand would not remain long enough bound to the receptor to activate estrogen action [94]. This proposal was all to change with the discovery of the pharmacological properties of 4-hydroxytamoxifen, a metabolite of tamoxifen then thought to be the principal metabolite of tamoxifen [96]. 4-Hydroxytamoxifen has a binding affinity for the ER equivalent to estradiols, so if it was possible to have high affinity antiestrogens, then low affinity was not the mechanism of antiestrogen action. The shape of the resulting complex was the key to efficacy and the subsequent modulation of signal transduction. 4-Hydroxytamoxifen was subsequently adopted as the standard laboratory antiestrogen in cell culture and 20 years later was used as an antiestrogenic ligand to be crystallized with the ligand-binding domain of the human ER [97].

In the 1970s, what was needed was a model cell system to study the structure-function relationships of ligands that bind to the ER. In this way, the intrinsic efficacy of the ligand ER complex could be deciphered, without concerns about pharmacokinetics and metabolism. The ER-positive breast cancer cell line MCF-7 had been described [98] but the fact that the cells apparently grew spontaneously in culture and would not respond to estradiol with growth but would when inoculated into athymic mice [99] led to considerable controversy in the field. Maybe estrogen was acting indirectly to promote breast cancer growth? Nevertheless, tamoxifen did block the spontaneous growth of MCF-7 cells and this blockade could be reversed with estradiol [100]. Interestingly enough, MCF-7 cells, or rather their ER, would be essential to create the first monoclonal antibodies to human ER [101, 102] and subsequently be the critical tool necessary to clone and sequence the human ER [103, 104].

The first cell system used to study the modulation of the ligand ER complex in vitro was primary cultures of the immature rat pituitary gland [105]. The target for the ER was the prolactin gene [22, 106]. The first publication validated the mechanism of actions of nonsteroidal antiestrogens at the ER to regulate estrogen-induced gene transcription as competitive inhibition of estradiol binding to the ER and that it was an advantage but not a requirement for an antiestrogen to be metabolically activated [106]. As with other drug receptor interactions, affinity and the intrinsic efficacy of the drug receptor complex are not interconnected for drug action. Numerous studies of structure-function relationships of triphenylethylenes described the structure-function relationships to modulate the ER complex between the extremes for estrogenic intrinsic efficacy and complete antiestrogen action [22, 107–111]. The structure-activity relationship [112] studies permitted the creation of a map of the hypothetical folding of the ER complex. However, it was the serendipitous advance in deciphering breast cancer cell replication in vitro that was to enhance the interpretation of all future laboratory studies.

In the mid-1980s, the Katzenellenbogen laboratory [113] made the critical discovery that ER-positive breast cancer cells had all been cultured in media containing high concentrations of a pH indicator, phenol red that contained a contaminant that was an estrogen (Fig. 1.7) [114, 115] (note: this is reminiscent of the anol-dianol controversy). Removal of the phenol red from media now permitted the structure-activity relationship studies of nonsteroidal antiestrogens to be extrapolated from prolactin gene modulation to the replication of breast cancer cell lines [116, 117].

However, the critical question to be addressed in molecular pharmacology was "what is the essential interaction of the antiestrogenic side chain with the ER that modulates estrogen-like and antiestrogen action?" A simple estrogen/antiestrogen

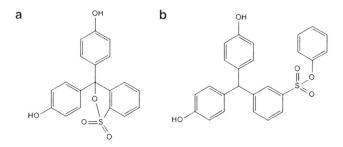

Fig. 1.7 pH indicator phenol red and contaminant bis(4-hydroxyphenyl)-[2-9phenoxy-sulfonul-phenyl]methane found in the growth medium that produced estrogenic effect of the MCF-7 cell line [114, 115]

model of the ER had been proposed as the "crocodile model" [118] with the jaws closed for estrogen action and the antiestrogen, a stick in the jaws to keep them open for antiestrogen action (Fig. 1.8). An antiestrogenic region (AER) that interacts with the appropriately positioned alkylaminoethoxy side chain on the ligand backbone had been proposed previously [22, 112, 118], but how to find it? Several advances were necessary before progress could occur. A model of acquired drug resistance to tamoxifen in athymic mice needed to be developed, the ER needed to be screened for mutations in drug resistant MCF-7 breast tumors, and ER needed to be stably transfected into ER-negative breast cancer cell and suitable gene modulated. All this was done to propose a hypothetical modulation of the antiestrogen ER complex prior to the crystallization of the ligand-binding domain with estradiol and raloxifene [119]. A biological clue was found in the human ER that would complement the structural knowledge of the ligand ER binding domain complex with functional information at a transforming growth factor-alpha (TGFα) gene target.

A mutation, asp 351 tyr, was noted in one MCF-7 tumor cell line with acquired resistance to tamoxifen [120]. The first transfection of the wild-type ER [121] into the ER-negative breast cancer cell line MDA-MB-231 eventually allowed any mutant ER to be transfected. The interaction of ERs with ligands could now be monitored at the estrogen-responsive binding domain with 4-hydroxytamoxifen and raloxifene [97, 119] indicating that while raloxifene's side chain shielded and possibly neutralized asp351, the side chain of tamoxifen was shorter and barely interacted with asp 351 [122–124]. To address the hypothesis that the side chain was preventing the interaction of asp 351 with activating function 1 (AF-1) motif of the ER, ER complex was interrogated using mutations of asp 351 and structural derivation of raloxifene [125–128] (Fig. 1.6). It was concluded that this amino acid was important to alter surface interactions with other co-regulators of hormone action.

The modulation of the ER complex through coactivator proteins went some way to explain SERM action, i.e., nonsteroidal antiestrogens switching on and switching off sites around a woman's body. But long before this concept was discovered and described in the mid-1980s [129], the literature was full of examples of the

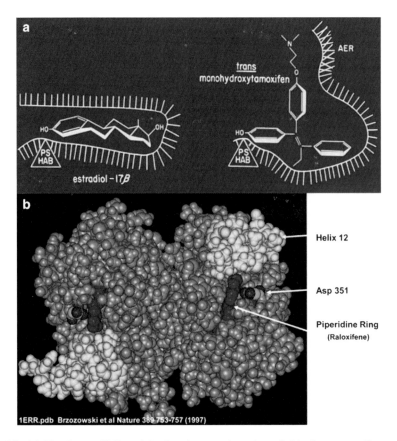

Fig. 1.8 (**a**) The "crocodile" model of antiestrogenic action of 4-hydroxytamoxifen and its interaction with the antiestrogenic region of the ER [118], (**b**) as well as the X-ray crystallography of the ligand-binding domain (LBD) of the ER interacting with the raloxifene piperidine ring via its Asp351 and thus producing an antagonistic conformation of the receptor and antiestrogenic biological effect (Front cover of [189])

species-specific pharmacology of nonsteroidal antiestrogens. We will illustrate this now but no adequate explanation has yet been offered or proven to explain the diverse pharmacology in different species.

Effect of Antiestrogens in Different Species

Lerner and coworkers [130] reported that the compound MER 25 antagonizes the actions of estradiol in rats and mice with no other demonstrable hormonal or antihormonal activity. In contrast, Emmens [131] found MER 25 to be only weakly active as an inhibitor of estradiol-stimulated vaginal cornification in the ovariecto-mized mouse. Nevertheless, the original claim of antiestrogenic activity has been adequately confirmed in a variety of interesting models. MER 25 inhibits diethyl-stilbestrol or estradiol-stimulated increases in the reticuloendothelial system [132] of the ovariectomized mouse. In the mature female rat, a large dose of MER 25 (20 mg) inhibits the estrogen-stimulated uterine ballooning observed at proestrus and doubling the dose also inhibits ovulation [133]. If MER 25 is administered after ovulation, there is inhibition of the estrogen-stimulated DNA, RNA, and protein synthesis that occurs during uterine decidualization [134]. The antiestrogenic action of MER 25 has also been reported at the level of the pituitary. Hypertrophy of the rat pituitary by continued estrogen administration is inhibited by the coadministration of MER 25 [135]. Similarly, estrogen-simulated prolactin release in the ovariectomized rat can be inhibited by large daily dose of MER 25 [136].

Although MER 25 is notable for its very low estrogenic activity in all species tested, some estrogenic responses in the uterus have been quantified. A single dose of MER 25 (5 mg) increases ovariectomized rat uterine glycogen, glucose, and percent water inhibition[137]. A striking short-lived increase in immature rat uterine glucose-6-phosphate dehydrogenase activity and a marked rise in uterine total lipid is observed after a single administration of MER 25 (10 mg) [138]. In ovariectomized mice, MER 25 has some estrogenic activity as evidenced by increases in uterine weight and a stimulation of the enzymes alkaline phosphatase and isocitrate dehydrogenase [76].

Overall, though, the pharmacology of MER 25 is established as an estrogen antagonist. Since the pharmacology of the related triphenylethylenes is so complex, this is presented in species-related groups.

Mouse

The antiestrogens based on triphenylethylene are generally considered to be estrogenic in the mouse. However, this statement is only true under precisely defined conditions. Tamoxifen (oral or SC) is typically estrogenic in the Allen-Doisy (vaginal smear) test using mature ovariectomized mice [75]. In comparative studies, tamoxifen [139, 140] and trioxifene [139] are estrogenic in the 3-day ovariectomized mouse uterine weight test. Similarly tamoxifen, ICI 47,699, enclomiphene, and zuclomiphene are fully uterotrophic in immature mice [141] and tamoxifen does not possess antiuterotrophic activity [142]. In contrast, nafoxidine [141] and trioxifene [139] are partially estrogenic with antiestrogenic properties in immature mice. It is of interest that trioxifene appears to be fully estrogenic in mature ovariectomized mice and antiestrogenic in immature mice, while tamoxifen is more estrogenic than trioxifene in both test systems [143]. Lee [143] pointed out that tamoxifen and nafoxidine are mitogenic in the ovariectomized mouse uterus and neither compound inhibits the mitogenic response to estrone. However, daily treatment of ovariectomized mice with tamoxifen for up to 14 days reduces estrone-stimulated uterine weight gain [144]. It is possible that the accumulation of tamoxifen may alter the pharmacology to produce an inhibitory effect.

In this context, SC administration of a large dose of tamoxifen (or related *p*-methoxylated compounds) to ovariectomized mice produces a short period of estrogenic activity followed by a prolonged antiestrogenic and antifertility response [20, 145, 146]. The validity of the vaginal smear technique to assay prolonged antiestrogenic activity was initially questioned [147] although there is agreement about the reduced effectiveness of tamoxifen to produce a fully cornified vaginal epithelium [148].

Rat

The pharmacology of antiestrogens in the rat is dependent upon the target tissue or biochemical end point being studied. For this reason the effects of antiestrogens in different organs will be considered.

All of the nonsteroidal antiestrogens are able to stimulate a partial estrogenic response in the immature and ovariectomized rat uterus. Histological comparisons of estrogen and antiestrogen-stimulated uteri have demonstrated selective differences in both cell stimulation and mitotic activity. CI628 [149], tamoxifen, 4-hydroxytamoxifen [150], and nafoxidine [151] stimulate an enormous increase in the size of luminal epithelial cells. Estradiol increases the incorporation of [^{3}H] thymidine [149] and the mitotic activity [152] in luminal epithelial cells, whereas antiestrogens are much less active [149, 150]. In general antiestrogens produce hypertrophy rather than hyperplasia of luminal epithelial cells.

Much research with antiestrogens has focused on the estrogen control mechanisms of pituitary function. This, in part, is because of the early clinical applications of both clomiphene and tamoxifen as agents for the induction of ovulation in subfertile women [153, 154]. Estrogen-stimulated prolactin release in ovariectomized rats [155] is partially inhibited by nafoxidine [156] and tamoxifen [157]. Studies [158] have demonstrated that in the intact rat the cyclical release of prolactin at proestrus is inhibited by continuous tamoxifen therapy. This is consistent with the finding that tamoxifen, 4-hydroxytamoxifen, and trioxifene inhibit estrogen-stimulated prolactin synthesis by rat pituitary cells in culture [22]. Similarly, tamoxifen inhibits the growth and secretion of prolactin by the estrogen-induced pituitary tumor 7315a [159]. Furthermore, tamoxifen sensitizes the pituitary tumor cells to the inhibitory effects of bromocriptine on prolactin secretion in vitro [160].

Tamoxifen [161–163] and enclomiphene [161] (zuclomiphene is inactive) inhibit ovulation by blocking estrogen action at the level of the hypothalamus and pituitary. Gonadotropin release is inhibited in male and female rats by large doses of clomiphene (mixed isomers) [57] but it is possible that the estrogenic *cis* isomer is predominantly responsible for these effects. The ability of centchroman and clomiphene (mixed isomers) to alter serum FSH, LH, and prolactin in male and female rats has been compared [164]. Clomiphene lowers LH in male rats, slightly increases LH in female rates, but causes a large increase in prolactin in both species.

Centchroman, with its rigid bicyclic structure, produces a similar effect to clomiphene on gonadotropin and prolactin levels in both sexes, although the compound is less estrogenic than clomiphene. Studies with the weakly estrogenic compound tamoxifen demonstrate that short-term (5 days) therapy of ovariectomized rats does not lower LH [165], whereas longer therapy (up to 4 weeks) results in a consistent decrease in LH levels [158]. Similarly, a large dose of tamoxifen is sufficiently estrogenic to decrease LH release in male rats [166].

Studies with rat pituitary cells in vitro demonstrates [167] that both estradiol and clomiphene (mixed isomers) sensitize the cells to the effects of LHRH (luteinizing hormone-releasing hormone). The antiestrogenic isomer enclomiphene is apparently only acting as an estrogen in this system. In contrast, Miller and Huang [168] observed that tamoxifen inhibits the estrogen sensitization of ovine pituitary cells to an LHRH analog. Furthermore, tamoxifen, CI628, and nafoxidine inhibit estrogen-stimulated LH release and reverse the inhibition of FSH release by estradiol in this system. To explain these contrasting results, it must be conceded that nothing is known about the pharmacology of antiestrogens in the sheep! Therefore, species differences may be responsible for differences in the action of the compounds. However, the fact that in vivo antiestrogens can cause increases or decreases in LH depending upon the physiological model used must point to the complex factors involved in the regulation of gonadotropin release.

Before considering other organ side effects of antiestrogens, one early observation with nonsteroidal estrogens in the pituitary is worthy of note. Continuous estradiol administration for several weeks can cause pituitary hypertrophy in the rat (F344), while administrating the estrogenic triphenylethylene TACE does not [37]. Of perhaps greater significance, TACE inhibits the hypertrophy of the pituitary produced by estradiol [169]. Current knowledge of the aberrant binding of triphenylethylene-based estrogen to the ER [1701, 171] may actually be the reason for the different carcinogenic actions of differently shaped estrogens.

Several estrogen-modulated synthetic events in the liver have been considered as potential sites of antiestrogen action. For convenience, and because the effects of antiestrogens are similar, the rat and primate liver will be considered together. Rat and monkey liver have a well-defined ER system [172, 173], suggesting a mechanism for the effects of estrogen and antiestrogen. The continuous treatment of ovariectomized immature rats with tamoxifen or estradiol increases the synthesis of renin substrate [174]. Similarly, a comparison of ethinyl estradiol and nafoxidine has demonstrated that both are full agonists in stimulating plasma renin substrate in mature female rats [175]. During tamoxifen therapy, breast cancer patients have elevated circulating levels of sex hormone-binding globulin (SHBG) [176]. This observation is of interest because SHBG synthesis in the liver in under estrogen control. Overall, it seems that only estrogenic effects have been described for antiestrogens in the mammalian liver.

Chick

Most studies with antiestrogens have focused on the effects in the oviduct and liver. The pharmacology of both tamoxifen [177] and 4-hydroxytamoxifen [178] in the oviduct is as a full antagonist. No estrogenic effects have been reported. In general, antiestrogens are full antagonists of estrogen action in the liver [179].

Conclusion

The purpose of our introductory chapter is to document the important evolution of knowledge about nonsteroidal synthetic estrogens that really laid the foundation for all future work on nonsteroidal antiestrogens and then selective ER modulators (SERMs).

The intense interest in a study of nonsteroidal antiestrogens in the laboratory during the 1960s and 1970s as antifertility agents in different species or as laboratory tools to dissect estrogen action in its target tissues now slowly started to evolve from reproduction research to targeted cancer therapeutics. Tamoxifen would soon no longer be a laboratory tool and pharmacological curiosity, but an orphan breast cancer drug in search of an optimal strategy to best be deployed in the clinic. This now becomes the theme of our book.

Postscript.   A series of chance meetings occurred at ICI Pharmaceuticals Division Alderley Park near my home in Cheshire. In 1967 I wanted to work in cancer research over my summer holiday (I had previously worked at the Yorkshire Cancer Research Campaign laboratory at Leeds University in the summer of 1966) so I went to ICI and I phoned up Dr. Steven Carter from the phonebook outside the laboratories in Alderley Park. He had just reported the unusual actions of cytochalasins in the journal Nature [180]. I asked him for a summer job and he asked me to set up an appointment. I said: "I'm outside ICI now," so he invited me in and the job was mine. Cytochalasins are a series of natural products but cytochalasin B caused polynuclear cells or at different concentration nuclear extrusion with a small cell membrane. This same natural product would later be used by Wayne Welshons to aid in discovering the actual location of the unoccupied ER [48, 181]. I had a great opportunity working in Steven Carter's laboratory on the electron microscopy of nuclear extrusion in mouse L cells. This was my introduction to ICI pharmaceuticals division. More importantly, I came to know Dora Richardson, the synthetic chemist who later would provide me with tamoxifen metabolites; Arthur (Walop) Walpole whose antifertility laboratory was opposite Steven Carter's; and Mike Barett, who was in charge of ICI's beta-blocker discovery program that was building on Jim Black's landmark discovery at ICI. Jim Black subsequently won the Nobel Prize in 1988 in Physiology and Medicine for "discoveries of important principles for drug treatment." Mike Barett's laboratory was next door to Steven Carter's. This again is where chance and opportunity take control, but you have to be ready to see the opportunity and be prepared to rise to the challenge. Mike Barett became the professor of Pharmacology at Leeds University. He apparently was impressed with my skill as a lecturer (I was a Ph.D. student at that time in the early 1970s) so he offered me a job as a lecturer in Pharmacology. I had no Ph.D. yet and no publications, but I was talent spotted!

I started my lifelong "love affair" with nonsteroidal estrogens and antiestrogens with the start of my Ph.D. thesis work entitled "A study of the oestrogenic and anti-oestrogenic activities of some substituted triphenylethylenes and triphenylethanes." I was supported by a Medical Research Council scholarship, which I only received by chance because I was originally on the waiting list. Someone declined their scholarship so there I was, a Ph.D. student in the Department of Pharmacology at the University of Leeds (1969–1972). I decided to study the ER with Dr. Edward Clark in the Department of Pharmacology at the University of Leeds. Dr. Jack Gorski had published an exciting series of reports showing that the ER could easily be extracted from the rat uterus and isolated by sucrose density gradient analysis. My project was going to be simple: I was to establish the new technique of sucrose density gradient analysis, isolate the receptor, and crystallize the protein with an estrogen and an antiestrogen. Through X-ray crystallography in the Astbury Department of Biophysics at the University of Leeds, we would establish the three-dimensional shape of the complexes to explain antiestrogenic action. The goal was to solve a fundamental question in pharmacology: What is the molecular mechanism of action for a drug? Progress was slow in establishing the receptor purification technique of sucrose gradient analysis, and I switched my thesis topic to study the structure-activity relationship of antiestrogens. As it turned out, this was a good, strategic decision, as it has taken the best efforts of the research community nearly 30 years to achieve success. The structure of the ER complex was solved by scientists at York University, England, in 1997. No one has yet succeeded in crystallizing the whole ER with an antiestrogen.

My study of failed contraceptives was less than inspiring as no one was recommending careers in a dead end. It was clear in the late 1960s that nonsteroidal antiestrogens would not be "morning-after pills." They were excellent in rats but did exactly the opposite in women. Also, as it turned out, the pharmaceutical industry chose to discontinue all their interest in these compounds because of too much toxicity or there was no money to be made. But chance meetings and my desire to be a part of developing a clinically useful drug for cancer would change that perspective.

The road to my Ph.D. was complicated in early 1972 as the university could not find an examiner. No one cared about failed contraceptives! Mike Barett solved the problem after Sir Charles Dodds declined with the words: "Sorry, I have not kept up with the literature during the past 20 years." He invited his former colleague Arthur Walpole to be my examiner, and after some grumbling by the university that it was inappropriate because "he was from industry," this set off a chain of events that would create tamoxifen as the gold standard for the treatment and prevention of breast cancer. This is the next chapter in our story as "Tamoxifen Goes Forward Alone."

During my Ph.D. studies, I learned all the names of the important players in estrogen action: Elwood Jensen, Jack Gorski, and Bill McGuire. Jensen and Gorski were world authorities on the ERs and my Ph.D. supervisor Ted Clark would often remark "look how many authors are on their papers; we cannot compete with these big groups." Bill McGuire was medically qualified and really drove the ER and progesterone receptor concept to predict the susceptibility of endocrine ablation into a clinical reality [182, 183]. Jensen and Gorski would eventually become my colleagues, coauthors, and then fellow members of the National Academy of Sciences. I remember well everyone congratulating Elwood Jensen at the pivotal meeting linking ER tumor level with response to ablative endocrine therapy in Bethesda, MD, in 1974 [184], when his election was announced. Elwood and I would receive the inaugural Dorothy P. Landon Award for translational research from the American Association for Cancer Research (AACR) in 2002, he for the ER target and me for the development of the "science of antiestrogens applied to cancer research" [185]. Bill McGuire and I would be close friends until his untimely death in 1992 [186–188]. Each of these prominent scientists gave me help and support in the early years of my career with invitations to their laboratories to talk about my "orphan drug tamoxifen" or with letters of recommendation. Each was important for my career development as a young scientist in the 1970s.

In closing Chap. 1, I wish to state that my focused interest in the pharmacology of nonsteroidal antiestrogens started with Leonard Lerner's discovery of MER 25. I was thrilled to meet him at meetings in Mont-Tremblant, Canada, of "Recent Progress in Hormone Research" started by Gregory Pincus of the Worcester Foundation. Len and I talked endlessly about a "group of forgotten drugs," nonsteroidal antiestrogens. Two enthusiasts. I was more than thrilled to receive the Bruce Cain Award with Len from the AACR in 1989 [125]. At that time something that was nothing, was being turned into something of medical significance.

References

1. Cook JW, Dodds EC, Hewett CL (1933) A synthetic oestrus-exciting compound. Nature 131:56
2. Jensen EV, Jacobson HI (1962) Basic guides to the mechanism of estrogen action. Recent Program Horm Res 18:387–414
3. Gorski J, Toft D, Shyamala G et al (1968) Hormone receptors: studies on the interaction of estrogen with the uterus. Recent Prog Horm Res 24:45–80
4. Jensen EV, DeSombre ER (1973) Estrogen-receptor interactions. Science 182:126–134
5. Allen E, Doisy EA (1923) An ovarian hormone. J Am Med Assoc 81:819–821
6. Kahnt LC, Doisy EA (1928) The vaginal smear method of assay of the ovarian hormone. Endocrinology 12:760–768
7. Emmens CW (1940/1941) Precursors of oestrogens. J Endocrinol 2:444–458
8. Emmens CW (1950) The intravaginal assay of naturally occurring oestrogens. J Endocrinol 6:302–307

9. Emmens CW (1942) Oestrogens and pro-oestrogens related to stilbene and triphenylethylene. J Endocrinol 3:168–173

10. Emmens CW (1947) Halogen-substituted oestrogens related to triphenylethylene. J Endocrinol 5:170–173

11. Martin L, Claringbold PJ (1958) A highly sensitive assay for oestrogens. Nature 181:620–621

12. Martin L (1960) The use of 2-3-5-triphenyltetrazolium chloride in the biological assay of oestrogens. J Endocrinol 20:187–197

13. Bulbring E, Burn JH (1935) The estimation of oestrin and of male hormone in oily solution. J Physiol 85:320–333

14. Lauson HD, Heller OG, Golden JB, Sevringhaus EL (1939) The immature rat uterus in the assay of estrogenic substances and a comparison of estradiol, estrone, and estriol. Endocrinology 24:35–44

15. Evans JS, Varney RF, Koch FC (1941) The mouse uterine weight method for the assay of estrogens. Endocrinology 28:747–752

16. Astwood EB (1938) A six-hour assay for the quantitative determination of estrogen. Endocrinology 23:25–31

17. Rubin BL, Dorfman AS, Black L, Dorfman RI (1951) Bioassay of estrogens using the mouse uterine response. Endocrinology 49:429–439

18. Terenius L (1965) Uptake of radioactive oestradiol in some organs of immature mice. The capacity and structural specificity of uptake studied with several steroid hormones. Acta Endocrinol (Copenh) 50:584–596

19. Terenius L (1966) Effect of synthetic oestrogens and analogues on the uptake of oestradiol by the immature mouse uterus and vagina. Acta Pharmacol Toxicol (Copenh) 24:89–100

20. Jordan VC (1975) Prolonged antioestrogenic activity of ICI 46, 474 in the ovariectomized mouse. J Reprod Fertil 42:251–258

21. Jordan VC, Naylor KE (1979) The binding of [3H]-oestradiol-17 beta in the immature rat uterus during the sequential administration of non-steroidal anti-oestrogens. Br J Pharmacol 65:167–173

22. Lieberman ME, Gorski J, Jordan VC (1983) An estrogen receptor model to describe the regulation of prolactin synthesis by antiestrogens in vitro. J Biol Chem 258:4741–4745

23. Dodds EC, Lawson W (1936) Synthetic oestrogenic agents without the phenanthrene nucleus. Nature 137:996

24. Dodds EC, Lawson W (1937) A simple aromatic oestrogenic agent with an activity of the same order as that of oestrone. Nature 139:627

25. Zondek B, Bergmann E (1938) Phenol methyl ethers as oestrogenic agents. Biochem J 32:641–645

26. Dodds EC, Lawson W (1937) Oestrogenic activity of p-hydroxy propenyl benzene (Anol). Nature 139:1068

27. Campbell NR, Dodds EC, Lawson W (1938) Oestrogenic activity of anol: a highly active phenol isolated from the byproducts. Nature 142:1121

28. Campbell NR, Dodds EC, Lawson W (1938) Oestrogenic activity of dianol, a dimeride of p-propenyl-phenol. Nature 141:78

29. Dodds E (1938) Biological effects of the synthetic oestrogenic substance 4:4'-dihydroxy-alpha:beta-diethylstilbene. Lancet 232:1389–1391

30. Dodds EC, Goldberg L, Lawson W, Robinson R (1938) Oestrogenic activity of certain synthetic compounds. Nature 141:247–248

31. Dodds EC, Golberg L, Lawson W, Robinson R (1938) Oestrogenic activity of esters of diethylstilbestrol. Nature 142:211–212

32. Dodds EC, Golberg L, Lawson W, Robinson R (1938) Oestrogenic activity of alkylated stilbestrols. Nature 142:34

33. Robson JM, Schonberg A (1937) Oestrous reactions, including mating, produced by triphenylethylene. Nature 140:196

34. Robson JM, Schonberg A, Fahim H (1938) Duration of action of natural and synthetic oestrogens. Nature 142:292–293
35. Robson JM, Schonberg A (1942) A new synthetic oestrogen with prolonged action when given orally. Nature 150:22–23
36. Robson JM, Ansari MY (1943) The fate of D.B.E. (alpha di-*p*-ethoxphenyl) (Beta-phenylbromoethylene) in the body. J Pharm Exptl Therap 79:340–345
37. Thompson CR, Werner HW (1951) Studies on estrogen tri-p-anisylchloroethylene. Proc Soc Exp Biol Med 77:494–497
38. Greenblatt RB, Brown NH (1952) The storage of estrogen in human fat after estrogen administration. Am J Obstet Gynecol 63:1361–1363
39. Thompson CR, Werner HW (1953) Fat storage of an estrogen in women following orally administered tri-p-anisylchloroethylene. Proc Soc Exp Biol Med 84:491–492
40. Haddow A, Watkinson JM, Paterson E, Koller PC (1944) Influence of synthetic oestrogens on advanced malignant disease. Br Med J 2:393–398
41. Kennedy BJ, Nathanson IT (1953) Effects of intensive sex steroid hormone therapy in advanced breast cancer. J Am Med Assoc 152:1135–1141
42. Dodds EC, Folley SJ, Glascock RF, Lawson W (1958) The excretion of microgram doses of hexoestrol by rabbits and rats. Biochem J 68:161–167
43. Glascock RF, Hoekstra WG (1959) Selective accumulation of tritium-labelled hexoestrol by the reproductive organs of immature female goats and sheep. Biochem J 72:673–682
44. Folca PJ, Glascock RF, Irvine WT (1961) Studies with tritium-labelled hexoestrol in advanced breast cancer. Comparison of tissue accumulation of hexoestrol with response to bilateral adrenalectomy and oophorectomy. Lancet 2:796–798
45. Tate AC, Jordan VC (1983) The estrogen receptor. In: Agarwal MK (ed) Textbook of Receptorology. Walter DeGruyter, Berlin, pp 381–463
46. Jordan VC, Tate AC, Lyman SD et al (1985) Rat uterine growth and induction of progesterone receptor without estrogen receptor translocation. Endocrinology 116:1845–1857
47. King WJ, Greene GL (1984) Monoclonal antibodies localize oestrogen receptor in the nuclei of target cells. Nature 307:745–747
48. Welshons WV, Lieberman ME, Gorski J (1984) Nuclear localization of unoccupied oestrogen receptors. Nature 307:747–749
49. Welshons WV, Cormier EM, Wolf MF et al (1988) Estrogen receptor distribution in enucleated breast cancer cell lines. Endocrinology 122:2379–2386
50. Lerner LJ (1981) The first non-steroidal antioestrogen- MER 25. In: Sutherland RL, Jordan VC (eds) Non steroidal antioestrogens. Academic, Sydney, pp 1–16
51. Segal SJ, Nelson WO (1958) An orally active compound with anti-fertility effects in rats. Proc Soc Exp Biol Med 98:431–436
52. Chang MC (1959) Degeneration of ova in the rat and rabbit following oral administration of 1-(p-2-diethylaminoethoxyphenyl)-1-phenyl-2-p-anisylethanol. Endocrinology 65:339–342
53. Barnes LE, Meyer RK (1962) Effects of ethamoxytriphetol, MRL-37, and clomiphene on reproduction in rats. Fertil Steril 13:472–480
54. Kistner RW, Smith OW (1959) Observations on the use of a nonsteroidal estrogen antagonist: MER 25. Surg Forum 10:725–729
55. Kistner RW, Smith OW (1961) Observations on the use of nonsteroidal estrogen antagonist: MER 25. Fertil Steril 12:121–141
56. Smith OW, Kistner RW (1963) Action of MER 25 and of clomiphene on the human ovary. JAMA 184:878–886
57. Holtkamp DE, Greslin JG, Root CA, Lerner LJ (1960) Gonadotrophin inhibiting and anti-fecundity effects of chloramiphene. Proc Soc Exp Biol Med 105:197–201
58. Davidson OW, Wada K, Segal SJ (1965) Effects of clomiphene at different stages of pregnancy in the rat. Implications regarding possible action mechanisms. Fertil Steril 16:195–201

59. Lednicer D, Babcock JC, Marlatt PE et al (1965) Mammalian antifertility agents. I. Derivatives of 2,3-diphenylindenes. J Med Chem 8:52–57
60. Lednicer D, Lyster SC, Duncan GW (1967) Mammalian antifertility agents. IV. Basic 3,4-dihydronaphthalenes and 1,2,3,4-tetrahydro-1-naphthols. J Med Chem 10:78–84
61. Lednicer D, Lyster SC, Aspergren BD, Duncan GW (1966) Mammalian antifertility agents. 3. 1-Aryl-2-phenyl-1,2,3,4-tetrahydro-1-naphthols, 1-aryl-2-phenyl-3,4-dihydronaphthalenes, and their derivatives. J Med Chem 9:172–176
62. Ray S, Grover PK, Kamboj VP et al (1976) Antifertility agents. 12. Structure-activity relationship of 3,4-diphenylchromenes and -chromans. J Med Chem 19:276–279
63. Greenwald GS (1965) Effects of a dihydronaphthalene derivative (U-11100a) on pregnancy in the rat. Fertil Steril 16:185–194
64. Harper MJ, Walpole AL (1967) Mode of action of I.C.I. 46,474 in preventing implantation in rats. J Endocrinol 37:83–92
65. Emmens CW (1970) Postcoital contraception. Br Med Bull 26:45–51
66. Emmens CW, Humphrey K, Martin L, Owen WH (1967) Antifertility properties of two non-oestrogenic steroids and MRL 37. Steroids 9:235–243
67. Palopoli FP, Feil VJ, Allen RE et al (1967) Substituted aminoalkoxytriarylhaloethylenes. J Med Chem 10:84–86
68. DiPietro DL, Sanders FJ, Goss DA (1969) Effect of *cis* and *trans* isomers of clomiphene citrate on uterine hexokinase activity. Endocrinology 84:1404–1408
69. Schulz KD, Haselmayer B, Holzel F (1971) The influence of clomid and its isomers on dimethylbenzanthracene-induced rat mammary tumors. In: Hubinot PO, Leroy F, Galand P (eds) Basic action of sex steroids on target organs. Karger, Basel
70. Self LW, Holtkamp DE, Kuhn WL (1967) Pituitary gonad related effects of isomers of clomiphene citrate. Fed Proc Fed Am Soc Exp Biol 26:534
71. Jordan VC, Haldemann B, Allen KE (1981) Geometric isomers of substituted triphenylethylenes and antiestrogen action. Endocrinology 108:1353–1361
72. Harper MJ, Walpole AL (1966) Contrasting endocrine activities of *cis* and *trans* isomers in a series of substituted triphenylethylenes. Nature 212:87
73. Bedford GR, Richardson DN (1966) Preparation and identification of *cis* and *trans* isomers of a substituted triarylethylene. Nature (London) 212:733
74. Kilbourn BT, Mais RHB, Owston PG (1968) Identification of isomers of a substituted triarylethylene: the crystal structure of 1-p-(2-dimethylaminoethoxyphenyl)-1,2-*cis*-diphenyl but-1-ene hydrobromide. Chem Commun 1:291
75. Harper MJ, Walpole AL (1967) A new derivative of triphenylethylene: effect on implantation and mode of action in rats. J Reprod Fertil 13:101–119
76. Collins DJ, Hobbs JJ, Emmens CW (1971) Antiestrogenic and antifertility compounds. 4. 1,1,2-triarylalkan-1-ols and 1,1,2-triarylalk-1-enes containing basic ether groups. J Med Chem 14:952–957
77. Callantine MR, Humphrey RR, Lee SL et al (1966) Action of an estrogen antagonist on reproductive mechanisms in the rat. Endocrinology 79:153–167
78. Jensen EV, Jacobson HI, Smith S et al (1972) The use of estrogen antagonists in hormone receptor studies. Gynecol Invest 3:108–123
79. Arbogast LY, DeSombre ER (1975) Estrogen-dependent in vitro stimulation of RNA synthesis in hormone-dependent mammary tumors of the rat. J Natl Cancer Inst 54:483–485
80. Salzer W (1946) Uber neue synthetische hochwirksame oestrogene. Hoppe-Seyler's Z. Physiol Chem 274:39–47
81. Silverman M, Bogert MT (1946) The synthesis of some indene and dihydronaphthalene derivatives related to stilbestrol. J Org Chem 11:34–49
82. Clark ER, Jordan VC (1976) Oestrogenic, anti-oestrogenic and fertility effects of some triphenylethanes and triphenylethylenes related to ethamoxytriphetol (MER 25). Br J Pharmacol 57:487–493

83. Abbott AC, Clark ER, Jordan VC (1976) Inhibition of oestradiol binding to oestrogen receptor proteins by a methyl-substituted analogue of tamoxifen. J Endocrinol 69:445–446

84. Robertson DW, Katzenellenbogen JA, Hayes JR, Katzenellenbogen BS (1982) Antiestrogen basicity–activity relationships: a comparison of the estrogen receptor binding and antiuterotrophic potencies of several analogues of (Z)-1,2-diphenyl-1-[4-[2-(dimethylamino)ethoxy]phenyl]-1-butene (tamoxifen, Nolvadex) having altered basicity. J Med Chem 25:167–171

85. Jones CD, Suarez T, Massey EH et al (1979) Synthesis and antiestrogenic activity of [3,4-dihydro-2-(4-methoxyphenyl)-1-naphthalenyl][4-[2-(1-pyrrolidinyl)ethoxy]-phe   nyl] methanone, methanesulfonic acid salt. J Med Chem 22:962–966

86. Kamboj VP, Setty BS, Chandra H et al (1977) Biological profile of centchroman–a new post-coital contraceptive. Indian J Exp Biol 15:1144–1150

87. Mukerjee SS, Sethi N, Srivastava GN et al (1977) Chronic toxicity studies of centchroman in rats and rhesus monkeys. Indian J Exp Biol 15:1162–1166

88. Dwani SAA, Saxena R, Setty BS, Gupta RC, Koll PL, Ray S, Anand N (1979) Seco-oestradiols and some non-steroidal estrogens: structural correlates of oestrogenic action. J Steroid Biochem 11:67

89. Saeed A, Durani N, Durani S et al (1984) Cis isomer of centchroman–a selective ligand for the microsomal antiestrogen binding site. Biochem Biophys Res Commun 125:346–352

90. Roy S, Datta JK (1976) Nature of estrogenic and anti-estrogenic actions of centchroman on rat uterus. Contraception 13:597–604

91. Toft D, Gorski J (1966) A receptor molecule for estrogens: isolation from the rat uterus and preliminary characterization. Proc Natl Acad Sci U S A 55:1574–1581

92. Toft D, Shyamala G, Gorski J (1967) A receptor molecule for estrogens: studies using a cell-free system. Proc Natl Acad Sci U S A 57:1740–1743

93. Jordan VC (2008) Tamoxifen: catalyst for the change to targeted therapy. Eur J Cancer 44:30–38

94. Korenman SG (1970) Relation between estrogen inhibitory activity and binding to cytosol of rabbit and human uterus. Endocrinology 87:1119–1123

95. Skidmore J, Walpole AL, Woodburn J (1972) Effect of some triphenylethylenes on oestradiol binding in vitro to macromolecules from uterus and anterior pituitary. J Endocrinol 52:289–298

96. Jordan VC, Collins MM, Rowsby L, Prestwich G (1977) A monohydroxylated metabolite of tamoxifen with potent antioestrogenic activity. J Endocrinol 75:305–316

97. Shiau AK, Barstad D, Loria PM et al (1998) The structural basis of estrogen receptor/coactivator recognition and the antagonism of this interaction by tamoxifen. Cell 95:927–937

98. Soule HD, Vazguez J, Long A et al (1973) A human cell line from a pleural effusion derived from a breast carcinoma. J Natl Cancer Inst 51:1409–1416

99. Shafie SM (1980) Estrogen and the growth of breast cancer: new evidence suggests indirect action. Science 209:701–702

100. Lippman ME, Bolan G (1975) Oestrogen-responsive human breast cancer in long term tissue culture. Nature 256:592–593

101. Greene GL, Fitch FW, Jensen EV (1980) Monoclonal antibodies to estrophilin: probes for the study of estrogen receptors. Proc Natl Acad Sci U S A 77:157–161

102. Greene GL, Nolan C, Engler JP, Jensen EV (1980) Monoclonal antibodies to human estrogen receptor. Proc Natl Acad Sci U S A 77:5115–5119

103. Greene GL, Gilna P, Waterfield M et al (1986) Sequence and expression of human estrogen receptor complementary DNA. Science 231:1150–1154

104. Green S, Walter P, Kumar V et al (1986) Human oestrogen receptor cDNA: sequence, expression and homology to v-erb-A. Nature 320:134–139

105. Lieberman ME, Maurer RA, Gorski J (1978) Estrogen control of prolactin synthesis in vitro. Proc Natl Acad Sci U S A 75:5946–5949

106. Lieberman ME, Jordan VC, Fritsch M et al (1983) Direct and reversible inhibition of estradiol-stimulated prolactin synthesis by antiestrogens in vitro. J Biol Chem 258:4734–4740

107. Jordan VC, Lieberman ME, Cormier E et al (1984) Structural requirements for the pharmacological activity of nonsteroidal antiestrogens in vitro. Mol Pharmacol 26:272–278

108. Jordan VC, Lieberman ME (1984) Estrogen-stimulated prolactin synthesis in vitro. Classification of agonist, partial agonist, and antagonist actions based on structure. Mol Pharmacol 26:279–285

109. Jordan VC, Koch R, Mittal S, Schneider MR (1986) Oestrogenic and antioestrogenic actions in a series of triphenylbut-1-enes: modulation of prolactin synthesis in vitro. Br J Pharmacol 87:217–223

110. Gottardis MM, Robinson SP, Satyaswaroop PG, Jordan VC (1988) Contrasting actions of tamoxifen on endometrial and breast tumor growth in the athymic mouse. Cancer Res 48:812–815

111. Jordan VC, Koch R (1989) Regulation of prolactin synthesis in vitro by estrogenic and antiestrogenic derivatives of estradiol and estrone. Endocrinology 124:1717–1726

112. Jordan VC (1984) Biochemical pharmacology of antiestrogen action. Pharmacol Rev 36:245–276

113. Berthois Y, Katzenellenbogen JA, Katzenellenbogen BS (1986) Phenol red in tissue culture media is a weak estrogen: implications concerning the study of estrogen-responsive cells in culture. Proc Natl Acad Sci U S A 83:2496–2500

114. Bindal RD, Carlson KE, Katzenellenbogen BS, Katzenellenbogen JA (1988) Lipophilic impurities, not phenolsulfonphthalein, account for the estrogenic activity in commercial preparations of phenol red. J Steroid Biochem 31:287–293

115. Bindal RD, Katzenellenbogen JA (1988) Bis(4-hydroxyphenyl)[2-(phenoxysulfonyl)phenyl] methane: isolation and structure elucidation of a novel estrogen from commercial preparations of phenol red (phenolsulfonphthalein). J Med Chem 31:1978–1983

116. Murphy CS, Langan-Fahey SM, McCague R, Jordan VC (1990) Structure-function relationships of hydroxylated metabolites of tamoxifen that control the proliferation of estrogen-responsive T47D breast cancer cells in vitro. Mol Pharmacol 38:737–743

117. Murphy CS, Parker CJ, McCague R, Jordan VC (1991) Structure-activity relationships of nonisomerizable derivatives of tamoxifen: importance of hydroxyl group and side chain positioning for biological activity. Mol Pharmacol 39:421–428

118. Jordan VC (1987) Laboratory models of breast cancer to aid the elucidation of antiestrogen action. J Lab Clin Med 109:267–277

119. Brzozowski AM, Pike AC, Dauter Z et al (1997) Molecular basis of agonism and antagonism in the oestrogen receptor. Nature 389:753–758

120. Wolf DM, Jordan VC (1994) The estrogen receptor from a tamoxifen stimulated MCF-7 tumor variant contains a point mutation in the ligand binding domain. Breast Cancer Res Treat 31:129–138

121. Jiang SY, Jordan VC (1992) Growth regulation of estrogen receptor-negative breast cancer cells transfected with complementary DNAs for estrogen receptor. J Natl Cancer Inst 84:580–591

122. Catherino WH, Wolf DM, Jordan VC (1995) A naturally occurring estrogen receptor mutation results in increased estrogenicity of a tamoxifen analog. Mol Endocrinol 9:1053–1063

123. Levenson AS, Catherino WH, Jordan VC (1997) Estrogenic activity is increased for an antiestrogen by a natural mutation of the estrogen receptor. J Steroid Biochem Mol Biol 60:261–268

124. Levenson AS, Jordan VC (1998) The key to the antiestrogenic mechanism of raloxifene is an 351 asp in estrogen receptor. Cancer Res 58:1872–1875

125. Schafer JI, Liu H, Tonetti DA, Jordan VC (1999) The interaction of raloxifene and the active metabolite of the antiestrogen EM-800 (SC 5705) with the human estrogen receptor. Cancer Res 59:4308–4313

126. MacGregor Schafer J, Liu H, Bentrem DJ et al (2000) Allosteric silencing of activating function 1 in the 4-hydroxytamoxifen estrogen receptor complex is induced by substituting glycine from aspartate at amino acid 351. Cancer Res 60:5097–5105

127. Liu H, Lee ES, Deb Los Reyes A et al (2001) Silencing and reactivation of the selective estrogen receptor modulator-estrogen receptor alpha complex. Cancer Res 61:3632–3639

128. Liu H, Park WC, Bentrem DJ et al (2002) Structure-function relationships of the raloxifene-estrogen receptor-alpha complex for regulating transforming growth factor-alpha expression in breast cancer cells. J Biol Chem 277:9189–9198

129. Lerner LJ, Jordan VC (1990) Development of antiestrogens and their use in breast cancer: eighth Cain memorial award lecture. Cancer Res 50:4177–4189

130. Lerner LJ, Holthaus FJ Jr, Thompson CR (1958) A non-steroidal estrogen antiagonist 1-(p-2-diethylaminoethoxyphenyl)-1-phenyl-2-p-methoxyphenyl   ethanol.   Endocrinology 63:295–318

131. Emmens CW, Cox RI, Martin L (1960) Oestrogen inhibition by steroids and other substances. J Endocrinol 20:198–209

132. Nicol T, Vernon-Roberts B, Quantock DC (1966) The effect of various anti-oestrogenic compounds on the reticulo-endothelial system and reproductive tract in the ovariectomized mouse. J Endocrinol 34:377–386

133. Shirley B, Wolinsky J, Schwartz NB (1968) Effects of a single injection of an estrogen antagonist on the estrous cycle of the rat. Endocrinology 82:959–968

134. Shelesnyak MC, Tic L (1963) Studies on the mechanism of decidualization. IV. Acta Endocrinol (Copenh) 42:465–472

135. Cutler A, Ober WB, Epstein JA, Kupperman HS (1961) The effect of 1-(p-2-diethylami-noethoxy-phenyl)-1-phenyl-2-panisyl ethanol upon rat pituitary and uterine responses to estrogen. Endocrinology 69:473–482

136. Jordan VC, Koerner S, Robison C (1975) Inhibition of oestrogen-stimulated prolactin release by anti-oestrogens. J Endocrinol 65:151–152

137. Wood JR, Wrenn TR, Bitman J (1968) Estrogenic and antiestrogenic effects of clomiphene, MER-25 and CN-55,945-27 on the rat uterus and vagina. Endocrinology 82:69–74

138. Harris DN, Lerner LJ, Hilf R (1968) The effects of progesterone and ethamoxytriphetol on estradiol-induced changes in the immature rat uterus. Trans N Y Acad Sci 30:774–782

139. Black LJ, Goode RL (1980) Uterine bioassay of tamoxifen, trioxifene and a new estrogen antagonist (LY117018) in rats and mice. Life Sci 26:1453–1458

140. Jordan VC, Rowsby L, Dix CJ, Prestwich G (1978) Dose-related effects of non-steroidal antioestrogens and oestrogens on the measurement of cytoplasmic oestrogen receptors in the rat and mouse uterus. J Endocrinol 78:71–81

141. Terenius L (1971) Structure-activity relationships of anti-oestrogens with regard to interaction with 17-beta-oestradiol in the mouse uterus and vagina. Acta Endocrinol (Copenh) 66:431–447

142. Terenius L (1970) Two modes of interaction between oestrogen and anti-oestrogen. Acta Endocrinol (Copenh) 64:47–58

143. Lee AE (1974) Effects of oestrogen antagonists on mitosis and (3H)oestradiol binding in the mouse uterus. J Endocrinol 60:167–174

144. Lee AE (1971) The limitations of using mouse uterine weight as an assay of oestrogen antagonism. Acta Endocrinol (Copenh) 67:345–352

145. Emmens CW (1971) Compounds exhibiting prolonged antioestrogenic and antifertility activity in mice and rats. J Reprod Fertil 26:175–182

146. Emmens CW, Carr WL (1973) Further studies of compounds exhibiting prolonged antioestrogenic and antifertility activity in the mouse. J Reprod Fertil 34:29–40

147. Martin L, Middleton E (1978) Prolonged oestrogenic and mitogenic activity of tamoxifen in the ovariectomized mouse. J Endocrinol 78:125–129

148. Martin L (1981) Effects of antiestrogens on cell proliferation in the rodent reproductive tract. In: Sutherland RL, Jordan VC (eds) Non-steroidal antiestrogens. Academic, Sydney, p 143

149. Kang YH, Anderson WA, DeSombre ER (1975) Modulation of uterine morphology and growth by estradiol-17beta and an estrogen antagonist. J Cell Biol 64:682–691
150. Jordan VC, Dix CJ (1979) Effect of oestradiol benzoate, tamoxifen and monohydroxy-tamoxifen on immature rat uterine progesterone receptor synthesis and endometrial cell division. J Steroid Biochem 11:285–291
151. Clark JH, Hardin JW, Padykula HA, Cardasis CA (1978) Role of estrogen receptor binding and transcriptional activity in the stimulation of hyperestrogenism and nuclear bodies. Proc Natl Acad Sci U S A 75:2781–2784
152. Kaye AM, Sheratzky D, Lindner HR (1972) Kinetics of DNA synthesis in immature rat uterus: age dependence and estradiol stimulation. Biochim Biophys Acta 261:475–486
153. Greenblatt RB, Barfield WE, Jungck EC, Ray AW (1961) Induction of ovulation with MRL/41. Preliminary report. JAMA 178:101–104
154. Klopper A, Hall M (1971) New synthetic agent for the induction of ovulation: preliminary trials in women. Br Med J 1:152–154
155. Chen CL, Meites J (1960) Effects of estrogen and progesterone on serum and pituitary prolactin levels in ovariectomized rats. Endocrinology 66:96
156. Heuson JC, Waelbroeck C, Legros N et al (1971) Inhibition of DMBA-induced mammary carcinogenesis in the rat by 2-br- -ergocryptine (CB 154), an inhibitor of prolactin secretion, and by nafoxidine (U-11, 100 A), an estrogen antagonist. Gynecol Invest 2:130–137
157. Jordan VC, Koerner S (1976) Tamoxifen as an anti-tumour agent: role of oestradiol and prolactin. J Endocrinol 68:305–311
158. Jordan VC, Dix CJ, Allen KE (1981) Effects of antioestrogens in carcinogen-induced rat mammary cancer. In: Sutherland RL, Jordan VC (eds) Non-steroidal anti-oestrogens. Academic, Sydney, pp 261–280
159. de Quijada M, Timmermans HA, Lamberts SW (1980) Tamoxifen suppresses both the growth of prolactin-secreting pituitary tumours and normal prolactin synthesis in the rat. J Endocrinol 86:109–116
160. de Quijada M, Timmermans HA, Lamberts SW, MacLeod RM (1980) Tamoxifen enhances the sensitivity of dispersed prolactin-secreting pituitary tumor cells to dopamine and bromo-criptine. Endocrinology 106:702–706
161. Labhsetwar AP (1970) Role of estrogens in ovulation: a study using the estrogen-antagonist, I.C.I. 46,474. Endocrinology 87:542–551
162. Bainbridge JG, Labhsetwar AP (1971) The role of oestrogens in spontaneous ovulation: location of site of action of positive feedback of oestrogen by intracranial implantation of the anti-oestrogen I.C.I. 46474. J Endocrinol 50:321–327
163. Billard R, McDonald PG (1973) Inhibition of ovulation in the rat by intrahypothalamic implants of an antioestrogen. J Endocrinol 56:585–590
164. Sheth AR, Vaidya RA, Arbatti NJ, Devi PK (1977) Effect of Centchroman on serum gonadotropins & prolactin in rats. Indian J Exp Biol 15:1191–1193
165. Dohler KDVSMA, Dohler U (1977) ICI46,474-lack of oestrogenic activity in the rat. ICRS Med Sci 5:185
166. Bartke A, Mason M, Dalterio S, Bex F (1978) Effects of tamoxifen on plasma concentrations of testosterone and gonadotrophins in the male rat. J Endocrinol 79:239–240
167. Hsueh AJ, Erickson GF, Yen SS (1978) Sensitisation of pituitary cells to luteinising hormone releasing hormone by clomiphene citrate in vitro. Nature 273:57–59
168. Miller WL, Huang ES (1981) Antiestrogens and ovine gonadotrophs: antagonism of estrogen-induced changes in gonadotropin secretions. Endocrinology 108:96–102
169. Segal SJ, Thompson CR (1956) Inhibition of estradiol-induced pituitary hypertrophy in rats. Proc Soc Exp Biol Med 91:623–625
170. Jordan VC, Schafer JM, Levenson AS et al (2001) Molecular classification of estrogens. Cancer Res 61:6619–6623
171. Bentrem D, Fox JE, Pearce ST et al (2003) Distinct molecular conformations of the estrogen receptor alpha complex exploited by environmental estrogens. Cancer Res 63:7490–7496

172. Aten RF, Weinberger MJ, Eisenfeld AJ (1980) Kinetics of in vivo nuclear translocation of the male and female rat liver estrogen receptors. Endocrinology 106:1127–1132
173. Aten RF, Dickson RB, Eisenfeld AJ (1979) Female and male green monkey liver estrogen receptor. Biochem Pharmacol 28:2445–2450
174. Bichon M, Bayard F (1979) Dissociated effects of tamoxifen and oestradiol-17 beta on uterus and liver functions. J Steroid Biochem 10:105–107
175. Kneifel MA, Katzenellenbogen BS (1981) Comparative effects of estrogen and antiestrogen on plasma renin substrate levels and hepatic estrogen receptors in the rat. Endocrinology 108:545–552
176. Sakai F, Cheix F, Clavel M et al (1978) Increases in steroid binding globulins induced by tamoxifen in patients with carcinoma of the breast. J Endocrinol 76:219–226
177. Sutherland R, Mester J, Baulieu EE (1977) Tamoxifen is a potent "pure" anti-oestrogen in chick oviduct. Nature 267:434–435
178. Binart N, Catelli MG, Geynet C et al (1979) Monohydroxytamoxifen: an antioestrogen with high affinity for the chick oviduct oestrogen receptor. Biochem Biophys Res Commun 91:812–818
179. Lazier CB, Capony F, Williams DL (1981) Antioestrogen action in chick liver: effects on oestrogen receptors in oestrogen-induced proteins. In: Sutherland RL, Jordan VC (eds) Non-steroidal antioestrogens. Academic, Sydney, pp 215–230
180. Carter SB (1967) Effects of cytochalasins on mammalian cells. Nature 213:261–264
181. Welshons WV, Grady LH, Judy BM et al (1993) Subcellular compartmentalization of MCF-7 estrogen receptor synthesis and degradation. Mol Cell Endocrinol 94:183–194
182. Clark GM, McGuire WL, Hubay CA et al (1983) Progesterone receptors as a prognostic factor in stage II breast cancer. N Engl J Med 309:1343–1347
183. Horwitz KB, McGuire WL (1975) Predicting response to endocrine therapy in human breast cancer: a hypothesis. Science 189:726–727
184. McGuire WL, Carbone PP, Vollmer EP (1975) Estrogen receptors in human breast cancer. Raven, New York
185. Jensen EV, Jordan VC (2003) The estrogen receptor: a model for molecular medicine. Clin Cancer Res 9:1980–1989
186. Jordan VC (1995) Third annual William L. McGuire Memorial Lecture. "Studies on the estrogen receptor in breast cancer"–20 years as a target for the treatment and prevention of cancer. Breast Cancer Res Treat 36:267–285
187. Wolf DM, Jordan VC (1993) William L. McGuire Memorial Symposium. Drug resistance to tamoxifen during breast cancer therapy. Breast Cancer Res Treat 27:27–40
188. Jordan VC (1995) Third Annual William L. McGuire Memorial Lecture. "Studies on the estrogen receptor in breast cancer" – 20 years as a target for the treatment and prevention of cancer. Breast Cancer Res Treat 36:267–185

Chapter 2
Tamoxifen Goes Forward Alone

Abstract Tamoxifen (ICI 46,474), the *trans* isomer of a substituted triphenyl-ethylene, was discovered in the fertility program at Imperial Chemical Industries, Pharmaceuticals Division, Cheshire, England. The plan was to use tamoxifen to regulate fertility, but this failed and interest refocused outside the company for applications to treat breast cancer. The initial application of the nonsteroidal antiestrogen was for the treatment of metastatic breast cancer in postmenopausal women and by the 1980s tamoxifen had replaced high-dose diethylstilbestrol therapy. Efficacy when compared with diethylstilbestrol was similar, but tamoxifen had fewer side effects. No other antiestrogens were developed by the pharmaceutical industry, as this was not considered a financially lucrative development strategy.

Introduction

History is lived forward but is written in retrospect. "We know the end before we consider the beginning and we can never wholly recapture what it was to know the beginning only" (C.V. Wedgewood, *William the Silent*). That is, unless one has lived through the evolving applications of tamoxifen.

Tamoxifen (ICI 46,474; Nolvadex), a nonsteroidal antiestrogen, started life as the endocrine treatment of choice for advanced breast cancer [1]. Adjuvant therapy with tamoxifen also proved to be effective [2] because a sustained survival advantage is noted for women with node-positive and node-negative disease. The Food and Drug Administration (FDA) approved the use of tamoxifen as an adjuvant therapy with chemotherapy (1986), as an adjuvant therapy alone (1988) in node-positive post-menopausal patients and pre- and postmenopausal node-negative patients with ER-positive disease (1990). Tamoxifen is used to treat breast cancer in men (1993). However, remarkably tamoxifen was also approved to reduce the risk of breast cancer in women at high risk (1998). Tamoxifen was also FDA approved for treatment of ductal carcinoma in situ (DCIS) (2000). No other cancer therapy is so widely approved and had so dramatic an impact on cancer care. Tamoxifen is,

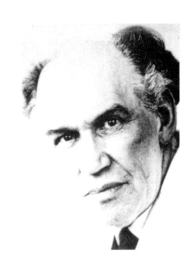

Fig. 2.1 Arthur Walpole who died suddenly on 2 July 1977. At the time of his death, he had retired as head of the Fertility Control Program at ICI's Pharmaceuticals Division at Alderley Park, near Macclesfield, Cheshire, but he had continued to work as a consultant on the joint research scheme between ICI and the Department of Pharmacology at the University of Leeds, England

however, one of those remarkable examples of a drug originally designed for one primary purpose that fails but is then steered by dedicated scientists toward a recognized secondary application where it becomes enormously successful.

The chief credit for the discovery of tamoxifen in 1962, and its subsequent application as an orphan drug treatment for metastatic breast cancer, must be given to Dr. Arthur L. Walpole (Fig. 2.1), then head of the fertility control program for Imperial Chemical Industries (ICI) Pharmaceuticals Division. Tamoxifen was identified as an effective postcoital contraceptive in rats [3–5] and there was a distinct possibility that antiestrogens could be developed as "morning-after" pills [6]. However, the basic pharmacology and physiology of ovulation and implantation are critically different in women and rats. When tamoxifen was tested in patients in preliminary clinical studies, it was found to induce ovulation rather than reduce fertility [7, 8] and so is marketed in some countries for the induction of ovulation in subfertile women [1].

The ovarian dependence of some breast cancers has long been recognized [9, 10] and the first antiestrogens [11, 12] were shown to be effective in their treatment, but the drugs then available were considered to be too toxic for chronic use [13–15] (Table 2.1). By the end of the 1960s, the direct role of estrogen in breast cancer growth was further substantiated with the description of ERs in breast tumors [18–20] and the subsequent clinical correlation with hormone dependency [21, 22]. However, clinical research with tamoxifen was not based on the ER but on proven antifertility activity as an antiestrogen in the rat. Walpole encouraged the clinical testing of the antiestrogen tamoxifen at the Christie Hospital and Holt Radium Institute in Manchester [16]. He had a long interest in cancer research [23] but also wanted to determine whether tamoxifen was an estrogen or an antiestrogen in humans because of the link between estrogens and breast cancer growth. A subsequent dose response study was published by Dr. Harold Ward [17]. But in 1972, ICI Pharmaceutical

Table 2.1 Comparison of the early chemical experience with antiestrogen as a treatment for metastatic breast cancer

Antiestrogen	Daily dose (mg)	Year	Response rate (%)	Toxicity
Ethamoxytriphetol	500–4,500	1960	25	Acute psychotic episodes
Clomiphene	100–300	1964–1974	34	Fear of cataracts
Nafoxidine	180–240	1976	31	Cataracts, ichthyosis, photophobia
Tamoxifen	20–40	1971–1973	31	Transient thrombocytopenia[a]

[a]"The particular advantage of this drug is the low incidence of troublesome side effects" [16]. "Side effects were usually trivial" [17]

Division chose to abandon clinical development because there would be no financial gain for the limited applications in the treatment of metastatic breast cancer where only one in three patients respond for, on average, 2 years [24].

This chapter will trace the "resurrection" and development of tamoxifen for the treatment of advanced breast cancer in postmenopausal patients and consider the unusual set of circumstances that set the stage for the subsequent success of tamoxifen as a long-term adjuvant therapy in patients with node-positive and node-negative disease. In 1990, the fashion was to change again with a plan to test the worth of tamoxifen as a preventive in women at risk for breast cancer [25–27]. Much of the basic laboratory work in animal models was conducted in the period 1974–1992. This produced a strong rationale to move forward with clinical trials and the meticulous evaluations of pharmacology of tamoxifen (Fig. 2.2). This is our story.

ICI 46,474: The Early Years

In 1958, Lerner and coworkers described the first nonsteroidal antiestrogen MER 25. The drug was tested in clinical trials but proved to be toxic at the high doses required [28]. A successor compound, clomiphene (also known as chloramiphene or MRL41) (Fig. 2.2), now known to be a mixture of two geometric isomers with opposing biological activities, was a postcoital contraceptive in rats but was developed only clinically as a fertility drug [29] (see Chap. 1).

To understand the obstacles that had to be overcome before the successful clinical development of tamoxifen, it is necessary to recapture the mood of the times in the 1950s/1960s. Coronary heart disease was a primary target for drug development and was proving to be a lucrative market. However, one product—triparanol (MER29) (Fig. 2.2)—was to become a cause *célèbre* and a major issue in the relationship between product safety and regulatory authorities. Indeed, this case was taught to Craig Jordan as an undergraduate at Leeds University, in the Pharmacology Department (1965–1969), to illustrate how drug development can go very wrong.

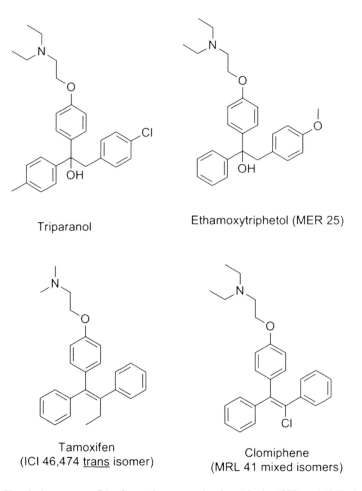

Fig. 2.2 Chemical structures of the first antiestrogens developed in the 1950s and 1960s, including tamoxifen

Triparanol was an orally active lipid-lowering agent developed by the Merrell Company during the 1960s [30]. Unfortunately, acute cataract formation was noted in young women treated with triparanol [31] and this ultimately led to the withdrawal of the medicine. The toxicity was linked to the accumulation of desmosterol as a consequence of the inhibition of cholesterol biosynthesis [32] (Fig. 2.3).

The punitive legal issues surrounding the withdrawal of triparanol forced the Merrell Company to avoid long-term treatments with any agents known to, or thought to, cause increases in the circulating levels of desmosterol. Triparanol [33], ethamoxytriphetol, and clomiphene [14] were all tested as treatments for breast cancer, but their potential to harm through cataract formation forced the Merrell Company to abandon work in the treatment of breast cancer. The administration of clomiphene for a few

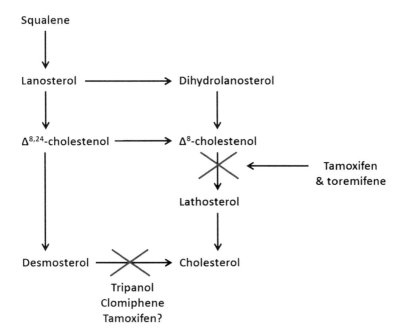

Fig. 2.3 The inhibition of cholesterol biosynthesis by triparanol, clomiphene, tamoxifen, and the chlorinated derivative of tamoxifen toremifene (see Chap. 3, Fig. 3.7)

days to induce ovulation was considered safe compared with the years of therapy necessary for breast cancer treatment.

Arthur Walpole, as head of the Fertility Control Program at ICI Pharmaceuticals Division Alderley Park, was already interested in the pharmacology of nonsteroidal estrogens and was asked to find a safer nonsteroidal antiestrogen in the early 1960s. Dora Richardson was the synthetic organic chemist for the program (Fig. 2.4) and a young reproductive endocrinologist Michael J. K. Harper conducted the antifertility studies in the rat model (Fig. 2.4). The discovery of ICI 46,474 with reduced concerns about desmosterol accumulation was an advance.

From the time that tamoxifen was first available in clinical practice (1973) until the late 1980s, there were remarkably few concerns about the toxicity of tamoxifen, because the side effects from chemotherapy, by contrast, were so severe. Only with the extended use of tamoxifen as an adjuvant therapy in node-negative women, and the proposed use of tamoxifen as a chemopreventive, was there a return to an evaluation of the toxicity of tamoxifen, both by laboratory studies and by the analysis of randomized clinical trials. Despite the fact that tamoxifen was considered safe for long-term adjuvant therapy in women with breast cancer, analysis of the prevention trials organized and run by the National Surgical Adjuvant Bowel and Breast Project (NSABP) would demonstrate a small increase in cataracts and cataract operations for women without disease taking tamoxifen to reduce breast cancer incidence [34, 35].

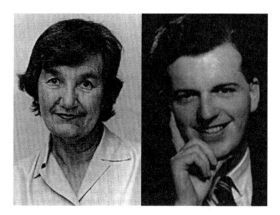

Fig. 2.4 (*Left*) Dora Richardson was a co-patent holder for ICI 46,474 and the organic chemist responsible for the synthesis of triphenylethylenes at ICI Pharmaceuticals. This photograph was taken on the occasion of her retirement in 1979. (*Right*) Mike Harper who discovered the opposing biological activities of the *cis* and *trans* isomers of substituted triphenylethylenes

ICI 46,474 was first synthesized by Dr. Dora Richardson at ICI Ltd., Pharmaceuticals Division (Fig. 2.4), and was shown to be an antifertility agent in rodents [4, 5]. Dr. Michael Harper (Fig. 2.4) [3] made the discovery that the geometric isomers of substituted triphenylethylenes have opposing biological properties: the *cis* isomer ICI 47,699 is an estrogen, whereas the *trans* isomer ICI 46,474 has antiestrogenic activity. Thus the structure of the drug can program the cells for estrogenic or antiestrogenic properties [36–38]. Another observation made by Harper and Walpole was that ICI 46,474 exhibits species specificity; in short-term tests, the compound is an estrogen in the mouse and an antiestrogen in the rat [3, 4]. The triphenylethylene derivative blocks the binding of [^{3}H]estradiol to ERs derived from both rat and mouse target tissues [39–42], but no completely satisfactory subcellular mechanism for the species difference of ICI 46,474 has yet been established. In fact, the situation is probably more complex than may at first be appreciated. The long-term administration of tamoxifen to ovariectomized mice results in an initial estrogen-like effect in the vagina [40] and the uterus [43], but as treatment progresses both the uterus and vagina become refractory to the effects of exogenous estrogen, and ICI 46,474 becomes a complete antiestrogen in the vagina.

Preliminary clinical studies with ICI 46,474 to treat advanced breast cancer in postmenopausal women were conducted by Mary Cole and coworkers [16] at the Christie Hospital in Manchester. The confirmation that ICI 46,474 could be used successfully as palliative in advanced disease but produces few side effects [17, 44] acted as a catalyst to encourage the study of the mode of action of the drug in animal tumor models. Indeed the conversation between the laboratory and the clinic became the hallmark for the successful development of tamoxifen.

Animal studies were first started in 1973 at the Worcester Foundation for Experimental Biology Shrewsbury, Massachusetts [45–50]. The dimethylbenzanthracene (DMBA)-induced rat mammary carcinoma model, originally described a decade earlier by the Nobel Laureate Professor Charles Huggins [51], was used to study the efficacy and mode of action of ICI 46,474 under controlled laboratory conditions. The model was considered to be state of the art, because no other hormone-dependent models were then available for study. Rob Nicholson, then a graduate student at the Tenovus Institute for Cancer Research in Cardiff, Wales, also selected the DMBA-induced rat mammary carcinoma model for this study of the antitumor actions of ICI 46,474 and related compounds [52]. These parallel research ventures fully described the antitumor activity of the antiestrogen in vivo [41, 48–50, 53, 54] at a time when the efficacy of tamoxifen was being established widely in breast cancer clinical trials [55].

ICI 46,474 to Tamoxifen

In 1973, Nolvadex, the ICI brand of tamoxifen (as its citrate salt), was approved for the treatment of breast cancer by the Committee on the Safety of Medicines in the United Kingdom. Similar approval was given in the United States for the treatment of advanced disease in postmenopausal women by the Food and Drug Administration on 30 December 1977. Nolvadex was available in more than 110 countries as the first-line endocrine therapy for the treatment of breast cancer [1]. To mark this achievement, ICI Pharmaceutical Division was presented with the Queen's Award for Technological Achievement by the Lord Lieutenant of Cheshire, Viscount Leverhulme, on 6 July 1978. The remarkable success of tamoxifen encouraged a closer examination of its pharmacology with a view to further development and wider applications.

The metabolism of tamoxifen in animals and patients was first described by Fromson and coworkers [56, 57]. The major metabolic route to be described was hydroxylation to form 4-hydroxytamoxifen, which was subsequently shown to have high binding affinity for the estrogen receptor and to be a potent antiestrogen in its own right [58] with antitumor properties in the DMBA model [59]. Indeed it is an advantage for the tamoxifen to be metabolically activated to 4-hydroxytamoxifen [60], but this is not a prerequisite for antiestrogen action. The metabolite was subsequently shown to localize in target tissues after the administration of radioactive tamoxifen to rats [61]. Originally, 4-hydroxytamoxifen was believed to be the major metabolite in patients [57], but Hugh Adam [62] at ICI Pharmaceutical Division demonstrated that N-desmethyltamoxifen is the principal metabolite found in patients. There is usually a blood level ratio of 2:1 for N-desmethyltamoxifen that has twice the plasma half-life of tamoxifen (14 days vs. 7 days) [63]. The ubiquitous use of tamoxifen resulted in the publication of numerous methods to estimate tamoxifen and its metabolites in serum (reviewed in [64]). The metabolites that have been identified in patients are shown in Fig. 2.5. The minor metabolites, metabolite Y [65], metabolite Z [66], and 4-hydroxy-N-desmethyltamoxifen [67], all contribute to the antitumor actions of tamoxifen, because they are all antiestrogens which inhibit the binding of estradiol to the ER. The metabolism of tamoxifen will be considered in more detail in Chap. 3.

The next significant advance came with the availability of hormone-dependent human breast cancer cells to study antitumor mechanisms in the laboratory.

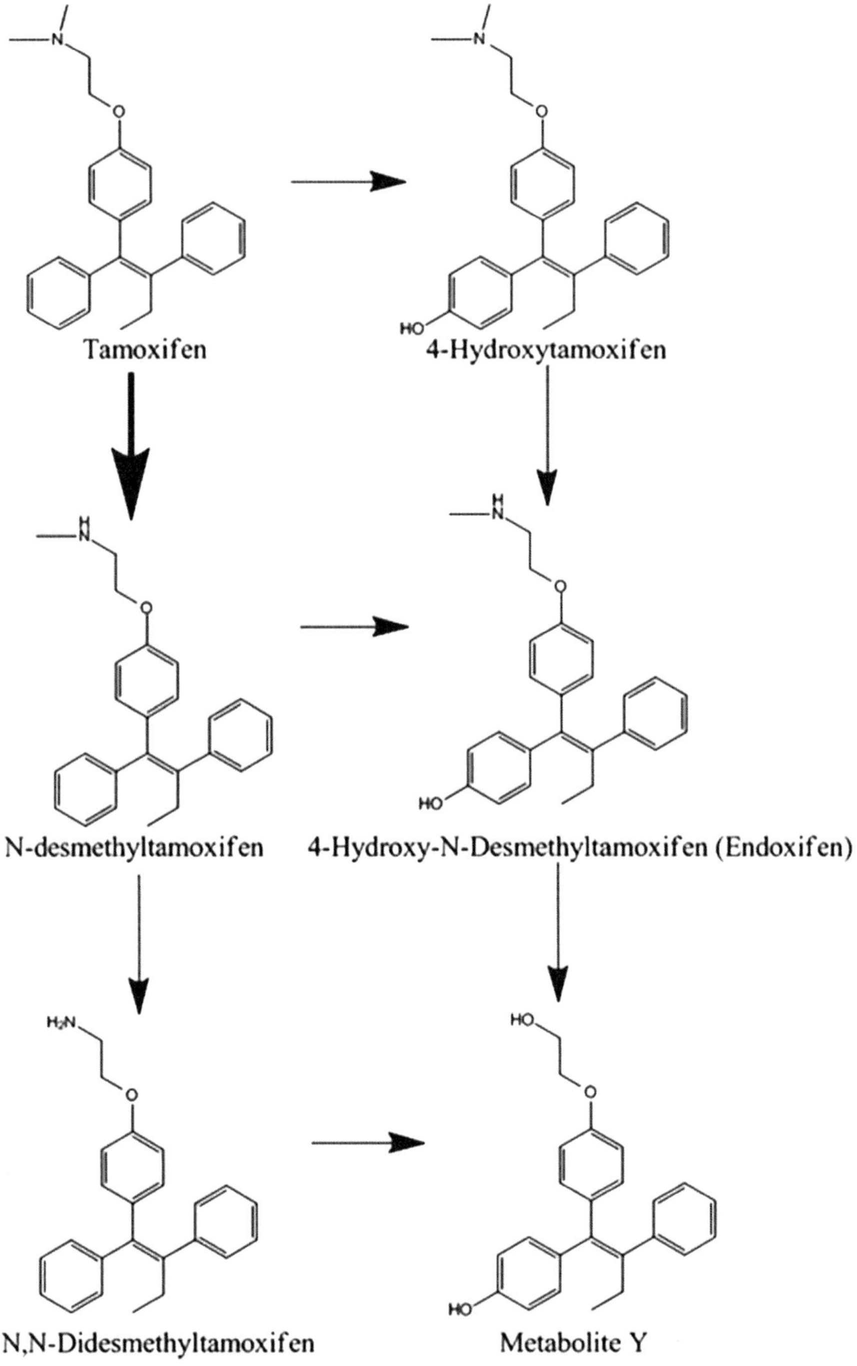

Fig. 2.5 The scheme of tamoxifen metabolism and the structures of its metabolites

Marc Lippman [68] was the first to describe the ability of tamoxifen to inhibit the growth of MCF-7 ER-positive breast cancer cells [69] in culture and to demonstrate that the addition of estrogen could reverse the action of tamoxifen. Nearly a decade later, Kent Osborne [70] and Rob Sutherland [71] independently described the blockade by tamoxifen of breast cancer cells at the G_1 phase of the cell cycle.

Studies with the heterotransplantation of MCF-7 cells into athymic mice demonstrated that, unlike estradiol, tamoxifen does not support the growth of tumors [72]. Tamoxifen [73] and its metabolites [74] will block estrogen-stimulated tumor growth. However, very high circulatory levels (2,300 pg/ml) of estradiol in a low-tamoxifen environment (40 ng/ml) can partly reverse the inhibitory actions of tamoxifen for MCF-7 tumor growth [75]. Overall, these studies of the reversibility of tamoxifen action could have implications for its extended adjuvant use in premenopausal women.

These significant biological advances propelled tamoxifen forward to become the only nonsteroidal estrogen antagonist that would become the "gold standard" for the endocrine therapy of breast cancer for two decades. But none of this seemed possible in the 1970s when ICI Pharmaceutical Division was chauffeuring thousands of rats from Alderley Park to Leeds University. This investment in independent academic research would convert an orphan drug to be multibillion GBP blockbuster that saved millions of women's lives [76]. What is amazing is that the early work occurred without patent protection, but that changed.

Patenting Problems

Adequate patent protection is required to develop an innovation in a timely manner. In 1962, ICI Pharmaceuticals Division filed a broad patent in the United Kingdom (UK) (Application number GB19620034989 19620913). The application stated, "The alkene derivatives of the invention are useful for the modification of the endocrine status in man and animals and they may be useful for the control of hormone-dependent tumours or for the management of the sexual cycle and aberrations thereof. They also have useful hypocholesterolaemic activity."

This was published in 1965 as UK Patent GB1013907, which described the innovation that different geometric isomers of substituted triphenylethylenes had either estrogenic or antiestrogenic properties [3]. Indeed, this observation was significant, because when scientists at Merrell subsequently described the biological activity of the separated isomers of their drug clomiphene, they inadvertently reversed the naming [77]. This was subsequently rectified [78].

Although tamoxifen was approved for the treatment of advanced breast cancer in postmenopausal women in 1977 in the United States (the year before ICI Pharmaceuticals Division received the Queen's Award for Technological Achievement in the UK), the patent situation was unclear. ICI Pharmaceuticals Division was repeatedly denied patent protection in the United States until the 1980s because of the perceived primacy of the earlier Merrell patents and because no advance (i.e., a safer, more specific drug) was recognized by the patent office in the United States. In other words, the clinical development advanced steadily for more than a decade in the United States without the assurance of exclusivity. This situation also illustrates how unlikely the usefulness of tamoxifen was considered to be by the medical advisors to the pharmaceutical industry in general. No other company chose to "steal" tamoxifen. Remarkably, when tamoxifen was hailed as the adjuvant endocrine treatment of choice for breast cancer by the National Cancer Institute in 1984 [79], the patent application, initially denied in 1984, was awarded through the court of appeals in 1985. This was granted with precedence to the patent dating back to 1965! So, at a time when worldwide patent protection was being lost, the patent protecting tamoxifen started a 17-year life in the United States. The unique and unusual legal situation did not go uncontested by generic companies, but AstraZeneca (as the ICI Pharmaceuticals Division is now called) rightly retained patent protection for their pioneering product, most notably, from Smalkin's decision in Baltimore, 1996 (Zeneca, Ltd. vs. Novopharm, Ltd.Civil Action No S95-163 United States District Court, D. Maryland, Northern Division, 14 March 1996).

Conclusion

The unprecedented advance of tamoxifen from the first unsure steps seems unbelievable but actually occurred. This situation was dependent on the correct, prepared individuals being at the right place at the right time to advance a pioneering medicine that saves lives.

Postscript. In September 1972, at the time of the examination of my Ph.D. thesis by Dr. Arthur Walpole, I was unaware that the research director at ICI Pharmaceutical Division had ordered the termination of the clinical development of tamoxifen. This was a financial decision based on nonprofitability. My understanding is that all of the clinical research on tamoxifen (then ICI 46,474) had been reviewed in March 1972 at a symposium at Alderley Park [24].

   The termination of tamoxifen's development toward registration and clinical use had resulted in Walpole requesting early retirement. Scientists at ICI Pharmaceutical Division did none of the laboratory work on tamoxifen as an antitumor agent; that was outsourced to me for a decade. But how did that happen?

   I had already been recruited to the faculty as a lecturer in Pharmacology at Leeds, but first I was required to spend a couple of years in the United States to obtain my BTA (Been to America, a colloquial acronym as a prestigious research qualification). It had been arranged that I would go to the Worcester Foundation for Experimental Biology (the home of the oral contraceptive) to work with Mike Harper, who had left ICI Pharmaceutical Division some years earlier and now headed an Agency for International Development Program, to create a once a month contraceptive based on prostaglandins (the new research fashion!). I remember my conversation with Mike Harper on the telephone as I stood in the corridor on the phone in the old Medical School in Leeds. He asked three questions: "Could you start in September

(1972)?" "Would $12,000 a year be acceptable?" and "Would you work on prosta-glandins?" "Yes, yes, yes," I replied and headed off to the library to find out what prostaglandins were!

Walpole, my committee, and I met for my examination in the Department of Pharmacology at the Leeds University in early September 1972. This had become a matter of urgency as I had to complete the examination, drive to Southampton to board the QEII, and then travel from New York to Worcester, MA, to be a visiting scientist for 2 years at the Worcester Foundation for Experimental Biology.

When I arrived to the Worcester Foundation in September 1972—incidentally not knowing anything about prostaglandins—I discovered that Mike Harper had accepted a job with the World Health Organization in Geneva. My new boss Ed Klaiber said: "Next week give me a plan of research you propose to complete here in the next two years" and "You can do anything you like as long as some of it includes prostaglandins." Armed with a brand new Ph.D. in "failed contraceptives" (a topic not designed to equip me for a research career!), I immediately found myself as an independent investigator and planned my work on prostaglandins. However, my new circumstances would also allow me to explore my passion—to develop a drug to treat breast cancer.

A phone call to Walpole started the process of turning ICI 46,474 into tamoxifen, the gold standard for the endocrine treatment of breast cancer for the next 30 years. Walpole informed me that ICI Pharmaceuticals Division had just acquired Stuart Pharmaceuticals in Wilmington, Delaware, and they had created a new company ICI Americas. Lois Trench, the drug monitor for tamoxifen, would be the individual involved in the investment in my laboratory at the Worcester Foundation with an unrestricted research grant to determine how best to use tamoxifen in the clinic. But how to start? I was a pharmacologist with experience in "failed contraceptive" not a cancer research scientist. It seems that the way forward depends upon a clear plan, enthusiasm, and who you meet.

The National Cancer Act was passed in 1971 in the United States and the "war on cancer" began. The president of the Worcester Foundation Mahlon Hoagland realized that the research resources of the foundation in reproductive endocrinology could be steered toward endocrine-dependent cancers with the right advisor on the Scientific Advisory Board. Dr. Elwood Jensen, director of the Ben May Laboratory for Cancer Research at the University of Chicago, was a pioneer in the identification of the ER in estrogen target tissues in the rat and the application of this knowledge for the identification of estrogen-dependent breast tumors in women with metastatic breast cancer. The absence of ER in the tumor meant that there was no possibility of a response to endocrine ablation. Jensen spent a couple of days at the foundation in late 1972 and we spent time together going over my thesis work. I told him of my plans for tamoxifen and he generously agreed to have his staff (or rather Silvia Smith) teach me techniques of ER analysis and most importantly his colleague Dr. Gene DeSombre to teach me the dimethylbenzanthracene (DMBA)-induced rat mammary carcinoma model. My visit to Chicago to learn the techniques was a dream come true!

Lois Trench arranged for me to receive a small collection of deep-frozen breast tumors so we started the program of translational research with the aid of Suzanne Koerner, a superb technician. Lois insisted I became a consultant to ICI Americas to encourage clinicians in oncology groups to study tamoxifen in clinical trial. I lectured to the members of the Eastern Cooperative Oncology Group Breast Committee at their meetings in Miami and Jasper National Park in 1974. Too many adventures there to fit in the limited space here, I am afraid! Lois, then sponsored me to present the first study on tamoxifen as a preventive of mammary cancer in rats at the International Steroid Hormone Congress in Mexico City in September 1974 [45] (more adventures with my boss Ed Klaiber in Acapulco).

The idea of publishing my emerging data for the treatment and prevention of breast cancer did not occur immediately. Nobody in the scientific or clinical community really cared about the development of another (more expensive) endocrine therapy of limited effectiveness. However, that perspective was to change. Eliahu Caspi called me to his office one day in July 1974 and announced he had been charged with the responsibility of evaluating my CV and bibliography to explore the possibility of me staying at the foundation as a staff member and not returning to Leeds University. He was rather frightening as an individual and stared at me across his desk. He reiterated that he had been told to interview me and evaluate my CV. He then said: "but you haven't got one as you have not published anything." After a stunned silence from me, I replied: "but I haven't discovered anything," to which he then gave me the best advice I had received about developing an academic career up to that point. "Tell them the story so far; each paper can be written within about 2 weeks and create a theme of interlocking research papers." I have followed his advice ever since.

I would like to recount an unanticipated honor that occurred by chance in 2002. At the commencement of the University of Massachusetts Medical School at the Mechanics Hall in Worcester in 2001, I was delivering my acceptance speech for an honorary Doctor of Science degree and told my Eliahu Caspi story about publication—emphasizing that if you don't publish, it never happened. A year later I was asked to deliver the inaugural Eliahu Caspi Memorial Lecture at the Worcester Foundation. It was then that I learned of the remarkable background of Dr. Caspi and had the pleasure of spending time with his accomplished family. As a young man in Poland, Caspi had survived a Russian prison camp, escaped to the emerging Israel, joined the Haganah (early Israeli Defense Forces), and then came to America to complete his Ph.D. at Clark University in Worcester. He then joined the Worcester Foundation having a distinguished career in glucocorticoid metabolism and synthesis until his death in May 2001.

References

1. Furr BJ, Jordan VC (1984) The pharmacology and clinical uses of tamoxifen. Pharmacol Ther 25:127–205
2. Group EBCTC (1992) Systematic treatment of early breast cancer by hormonal, cytotoxic, or immune therapy. 133 randomised trials involving 31,000 recurrences and 24,000 deaths among 75,000 women. Lancet 339:1–15, and 71–85

3. Harper MJ, Walpole AL (1966) Contrasting endocrine activities of *cis* and *trans* isomers in a series of substituted triphenylethylenes. Nature 212:87
4. Harper MJ, Walpole AL (1967) A new derivative of triphenylethylene: effect on implantation and mode of action in rats. J Reprod Fertil 13:101–119
5. Harper MJ, Walpole AL (1967) Mode of action of I.C.I. 46,474 in preventing implantation in rats. J Endocrinol 37:83–92
6. Emmens CW (1970) Postcoital contraception. Br Med Bull 26:45–51
7. Klopper A, Hall M (1971) New synthetic agent for the induction of ovulation: preliminary trials in women. Br Med J 1:152–154
8. Williamson JG, Ellis JD (1973) The induction of ovulation by tamoxifen. J Obstet Gynaecol Br Commonw 80:844–847
9. Beatson GT (1896) On the treatment of inoperable cases of carcinoma of the mamma: suggestions for a new method of treatment with illustrative cases. Lancet 2:104–107
10. Boyd S (1900) On oophorectomy in cancer of the breast. Br Med J 2:1161–1167
11. Lerner LJ, Holthaus FJ Jr, Thompson CR (1958) A non-steroidal estrogen antiagonist 1-(p-2-diethylaminoethoxyphenyl)-1-phenyl-2-p-methoxyphenyl ethanol. Endocrinology 63:295–318
12. Holtkamp DE, Greslin JG, Root CA, Lerner LJ (1960) Gonadotrophin inhibiting and anti-fecundity effects of chloramiphene. Proc Soc Exp Biol Med 105:197–201
13. Kistner RW, Smith OW (1959) Observations on the use of nonsteroidal estrogen antagonist: MER 25. Surg Forum 10:725–729
14. Herbst AL, Griffiths CT, Kistner RW (1964) Clomiphene sitrate (Nsc-35770) in disseminated mammary carcinoma. Cancer Chemother Rep 43:39–41
15. Legha SS, Slavik M, Carter SK (1976) Nafoxidine–an antiestrogen for the treatment of breast cancer. Cancer 38:1535–1541
16. Cole MP, Jones CT, Todd ID (1971) A new anti-oestrogenic agent in late breast cancer. An early clinical appraisal of ICI46474. Br J Cancer 25:270–275
17. Ward HW (1973) Anti-oestrogen therapy for breast cancer: a trial of tamoxifen at two dose levels. Br Med J 1:13–14
18. Sander S (1968) The in vitro uptake of oestradiol in biopsies from 25 breast cancer patients. Acta Pathol Microbiol Scand 74:301–302
19. Johansson H, Terenius L, Thoren L (1970) The binding of estradiol-17beta to human breast cancers and other tissues in vitro. Cancer Res 30:692–698
20. Korenman SG, Dukes BA (1970) Specific estrogen binding by the cytoplasm fof human breast carcinoma. J Clin Endocrinol Metab 30:639–645
21. Jensen EV, Block GE, Smith S et al (1971) Estrogen receptors and breast cancer response to adrenalectomy. Natl Cancer Inst Monogr 34:55–70
22. McGuire WLCP, Vollmer EP (1975) Estrogen receptors in human breast cancer. Raven, New York
23. Jordan VC (1988) The development of tamoxifen for breast cancer therapy: a tribute to the late Arthur L. Walpole. Breast Cancer Res Treat 11:197–209
24. Jordan VC (2006) Tamoxifen (ICI46,474) as a targeted therapy to treat and prevent breast cancer. Br J Pharmacol 147(Suppl 1):S269–S276
25. Powles TJ, Hardy JR, Ashley SE et al (1989) A pilot trial to evaluate the acute toxicity and feasibility of tamoxifen for prevention of breast cancer. Br J Cancer 60:126–131
26. Powles TJ, Tillyer CR, Jones AL et al (1990) Prevention of breast cancer with tamoxifen–an update on the Royal Marsden Hospital pilot programme. Eur J Cancer 26:680–684
27. Fisher B (1992) The evolution of paradigms for the management of breast cancer: a personal perspective. Cancer Res 52:2371–2383
28. Lerner LJ (1981) The first nonsteroidal antioestrogen-MER 25. In: Sutherland RL, Jordan VC (eds) Non-steroidal antioestrogens: molecular pharmacology and antitumour activity. Academic, Sydney, pp 1–16
29. Clark JH, Markaverich BM (1982) The agonistic-antagonistic properties of clomiphene: a review. Pharmacol Ther 15:467–519

30. Hollander W, Chobanian AV, Wilkins RW (1960) The effects of triparanol (MER-29) in subjects with and without coronary artery disease. JAMA 174:5–12
31. Laughlin RC, Carey TF (1962) Cataracts in patients treated with triparanol. JAMA 181:339–340
32. Avigan J, Steinberg D, Vroman HE et al (1960) Studies of cholesterol biosynthesis. I. The identification of desmosterol in serum and tissues of animals and man treated with MER-29. J Biol Chem 235:3123–3126
33. Kraft RO (1962) Triparanol in the treatment of disseminated mammary carcinoma. Cancer Chemother Rep 25:113–115
34. Fisher B, Costantino JP, Wickerham DL et al (2005) Tamoxifen for the prevention of breast cancer: current status of the National Surgical Adjuvant Breast and Bowel Project P-1 study. J Natl Cancer Inst 97:1652–1662
35. Fisher B, Costantino JP, Wickerham DL et al (1998) Tamoxifen for prevention of breast cancer: report of the National Surgical Adjuvant Breast and Bowel Project P-1 Study. J Natl Cancer Inst 90:1371–1388
36. Lieberman ME, Gorski J, Jordan VC (1983) An estrogen receptor model to describe the regulation of prolactin synthesis by antiestrogens in vitro. J Biol Chem 258:4741–4745
37. Jordan VC, Koch R, Langan S, McCague R (1988) Ligand interaction at the estrogen receptor to program antiestrogen action: a study with nonsteroidal compounds in vitro. Endocrinology 122:1449–1454
38. Murphy CS, Langan-Fahey SM, McCague R, Jordan VC (1990) Structure-function relationships of hydroxylated metabolites of tamoxifen that control the proliferation of estrogen-responsive T47D breast cancer cells in vitro. Mol Pharmacol 38:737–743
39. Skidmore J, Walpole AL, Woodburn J (1972) Effect of some triphenylethylenes on oestradiol binding in vitro to macromolecules from uterus and anterior pituitary. J Endocrinol 52:289–298
40. Jordan VC (1975) Prolonged antioestrogenic activity of ICI 46, 474 in the ovariectomized mouse. J Reprod Fertil 42:251–258
41. Jordan VC, Jaspan T (1976) Tamoxifen as an anti-tumour agent: oestrogen binding as a predictive test for tumour response. J Endocrinol 68:453–460
42. Terenius L (1970) Two modes of interaction between oestrogen and anti-oestrogen. Acta Endocrinol (Copenh) 64:47–58
43. Jordan VC, Lababidi MK, Mirecki DM (1990) Anti-oestrogenic and anti-tumour properties of prolonged tamoxifen therapy in C3H/OUJ mice. Eur J Cancer 26:718–721
44. O'Halloran MJ, Maddock PG (1974) I.C.I. 46,474 in breast cancer. J Ir Med Assoc 67:38–39
45. Jordan VC (1974) Antitumor activity of the antiestrogen ICI 46,474 (tamoxifen) in the dimethylbenzanthracene (DMBA)-induced rat mammary carcinoma model. J Steroid Biochem 5:354
46. Jordan VC (1974) The antiestrogen tamoxifen (ICI 46,474) as an antitumor agent. In: Proceedings of the Eastern cooperative oncology group, Miami
47. Jordan VC (1974) Tamoxifen: mechanism of antitumor activity in animals and man. In: Proceedings of the Eastern cooperative oncology group, Jasper
48. Jordan VC (1976) Effect of tamoxifen (ICI 46,474) on initiation and growth of DMBA-induced rat mammary carcinomata. Eur J Cancer 12:419–424
49. Jordan VC, Koerner S (1975) Tamoxifen (ICI 46,474) and the human carcinoma 8S oestrogen receptor. Eur J Cancer 11:205–206
50. Jordan VC, Koerner S (1976) Tamoxifen as an anti-tumour agent: role of oestradiol and prolactin. J Endocrinol 68:305–311
51. Huggins C, Grand LC, Brillantes FP (1961) Mammary cancer induced by a single feeding of polymucular hydrocarbons, and its suppression. Nature 189:204–207
52. Nicholson RI, Golder MP (1975) The effect of synthetic anti-oestrogens on the growth and biochemistry of rat mammary tumours. Eur J Cancer 11:571–579
53. Jordan VC, Dowse LJ (1976) Tamoxifen as an anti-tumour agent: effect on oestrogen binding. J Endocrinol 68:297–303

54. Nicholson RI, Golder MP, Davies P, Griffiths K (1976) Effects of oestradiol – 17beta and tamoxifen on total and accessible cytoplasmic oestradiol – 17beta receptors in DMBA-induced rat mammary tumours. Eur J Cancer 12:711–717
55. Tamoxifen Workshop (1976) Proceedings of the annual spring meeting of the primary breast cancer therapy group, Key Biscayne, p 1409: 66
56. Fromson JM, Pearson S, Bramah S (1973) The metabolism of tamoxifen (I.C.I. 46,474). I. In laboratory animals. Xenobiotica 3:693–709
57. Fromson JM, Pearson S, Bramah S (1973) The metabolism of tamoxifen (I.C.I. 46,474). II. In female patients. Xenobiotica 3:711–714
58. Jordan VC, Collins MM, Rowsby L, Prestwich G (1977) A monohydroxylated metabolite of tamoxifen with potent antioestrogenic activity. J Endocrinol 75:305–316
59. Jordan VC, Allen KE (1980) Evaluation of the antitumour activity of the non-steroidal antioestrogen monohydroxytamoxifen in the DMBA-induced rat mammary carcinoma model. Eur J Cancer 16:239–251
60. Allen KE, Clark ER, Jordan VC (1980) Evidence for the metabolic activation of non-steroidal antioestrogens: a study of structure-activity relationships. Br J Pharmacol 71:83–91
61. Borgna JL, Rochefort H (1981) Hydroxylated metabolites of tamoxifen are formed in vivo and bound to estrogen receptor in target tissues. J Biol Chem 256:859–868
62. Adam HK, Douglas EJ, Kemp JV (1979) The metabolism of tamoxifen in human. Biochem Pharmacol 28:145–147
63. Patterson JS, Settatree RS, Adam HK, Kemp JV (1980) Serum concentrations of tamoxifen and major metabolite during long-term nolvadex therapy, correlated with clinical response. Eur J Cancer 1:89–92
64. Jordan VC, Murphy CS (1990) Endocrine pharmacology of antiestrogens as antitumor agents. Endocr Rev 11:578–610
65. Jordan VC, Bain RR, Brown RR et al (1983) Determination and pharmacology of a new hydroxylated metabolite of tamoxifen observed in patient sera during therapy for advanced breast cancer. Cancer Res 43:1446–1450
66. Kemp JV, Adam HK, Wakeling AE, Slater R (1983) Identification and biological activity of tamoxifen metabolites in human serum. Biochem Pharmacol 32:2045–2052
67. Lien EA, Solheim E, Lea OA et al (1989) Distribution of 4-hydroxy-N-desmethyltamoxifen and other tamoxifen metabolites in human biological fluids during tamoxifen treatment. Cancer Res 49:2175–2183
68. Lippman ME, Bolan G (1975) Oestrogen-responsive human breast cancer in long term tissue culture. Nature 256:592–593
69. Brooks SC, Locke ER, Soule HD (1973) Estrogen receptor in a human cell line (MCF-7) from breast carcinoma. J Biol Chem 248:6251–6253
70. Osborne CK, Boldt DH, Clark GM, Trent JM (1983) Effects of tamoxifen on human breast cancer cell cycle kinetics: accumulation of cells in early G1 phase. Cancer Res 43:3583–3585
71. Sutherland RL, Green MD, Hall RE et al (1983) Tamoxifen induces accumulation of MCF 7 human mammary carcinoma cells in the G0/G1 phase of the cell cycle. Eur J Cancer Clin Oncol 19:615–621
72. Shafie SM, Grantham FH (1981) Role of hormones in the growth and regression of human breast cancer cells (MCF-7) transplanted into athymic nude mice. J Natl Cancer Inst 67:51–56
73. Osborne CK, Hobbs K, Clark GM (1985) Effect of estrogens and antiestrogens on growth of human breast cancer cells in athymic nude mice. Cancer Res 45:584–590
74. Gottardis MM, Robinson SP, Jordan VC (1988) Estradiol-stimulated growth of MCF-7 tumors implanted in athymic mice: a model to study the tumoristatic action of tamoxifen. J Steroid Biochem 30:311–314
75. Iino Y, Wolf DM, Langan-Fahey SM et al (1991) Reversible control of oestradiol-stimulated growth of MCF-7 tumours by tamoxifen in the athymic mouse. Br J Cancer 64:1019–1024
76. Jordan VC (2008) Tamoxifen: catalyst for the change to targeted therapy. Eur J Cancer 44: 30–38

77. Palopoli FP, Feil VJ, Allen RE et al (1967) Substituted aminoalkoxytriarylhaloethylenes. J Med Chem 10:84–86
78. Ernst S, Hite G, Cantrell JS et al (1976) Stereochemistry of geometric isomers of clomiphene: a correction of the literature and a reexamination of structure-activity relationships. J Pharm Sci 65:148–150
79. Consensus conference (1985) Adjuvant chemotherapy for breast cancer. JAMA 254:3461–3463

Chapter 3
Metabolites of Tamoxifen as the Basis of Drug Development

Abstract By the early 1970s, a number of metabolites of tamoxifen had been identified in animals and following administration to a few patients. The hydroxylated metabolite of tamoxifen, 4-hydroxytamoxifen, proved to be the most interesting. The discovery of its high binding affinity for the estrogen receptor made it a new laboratory tool for all future in vitro studies of antiestrogen action and also provided the clue for all future structure-function relationships studies of new antiestrogens. These compounds would subsequently be developed as selective estrogen receptor modulators (SERMs). Tamoxifen is a prodrug but it is the metabolite 4-hydroxy-N-desmethyltamoxifen or endoxifen that has attracted pharmacogenetic interest. Mutations of the CYP2D6 gene control endoxifen production and have been associated with drug efficacy in some clinical trials.

Introduction

Tamoxifen is believed to be a prodrug and can be metabolically activated to 4-hydroxytamoxifen [1–4] or alternatively can be metabolically routed via N-desmethyltamoxifen to 4-hydroxy-N-desmethyltamoxifen [5, 6] (endoxifen) (Fig. 3.1). The hydroxylated metabolites of tamoxifen have a high binding affinity for the ER [1, 7]. The finding that the CYP2D6 subtype of cytochrome P450 activates tamoxifen to endoxifen [8] has implications for cancer therapeutics. It has been proposed that women with enzyme variants that cannot make endoxifen may not have as successful an outcome with tamoxifen therapy. Alternatively, women who have a wild-type enzyme may make high levels of the potent antiestrogen endoxifen and experience hot flashes. As a result, these women may take selective serotonin reuptake inhibitors (SSRIs) to ameliorate hot flashes but there are potential pharmacological consequences to this strategy. Some of the SSRIs are metabolically altered by the CYP2D6 enzyme [9]. It is therefore possible to envision a drug interaction whereby SSRIs block the metabolic activation of tamoxifen.

P.Y. Maximov et al., *Tamoxifen*, Milestones in Drug Therapy,
DOI 10.1007/978-3-0348-0664-0_3, © Springer Basel 2013

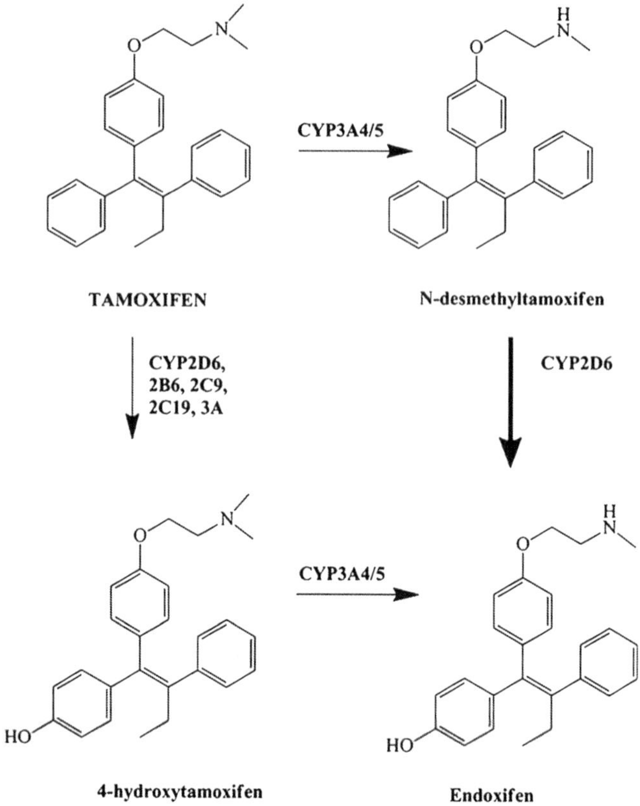

Fig. 3.1 The metabolic activation of tamoxifen to phenolic metabolites that have a high binding activity for the human ER. Both 4-hydroxytamoxifen and endoxifen are potent antiestrogens in vitro

This chapter will describe the scientific twists and turns that tamoxifen and its metabolites have taken over the past 30 years. The story is naturally dependent on the fashions in therapeutic research at the time. What seems obvious to us as a successful research strategy today, with millions of women taking tamoxifen, was not so 30 years ago at the beginning when the clinical community and pharmaceutical industry did not see "antihormones" as a priority at all for drug development [10]. In 1972, tamoxifen was declared an orphan drug with little prospect of successful clinical development [11].

Basic Mechanisms of Tamoxifen Metabolism

The original survey of the putative metabolites of tamoxifen was conducted in the laboratories of ICI Pharmaceuticals Division and published in 1973 [12]. A number of hydroxylated metabolites were noted (Fig. 3.2) following the administration of

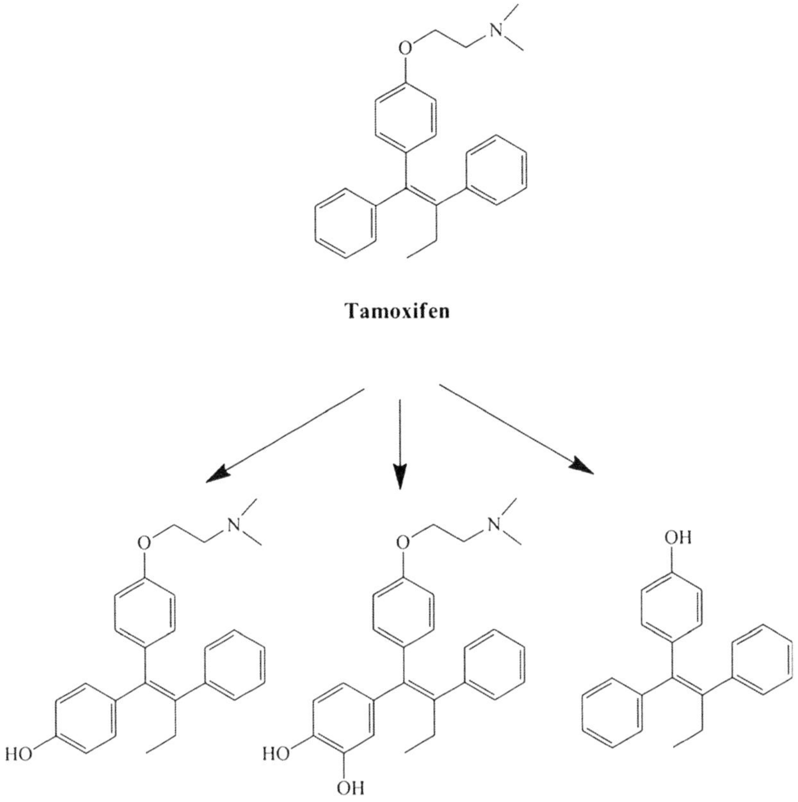

Tamoxifen

4-hydroxytamoxifen   **3,4-dihydroxytamoxifen**   **Metabolite E**
(Metabolite B)   **(Metabolite D)**

Fig. 3.2 The original hydroxylated metabolites of tamoxifen noted in animals by Fromson and coworkers [12]

[14]C-labeled tamoxifen to various species (rat, mouse, monkey, and dog). The major route of excretion of radioactivity was in the feces. The rat and dog studies showed that up to 53 % of the radioactivity derived from tamoxifen was excreted via the bile and up to 69 % of this was reabsorbed via an enterohepatic recirculation until elimination eventually occurs [12]. The hydroxylated metabolites are excreted as glucuronides. However, no information about their biological activity was available until the finding that 4-hydroxytamoxifen had a binding affinity for the ER equivalent to 17β estradiol [1]. Similarly, 3, 4-dihydroxytamoxifen (Fig. 3.2) bound to the human ER but interestingly enough, 3, 4-dihydroxytamoxifen was not significantly estrogen-like in the rodent uterus despite being antiestrogenic [1, 4].

Additional studies on the metabolism of tamoxifen in four women [13] identified 4-hydroxytamoxifen as the primary metabolite using a thin layer chromatographic technique to identify ^{14}C-labeled metabolites. This assumption, coupled with the

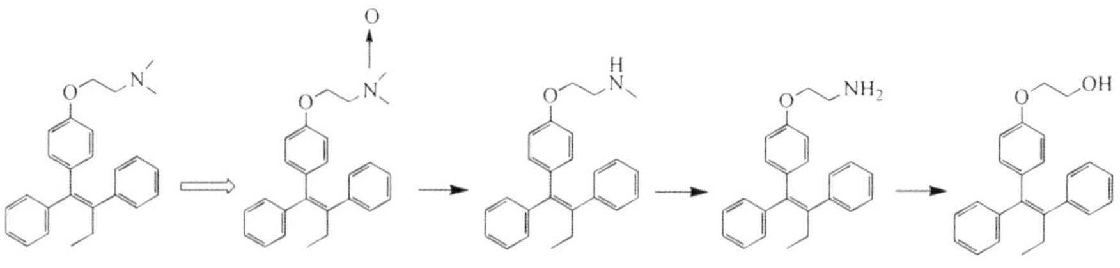

Fig. 3.3 The serial metabolic dimethylation and deamination of the antiestrogenic side chain of tamoxifen. Each of the metabolites is a weak antiestrogen with poor binding affinity for the ER

potent antiestrogenic actions of 4-hydroxytamoxifen [1] and the conclusion that it was an advantage, but not a requirement for tamoxifen to be metabolically activated [2, 14], seemed to confirm the idea that 4-hydroxytamoxifen was the active metabolite that bound in rat estrogen target tissues to block estrogen action [3]. However, the original analytical methods used to identify 4-hydroxytamoxifen as the major metabolite in humans were flawed [15] and subsequent studies identified N-desmethyltamoxifen (Fig. 3.3) as the major metabolite circulating in human serum [16]. The metabolite was found to be further demethylated to N-desdimethyltamoxifen (metabolite Z) [17] and then deaminated to metabolite Y, a glycol derivative of tamoxifen [18, 19]. The metabolites (Fig. 3.3) that are not hydroxylated at the 4 position of tamoxifen (equivalent to the three phenolic hydroxyl of estradiol) are all weak antiestrogens that would each contribute to the overall antitumor actions of tamoxifen at the ER based on their relative binding affinities for the ER and their actual concentrations locally.

At the end of the 1980s, the identification of another metabolite tamoxifen 4-hydroxy-N-desmethyltamoxifen in animals [20] and man [5, 6] was anticipated but viewed as obvious and uninteresting. The one exception that was of interest was metabolite E (Fig. 3.2) identified in the dog [12]. This phenolic metabolite without the dimethylaminoethyl side chain is a full estrogen [19, 21]. The dimethylaminoethoxy side chain of tamoxifen is necessary for antiestrogenic action [21].

It is not a simple task to study the actions of metabolites in vivo. Problems of pharmacokinetics, absorption, and subsequent metabolism all conspire to confuse the interpretation of data. Studies in vitro using cell systems of estrogen target tissues were defined and refined in the early 1980s to create an understanding of the actual structure-function relationships of tamoxifen metabolites. Systems were developed to study the regulation of the prolactin gene in primary cultures of immature rat pituitary gland cells [14, 22] or cell replication in ER-positive breast cancer cells [23–26]. Overall, these models were used to describe the importance of a phenolic hydroxyl to tether the triphenylethylenes appropriately in the ligand-binding domain of the ER and to establish the appropriate positioning of an "antiestrogenic" side chain in the "antiestrogen region" of the ER [22] to modulate gene activation and growth [14, 22, 27–30]. These structure-function studies that created hypothetical models of the ligand-ER complex were rapidly advanced with the first reports of the X-ray crystallography of the estrogen, 4-hydroxytamoxifen [31], or raloxifene ER ligand-binding domain [32] complexes. The ligand-receptor protein interaction was subsequently interrogated by examining the interaction of the specific amino acid asp 351 with the antiestrogenic side chain of the ligand [33]. A mutation was found as the dominant ER species in a tamoxifen-stimulated breast tumor grown in athymic mice [33, 34]. The structure-function relationships studies, that modulated estrogen action at a transforming growth factor-alpha gene target, demonstrated that the ligand shape would ultimately program the shape of the ER complex in a target tissue [35–39]. This concept is at the heart of metabolite pharmacology and is required to switch on and switch off target sites around the body. The other piece of the mechanism of the SERM puzzle that was eventually solved was the need for another player to partner with the ER complex. Coactivators [40] can enhance the estrogen-like effects of compounds at a target site [41]. However, in the early 1990s, the molecular and clinical use of this knowledge with the development and application of SERMs was in the future [42].

It is clear from this background about the early development of tamoxifen and the fact that tamoxifen was considered to be such a safe drug in comparison to other cytotoxic agents used in therapy during the 1970s and 1980s that there was little enthusiasm for in-depth studies of tamoxifen metabolism. However, this perspective was to change in the 1990s with the widespread use of tamoxifen as the gold standard for the treatment and prospect of clinical trials to evaluate the worth of tamoxifen for the prevention of breast cancer.

The urgent focus of translational research in the early 1990s was to discover why tamoxifen was a complete carcinogen in rat liver [43, 44] and to determine whether there was a link between metabolism and the development of endometrial cancer noted in very small but significant numbers of postmenopausal women taking adjuvant tamoxifen [45, 46].

All interest in the metabolism of tamoxifen focused on the production of DNA adducts [47] that were responsible for rat liver carcinogenesis and, at the time, believed to be potentially responsible for carcinogenesis in humans [48]. Although many candidates were described [49–52], the metabolite found to be responsible for the initiation of rat liver carcinogenesis is α-hydroxytamoxifen [53–57] (Fig. 3.4). α-Hydroxytamoxifen has been resolved into R-(+) and S-(−)enantiomers. Metabolism by rat liver microsomes gave equal amounts of the two forms, but in hepatocytes the R form gave 8× the level of DNA adducts as the S form. As both had the same chemical reactivity toward DNA, Osborne et al. [58] suggested that the R form was a better sulfotransferase substrate. This enzyme is believed to catalyze DNA adduct formation. Subsequently, Osborne et al. [59] conducted studies with alpha-hydroxy-N-desmethyltamoxifen; the R-(+) gave 10× the level of adducts in rat hepatocytes as the S-(−).

There were reasonable concerns that the hepatocarcinogenicity of tamoxifen in rats would eventually translate to humans but fortunately this is now known to be untrue [60]. The demonstration of carcinogenesis in the rat liver appears to be related to poor DNA repair mechanisms in the inbred strains of rats. In contrast, it appears that the absence of liver carcinogenesis in women exposed to tamoxifen

α-hydroxytamoxifen   Tamoxifen-DNA adduct at deoxyguanosine

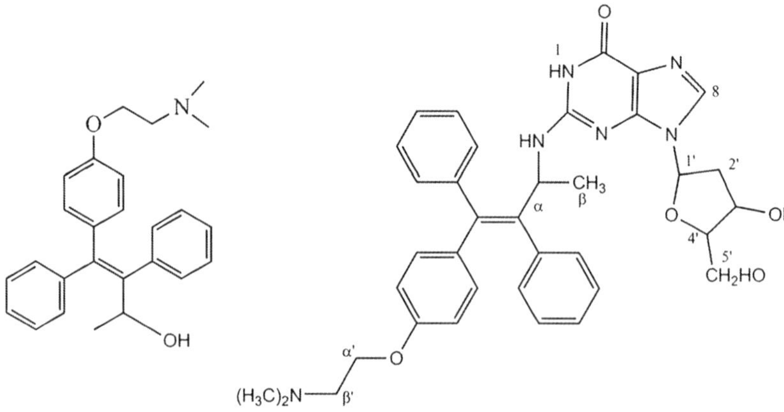

Fig. 3.4 The putative metabolite of tamoxifen, α- hydroxytamoxifen, that produces DNA adducts through covalent binding to deoxyguanosine in the rat liver

[61] is believed to result from the sophisticated mechanisms of DNA repair inherent in human cells. These concepts are described in more detail in Chap. 6.

The questions that next needed to be addressed were: Can improvements be made to the tamoxifen molecule? What happens to tamoxifen in patients?

Metabolic Mimicry

The demonstration [1, 2] that the class of compounds referred to as nonsteroidal antiestrogens were metabolically activated to compounds with high binding affinity for the ER created additional opportunities for the medicinal chemists within the pharmaceutical industry to develop new agents. An initial attempt was 3-hydroxytamoxifen (droloxifene) that was evaluated extensively in clinical trials. Those trials have been reviewed [62] but no advantages over tamoxifen were found. It is important to note that all studies used higher doses compared to tamoxifen. This emphasizes the principle that because droloxifene is a hydroxylated compound, it is excreted more rapidly.

Drug discovery accelerated once the nonsteroidal antiestrogens [63] were recognized to be SERMs [64–66] and had applications not only for the treatment and prevention of breast cancer but also as potential agents to treat osteoporosis and coronary heart disease [67, 68]. The reader is referred to other recent review articles to obtain further details of new medicines under investigation [67, 68] but some current examples are worthy of note and will be mentioned briefly. Compounds of interest that have their structural origins from metabolites of nonsteroidal antiestrogens are summarized in Fig. 3.5.

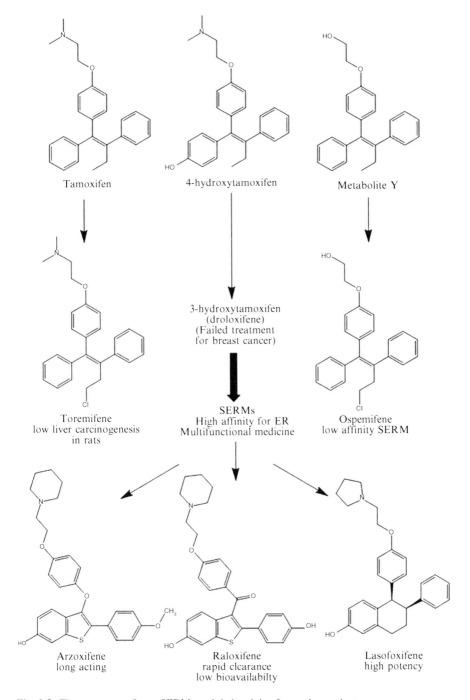

Fig. 3.5 The structures of new SERMs and their origins from other antiestrogens

Raloxifene is an agent that originally was destined to be a drug to treat breast cancer but it failed in that application [69]. It appears that the pharmacokinetics and bioavailability of raloxifene are a challenge. Only about 2 % of administered raloxifene is bioavailable [70] but despite this, the drug is known to have a reasonable biological half-life of 27 h. The reason for this disparity is that raloxifene is a polyphenolic drug that can be glucuronidated and sulfated by bacteria in the gut so the drug cannot be absorbed [71, 72]. This phase II metabolism in turn controls enterohepatic recirculation and ultimately impairs the drug from reaching and interacting with receptors in the target. This concern has been addressed with the development of the long-acting raloxifene derivative arzoxifene that is known to be superior to raloxifene as a chemopreventive in rat mammary carcinogenesis [73]. One of the phenolic groups (Fig. 3.5) is methylated to provide protection from phase II metabolism.

Nevertheless, arzoxifene has not performed well as a treatment for breast cancer [74, 75]; higher doses are less effective than lower doses. These data imply that effective absorption is impaired by phase III metabolism. That being said, the results of trials evaluating the effects of arzoxifene as a drug to treat osteoporosis have been completed [76–78].

Unfortunately, the bioavailability of phenolic drugs is also dependent on phase II metabolism to inactive conjugates in the target tissue. 4-Hydroxytamoxifen [1] is only sulfated by three of seven sulfotransferase isoforms, whereas raloxifene is sulfated by all seven [79]. Maybe local phase II metabolism plays a role in neutralizing the antiestrogen action of raloxifene in the breast? Falany et al. [79] further report that SULT1E1, that sulfates raloxifene in the endometrium, is only expressed in the secretory phase. In contrast, 4- hydroxytamoxifen is sulfated at all stages of the uterine cycle.

Lasofoxifene is a diaryltetrahydronaphthalene derivative referred to as CP336156 [80] that has been reported to have high binding affinity for ER and have potent activity in preserving bone density in the rat [81, 82]. The structure of CP336156 is reminiscent of the putative antiestrogenic metabolic route for nafoxidine [83] (Chap. 1, Fig. 1.4) that failed to become a breast cancer drug because of unacceptable side effects [84]. CP336156 is the l enantiomer that has 20 times the binding affinity for the ER as the d enantiomer. Studies demonstrate that the l enantiomer had twice the bioavailability of the d enantiomer. The authors [80] ascribed the difference to enantioselective glucuronidation of the d isomer. An evaluation of CP336156 in the prevention and treatment of rat mammary tumors induced by N-nitroso-N-methylurea shows activity similar to that of tamoxifen [85].

Ospemifene or deaminohydroxytoremifene is related to metabolite Y formed by the deamination of tamoxifen [19]. Metabolite Y has a very low binding affinity for the ER [19, 86] and has weak antiestrogenic properties compared with tamoxifen. Ospemifene is a known metabolite of toremifene (4-chlorotoremifene) but unlike tamoxifen, there is little carcinogenic potential in animals [87]. It is possible that the large chlorine atom on the 4 position of toremifene and ospemifene reduces α-hydroxylation to the ultimate carcinogen related to α-hydroxytamoxifen (Fig. 3.5). Deaminohydroxytoremifene has very weak estrogenic and antiestrogenic

properties in vivo [88] but demonstrates SERM activity in bone and lowers cholesterol. The compound is proposed to be used as a preventative for osteoporosis.
Preliminary clinical data in healthy men and postmenopausal women demonstrate
pharmacokinetics suitable for daily dosing between 25 and 200 mg [89]. Interestingly enough, unlike raloxifene, ospemifene has a strong estrogen-like action in the
vagina but neither ospemifene nor raloxifene affects endometrial histology [90, 91].

Overall, the goal of developing a bone-specific agent is reasonable, but the key to
commercial success will be the prospective demonstration of the prevention of
breast and endometrial cancer as beneficial side effects. This remains a possibility
based on prevention studies completed in the laboratory [92, 93].

Tamoxifen Metabolism Today

During the past decade, there has been considerable interest in the pharmaco-
genetics of tamoxifen-metabolizing enzymes in humans. The central hypothesis is
that aberrant genes responsible for the metabolic activation of tamoxifen will
influence therapeutics.

A comprehensive evaluation of the sequential biotransformation of tamoxifen
has been completed by Desta and coworkers [8]. They used human liver
microsomes and experiments with specifically expressed human cytochrome
P450s to identify the prominent enzymes involved in phase I metabolism. Their
results are summarized in Fig. 3.1 with the relevant CYP genes indicated for
the metabolic transformations. The authors make a strong case that
N-desmethyltamoxifen, the principal metabolite of tamoxifen that accumulates
in the body, is converted to endoxifen by the enzyme variant CYP2D6. The
CYP2D6 enzyme is also important to produce the potent primary metabolite
4-hydroxytamoxifen (this was first reported by David Kupfer at the Worcester
Foundation 15 years ago! [94]), but the metabolite can also be formed by other
enzymes: CYP2B6, CYP2C9, CY2C19, and CYP3A4.

The CYP2D6 phenotype is defined as the metabolic ratio (MR) by dividing the
concentration of an unchanged probe drug, known to be metabolized by the
CYP2D6 gene product, by the concentration of the relevant metabolite at a specific
time. These measurements have resulted in the division of the CYP2D6 phenotype
in four metabolic classes: poor metabolizers (PM), intermediate metabolizers (IM),
extensive metabolizers (EM), and ultrarapid metabolizers (UM). Over 80 different
single-nucleotide polymorphisms have been identified but there are inconsistencies
in the precise definitions of ascribing a genotype to a phenotype [95, 96]. Bradford
[96] and Raimundo and coworkers [97] have described the frequency of common
alleles for CYP2D6. Pertinent to the current discussion of tamoxifen metabolism,
the CYP2D6*4 allele [98] is estimated to have a frequency of 12–23 % in
Caucasians, 1.2–7 % in black Africans, and 0–2.8 % in Asians [95, 96]. A lower
estimate of (<10 %) of the PM phenotype is presented by Bernard and
coworkers [99].

The molecular pharmacology of endoxifen has been reported [7, 100, 101]. Endoxifen and 4-hydroxytamoxifen were equally potent at inhibiting estrogen-stimulated growth of ER-positive breast cancer cells MCF-7, T47D, and BT474. Both metabolites are significantly superior in vitro to tamoxifen the parent drug. Additionally, the estrogen-responsive genes pS2 and progesterone receptor were both blocked to an equivalent degree by endoxifen and 4-hydroxytamoxifen [100, 101]. Lim and coworkers [101] have extended the comparison of endoxifen and 4-hydroxytamoxifen in MCF-7 cells by comparing and contrasting global gene regulation using the Affymetrix U133A Gene Chip Array. There were 4,062 total genes that were either up- or downregulated by estradiol, whereas, in the presence of estradiol, 4-hydroxytamoxifen or endoxifen affected 2,444 and 2,390 genes, respectively. Overall, the authors [101] demonstrated good correlation between RT-PCR and select genes from the microarray and concluded that the global effects of endoxifen and 4-hydroxytamoxifen were similar.

Stearns and coworkers [102] and Jin and coworkers [103] have confirmed and significantly extended Lien's original identification of endoxifen and observation [5, 6] that there are usually higher circulating levels of endoxifen than 4-hydroxytamoxifen in patients receiving adjuvant tamoxifen therapy. However, Flockhart's group [102] has advanced the pharmacogenomics and drug interactions surrounding tamoxifen therapy that should be a consideration in the antihormonal treatment of breast cancer.

The ubiquitous use of tamoxifen for the treatment of node-negative women [104] during the 1990s, the use of tamoxifen plus radiotherapy following lumpectomy for the treatment of ductal carcinoma in situ (DCIS) [105], as well as the option to use tamoxifen for chemoprevention in high-risk pre- and postmenopausal women [106] enhanced awareness of the menopausal side effects experienced by women when taking tamoxifen. Up to 45 % of women with hot flashes grade them as severe [106]; therefore, there have been efforts to improve quality of life. Treatments with the SSRIs are popular [102, 107, 108] (Fig. 3.6). The SSRIs are twice as effective as the "placebo" effect at reducing menopausal symptoms in randomized clinical trials [107–109], so there is naturally an increased usage of SSRIs with long-term tamoxifen treatment to maintain compliance. Unfortunately, the metabolism of tamoxifen to hydroxylated metabolites [94, 110, 111] and the metabolism of SSRIs [9, 112–115] both occur via the CYP2D6 gene product. Indeed Stearns and coworkers [102] showed that the paroxetine reduced the levels of endoxifen during adjuvant tamoxifen therapy and endoxifen levels decrease by 64 % in women with wild-type CYP2D6 enzyme. Patients were examined who were taking venlafaxine, sertraline, and paroxetine and compared with those women who were homozygotes for the CYP2D6*4/*4 inactive genotype. Patients with the wild-type gene who took the most potent inhibitor paroxetine had serum levels of endoxifen equivalent to the patients with the aberrant CYP2D6 gene. In fact, the clinical data were consistent with the inhibition constants for the inhibition of CYP2D6 by paroxetine (potent), fluoxetine, sertraline, citalopram (intermediate), and venlafaxine (weak) which are 0.05, 0.17, 1.5, 7, and 33 μmol/l, respectively.

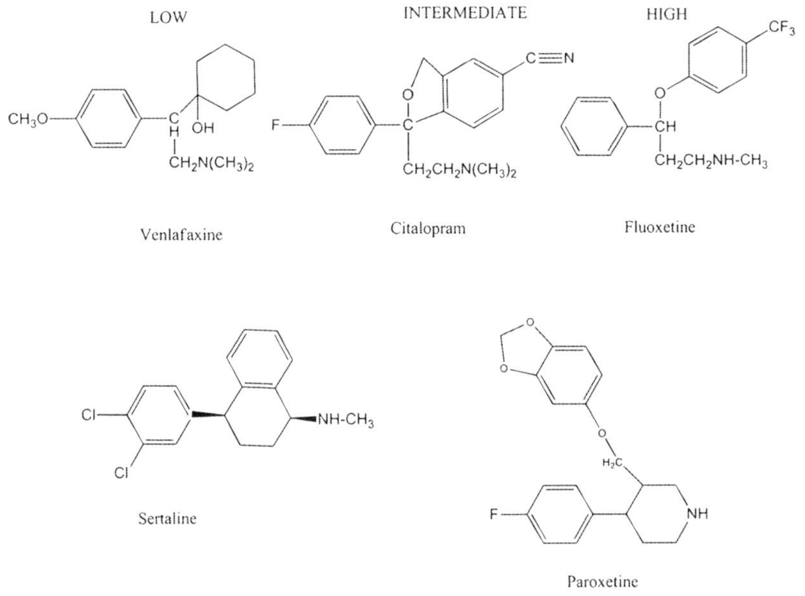

Fig. 3.6 The structures of selective serotonin reuptake inhibitors (SSRIs) that have low interme-diate to high affinity for the CYP2D6 enzyme system. High affinity binders for CYP2D6 block the metabolic activation of tamoxifen to endoxifen (Fig. 3.1)

The CYP2D6 gene product that is fully functional (wild type) is classified as the CYP2D6*1. A large number of alleles are associated with no enzyme activity or reduced activity. Conversely, high metabolizers can have multiple copies of the CYP2D6 allele [116]. A recent study by Borges and coworkers [117] continues to expand our understanding of the detrimental effect of CYP2D6 variants plus concomitant administration of SSRIs on endoxifen levels. But, it is the clinical correlations with tumor responses and side effects that are of importance if pharmacogenomics is to be truly relevant in breast cancer therapy.

Clinical Correlations

The metabolic activation of tamoxifen to endoxifen by the CYP2D6 enzyme system still remains controversial to plan the treatment of patients with breast cancer. Since the discovery and description of the pharmacological properties of endoxifen, retrospective clinical trials were examined to determine the pharmacological rele-vance of endoxifen. The results of clinical trials, however, vary. Clinical investiga-tion by Dieudonne and coworkers [118] have shown that patients with CYP2D6*4/ *4 homozygous mutation, which reduces the levels of endoxifen in patients' plasma, are still responding to tamoxifen treatment and tamoxifen still has an effect on endometrial tissue and elevated the plasma levels of FSH and SHBG in those patients to the levels found in general tamoxifen-treated population. Study by Schroth and coworkers [119] have shown that there was an association of CYP2D6 genotype and clinical outcome for breast cancer patients, in particular the presence of two wild-type alleles correlated with better clinical outcomes and presence of mutant alleles with worse outcomes. Study by Kiyotani and coworkers [120] showed also that there is a significant correlation between the presence of risk alleles of CYP2D6, which are associated with lower plasma levels of endoxifen, and significantly lower recurrence-free survival in breast cancer patients that were taking tamoxifen as monotherapy. Study by Lammers and coworkers [121] also has demonstrated correlation between the overall survival of breast cancer patients that were taking tamoxifen 40 mg daily with poor metabolizer genotype, compared to patients with extensive metabolizer genotype. A study by Madlensky and coworkers [122] has shown that there is no association between breast cancer outcomes and the concentrations of 4-hydroxytamoxifen or endoxifen; however, they have demonstrated a threshold of endoxifen concentration, below which there is an increase in breast cancer recurrence rate and that about 80 % of patients are above that threshold. Interestingly, their threshold concentration of endoxifen is equivalent to concentrations found in patients with poor metabolizer genotype. In the study by Lash and coworkers [123], it was shown that there is virtually no correlation between recurrence rates of breast cancer in patients and the presence of one or two functional alleles. However, in 2012 results of studies from Arimidex, Tamoxifen, Alone or in Combination (ATAC) and Breast International Group (BIG) I-98 trails were published [124, 125]. The results concurrently showed no association between the recurrence rates and the genotypes of the postmenopausal patients taking tamoxifen alone or in combination with aromatase inhibitor. The results of the trials have sparked a controversy [126]. One thing that is certain is that endoxifen plasma levels do vary in patients taking tamoxifen depending on their metabolic genotype [127, 128]. It should be noted that in some of the trials the patients were postmenopausal or had previous chemotherapy. In 2012, we simulated the estrogen environment of postmenopausal women in vitro and test the antiestrogenic properties of tamoxifen and its metabolites in physiological concentrations on a panel of ER-positive human breast cancer cell lines (MCF-7, T47D, ZR-75-1, and BT474). The concentrations of estrogens (E1/E2) used to simulate postmenopausal women treated with tamoxifen were obtained from published studies [129, 130], as well as the concentrations of tamoxifen and its metabolites (N-desmethyltamoxifen, 4-hydroxytamoxifen, and endoxifen) based on the CYP2D6 genotype in postmenopausal breast cancer patients [128]. Our results demonstrate that irrespective of CYP2D6 genotype (extensive, intermediate, or poor metabolizers (EM, IM, and PM, respectively)), tamoxifen and its primary metabolites (N-desmethyltamoxifen and 4-hydroxytamoxifen) are able to inhibit completely the estrogen-stimulated growth of breast cancer cells in vitro. Additional endoxifen in any concentration corresponding to CYP2D6 genotype was not able to increase the antiestrogenic effect of tamoxifen and its primary metabolites. Moreover, we demonstrate that 4-hydroxytamoxifen is absolutely essential for inhibition of estrogen action. Based on our results, we can conclude that endoxifen is pharmacologically supportive but not essential for any genotype of CYP2D6 in a postmenopausal setting.

However, little is known on the role on the antiestrogenic impact of endoxifen in premenopausal women that are treated with tamoxifen. We have simulated premenopausal estrogen environment in vitro and used the same concentrations of tamoxifen and its metabolites found in different CYP2D6 genotypes. Our results show that tamoxifen and its primary metabolites are able to inhibit partially the estrogenic effect in the same panel of ER-positive human breast cancer cell lines; however, the addition of endoxifen, unlike in postmenopausal simulation, further inhibits the estrogens. Interestingly, the higher concentrations of endoxifen associated with EM and IM genotypes are inhibiting estrogens better, than at lower concentrations as found patients with PM genotype. It should be noted that addition of endoxifen at PM concentrations does not increase the antiestrogenic properties of tamoxifen and its primary metabolites in vitro. It was shown that the increase of tamoxifen dose in breast cancer patients increases the plasma levels of endoxifen [131–133]. In particular, it was shown by Irvin and coworkers [131] that the increase of tamoxifen dose to 40 mg daily administered by patients with IM and PM genotype increased the plasma levels of endoxifen. Using these levels of increased tamoxifen and its metabolites, we have simulated the average premenopausal estrogen setting in vitro and assessed the pharmacological impact of increased concentrations of endoxifen in IM and PM setting. Our results show that biologically there is no significant difference after treatments with tamoxifen primary metabolites and endoxifen at concentrations corresponding to 20 and 40 mg/daily. Interestingly, none of the tamoxifen treatments were able to fully inhibit the estrogen action in MCF-7 and T47D cells in the premenopausal setting; increasing the concentrations of endoxifen to levels higher than physiological was able to fully inhibit estrogen action. We conclude that endoxifen thus contributes to inhibition of estrogen action and growth of ER-positive breast cancer cells; however, endoxifen plays a supportive in a situation following chemotherapy in premenopausal patients.

Postscript. On my return from the United States to Leeds University in 1974, I was supported by the ICI Pharmaceutical Division Clinical Department and the Yorkshire Cancer Campaign. In 1975, I initially wished to study the hydroxylated metabolites of tamoxifen for two reasons: (1) would the metabolites be estrogens if low affinity was important for antiestrogenic activity or (2) would potent antiestrogen effects of the metabolites explain the potent antiestrogenic properties of tamoxifen in rats but the really weak antiestrogenic activity to block ER in vitro. Dora Richardson gave me their limited supply of the precious metabolites monohydroxytamoxifen (metabolite B) and dihydroxytamoxifen (metabolite D).

My students at Leeds University Clive Dix and Margaret Collins took the leading roles in discovering the pharmacological properties of 4-hydroxytamoxifen (the correct name of metabolite B). I recall telling Clive Dix to redo all ligand-binding experiments of 4-hydroxytamoxfien competition inhibiting the binding of

[^{3}H]estradiol to rat uterine cytosolic ER. "Look Clive, there are no reports of a nonsteroidal antiestrogens binding to the ER with the same affinity as estradiol- learn to do your serial dilutions properly!" He was correct and it was an important discovery. When we discovered the potent antiestrogenic properties of 4-hydroxytamoxifen, I was informed by Sandy Todd at ICI Pharmaceutical Division that there were no patents for the metabolites. The scientists at ICI had clearly never believed the clinical development process would take off, as it did in the early 1970s with animal data to support clinical trials. A rule at ICI that all drug metabolites for a drug in active development and marketing had to be patented had been broken (remember the program was terminated in 1972). As a result, in 1976, I agreed to write up our paper, lodge it with ICI staff at ICI Pharmaceutical Division, and delay publishing until a patent was obtained for 4-hydroxytamoxifen. This occurred 1 year later. I also voluntarily agreed to not talk about our work in 1976 as it was important to get tamoxifen FDA approved in the United States. In 1976, I set off to Key Biscayne to the NSABP meeting to tell them all about tamoxifen [134].

What happened to 4-hydroxytamoxifen? It became the antiestrogen of choice for all laboratory studies in vitro for the next 30 years, but we also showed it was not the product to be developed instead of tamoxifen [135]. If tamoxifen was a prodrug, then 4-hydroxytamoxifen could be the active agent. The patent for 4-hydroxytamoxifen was sold to Besins International and a French physician Dr. Maurvais Jarvais, who advanced the proposal that breast cancer and breast pain could be resolved with a daily preparation rubbed on the breast [136]. Clinical trials have addressed this issue over the past 30 years.

I was subsequently awarded a Leeds University/ICI Pharmaceutical Division Joint Research scheme to evaluate the therapeutic potential of 6,7 alpha-substituted estradiol alkylated derivatives. We had discovered that substitution of the 6 and 7 positions of estradiol still retained significant binding affinity of the ligand for the receptor. The idea was to use the estradiol as the carrier molecule for an alkylating moiety to be delivered to the DNA precisely and kill ER-positive breast cancers. Alternatively, we could radiolabel the estradiol and subsequently discover the sites for estrogen-regulated genes. Neither of these ideas were successful. We published our findings [137] but did not follow up the 7-substituted estradiol with a $(CH_2)_{10}$ side chain. The further development of the idea was to result in the pure antiestrogen fulvestrant [138], but this was entirely the discovery of the Pharma- ceutical Industry, with Alan Wakeling and his team.

We will find out what happened to the idea of estradiol with a long side chain at position 7 in Chap. 5.

References

1. Jordan VC, Collins MM, Rowsby L, Prestwich G (1977) A monohydroxylated metabolite of tamoxifen with potent antioestrogenic activity. J Endocrinol 75:305–316
2. Allen KE, Clark ER, Jordan VC (1980) Evidence for the metabolic activation of non-steroidal antioestrogens: a study of structure-activity relationships. Br J Pharmacol 71:83–91

3. Borgna JL, Rochefort H (1981) Hydroxylated metabolites of tamoxifen are formed in vivo and bound to estrogen receptor in target tissues. J Biol Chem 256:859–868

4. Jordan VC, Dix CJ, Naylor KE et al (1978) Nonsteroidal antiestrogens: their biological effects and potential mechanisms of action. J Toxicol Environ Health 4:363–390

5. Lien EA, Solheim E, Kvinnsland S, Ueland PM (1988) Identification of 4-hydroxy-N-desmethyltamoxifen as a metabolite of tamoxifen in human bile. Cancer Res 48:2304–2308

6. Lien EA, Solheim E, Lea OA et al (1989) Distribution of 4-hydroxy-N-desmethyltamoxifen and other tamoxifen metabolites in human biological fluids during tamoxifen treatment. Cancer Res 49:2175–2183

7. Johnson MD, Zuo H, Lee KH et al (2004) Pharmacological characterization of 4-hydroxy-N-desmethyl tamoxifen, a novel active metabolite of tamoxifen. Breast Cancer Res Treat 85:151–159

8. Desta Z, Ward BA, Soukhova NV, Flockhart DA (2004) Comprehensive evaluation of tamoxifen sequential biotransformation by the human cytochrome P450 system in vitro: prominent roles for CYP3A and CYP2D6. J Pharmacol Exp Ther 310:1062–1075

9. Crewe HK, Lennard MS, Tucker GT et al (1992) The effect of selective serotonin re-uptake inhibitors on cytochrome P4502D6 (CYP2D6) activity in human liver microsomes. Br J Clin Pharmacol 34:262–265

10. Jordan VC, Brodie AM (2007) Development and evolution of therapies targeted to the estrogen receptor for the treatment and prevention of breast cancer. Steroids 72:7–25

11. Jordan VC (2003) Tamoxifen: a most unlikely pioneering medicine. Nat Rev Drug Discov 2:205–213

12. Fromson JM, Pearson S, Bramah S (1973) The metabolism of tamoxifen (I.C.I. 46,474). I. In laboratory animals. Xenobiotica 3:693–709

13. Fromson JM, Pearson S, Bramah S (1973) The metabolism of tamoxifen (I.C.I. 46,474). II. In female patients. Xenobiotica 3:711–714

14. Lieberman ME, Jordan VC, Fritsch M et al (1983) Direct and reversible inhibition of estradiol-stimulated prolactin synthesis by antiestrogens in vitro. J Biol Chem 258:4734–4740

15. Adam HK, Gay MA, Moore RH (1980) Measurement of tamoxifen in serum by thin-layer densitometry. J Endocrinol 84:35–42

16. Adam HK, Douglas EJ, Kemp JV (1979) The metabolism of tamoxifen in humans. Biochem Pharmacol 27:145–147

17. Kemp JV, Adam HK, Wakeling AE, Slater R (1983) Identification and biological activity of tamoxifen metabolites in human serum. Biochem Pharmacol 32:2045–2052

18. Bain RR, Jordan VC (1983) Identification of a new metabolite of tamoxifen in patient serum during breast cancer therapy. Biochem Pharmacol 32:373–375

19. Jordan VC, Bain RR, Brown RR et al (1983) Determination and pharmacology of a new hydroxylated metabolite of tamoxifen observed in patient sera during therapy for advanced breast cancer. Cancer Res 43:1446–1450

20. Robinson SP, Langan-Fahey SM, Jordan VC (1989) Implications of tamoxifen metabolism in the athymic mouse for the study of antitumor effects upon human breast cancer xenografts. Eur J Cancer Clin Oncol 25:1769–1776

21. Jordan VC, Gosden B (1982) Importance of the alkylaminoethoxy side-chain for the estrogenic and antiestrogenic actions of tamoxifen and trioxifene in the immature rat uterus. Mol Cell Endocrinol 27:291–306

22. Lieberman ME, Gorski J, Jordan VC (1983) An estrogen receptor model to describe the regulation of prolactin synthesis by antiestrogens in vitro. J Biol Chem 258:4741–4745

23. Katzenellenbogen JA, Carlson KE, Katzenellenbogen BS (1985) Facile geometric isomerization of phenolic non-steroidal estrogens and antiestrogens: limitations to the interpretation of experiments characterizing the activity of individual isomers. J Steroid Biochem 22:589–596

24. Katzenellenbogen BS, Norman MJ, Eckert RL et al (1984) Bioactivities, estrogen receptor interactions, and plasminogen activator-inducing activities of tamoxifen and hydroxy-tamoxifen isomers in MCF-7 human breast cancer cells. Cancer Res 44:112–119

25. Berthois Y, Katzenellenbogen JA, Katzenellenbogen BS (1986) Phenol red in tissue culture media is a weak estrogen: implications concerning the study of estrogen-responsive cells in culture. Proc Natl Acad Sci U S A 83:2496–2500

26. Murphy CS, Meisner LF, Wu SQ, Jordan VC (1989) Short- and long-term estrogen deprivation of T47D human breast cancer cells in culture. Eur J Cancer Clin Oncol 25:1777–1788

27. Jordan VC, Lieberman ME, Cormier E et al (1984) Structural requirements for the pharmacological activity of nonsteroidal antiestrogens in vitro. Mol Pharmacol 26:272–278

28. Jordan VC, Koch R, Mittal S, Schneider MR (1986) Oestrogenic and antioestrogenic actions in a series of triphenylbut-1-enes: modulation of prolactin synthesis in vitro. Br J Pharmacol 87:217–223

29. Murphy CS, Langan-Fahey SM, McCague R, Jordan VC (1990) Structure-function relationships of hydroxylated metabolites of tamoxifen that control the proliferation of estrogen-responsive T47D breast cancer cells in vitro. Mol Pharmacol 38:737–743

30. Murphy CS, Parker CJ, McCague R, Jordan VC (1991) Structure-activity relationships of nonisomerizable derivatives of tamoxifen: importance of hydroxyl group and side chain positioning for biological activity. Mol Pharmacol 39:421–428

31. Shiau AK, Barstad D, Loria PM et al (1998) The structural basis of estrogen receptor/coactivator recognition and the antagonism of this interaction by tamoxifen. Cell 95:927–937

32. Brzozowski AM, Pike AC, Dauter Z et al (1997) Molecular basis of agonism and antagonism in the oestrogen receptor. Nature 389:753–758

33. Wolf DM, Jordan VC (1994) The estrogen receptor from a tamoxifen stimulated MCF-7 tumor variant contains a point mutation in the ligand binding domain. Breast Cancer Res Treat 31:129–138

34. Wolf DM, Jordan VC (1994) Characterization of tamoxifen stimulated MCF-7 tumor variants grown in athymic mice. Breast Cancer Res Treat 31:117–127

35. MacGregor Schafer J, Liu H, Bentrem DJ et al (2000) Allosteric silencing of activating function 1 in the 4-hydroxytamoxifen estrogen receptor complex is induced by substituting glycine for aspartate at amino acid 351. Cancer Res 60:5097–5105

36. Levenson AS, Jordan VC (1998) The key to the antiestrogenic mechanism of raloxifene is amino acid 351 (aspartate) in the estrogen receptor. Cancer Res 58:1872–1875

37. Liu H, Lee ES, Deb Los Reyes A et al (2001) Silencing and reactivation of the selective estrogen receptor modulator-estrogen receptor alpha complex. Cancer Res 61:3632–3639

38. Levenson AS, Catherino WH, Jordan VC (1997) Estrogenic activity is increased for an antiestrogen by a natural mutation of the estrogen receptor. J Steroid Biochem Mol Biol 60:261–268

39. Liu H, Park WC, Bentrem DJ et al (2002) Structure-function relationships of the raloxifene-estrogen receptor-alpha complex for regulating transforming growth factor-alpha expression in breast cancer cells. J Biol Chem 277:9189–9198

40. Onate SA, Tsai SY, Tsai MJ, O'Malley BW (1995) Sequence and characterization of a coactivator for the steroid hormone receptor superfamily. Science 270:1354–1357

41. Jordan VC, O'Malley BW (2007) Selective estrogen-receptor modulators and antihormonal resistance in breast cancer. J Clin Oncol 25:5815–5824

42. Jordan VC, Gapstur S, Morrow M (2001) Selective estrogen receptor modulation and reduction in risk of breast cancer, osteoporosis, and coronary heart disease. J Natl Cancer Inst 93:1449–1457

43. Greaves P, Goonetilleke R, Nunn G et al (1993) Two-year carcinogenicity study of tamoxifen in Alderley Park Wistar-derived rats. Cancer Res 53:3919–3924

44. Hard GC, Iatropoulos MJ, Jordan K et al (1993) Major difference in the hepatocarcinogenicity and DNA adduct forming ability between toremifene and tamoxifen in female Crl: CD(BR) rats. Cancer Res 53:4534–4541

45. Fornander T, Rutqvist LE, Cedermark B et al (1989) Adjuvant tamoxifen in early breast cancer: occurrence of new primary cancers. Lancet 1:117–120

46. Fisher B, Costantino JP, Redmond CK et al (1994) Endometrial cancer in tamoxifen-treated breast cancer patients: findings from the National Surgical Adjuvant Breast and Bowel Project (NSABP) B-14. J Natl Cancer Inst 86:527–537

47. Han XL, Liehr JG (1992) Induction of covalent DNA adducts in rodents by tamoxifen. Cancer Res 52:1360–1363

48. Rutqvist LE, Johansson H, Signomklao T et al (1995) Adjuvant tamoxifen therapy for early stage breast cancer and second primary malignancies. Stockholm Breast Cancer Study Group. J Natl Cancer Inst 87:645–651

49. Styles JA, Davies A, Lim CK et al (1994) Genotoxicity of tamoxifen, tamoxifen epoxide and toremifene in human lymphoblastoid cells containing human cytochrome P450s. Carcinogenesis 15:5–9

50. Lim CK, Yuan ZX, Lamb JH et al (1994) A comparative study of tamoxifen metabolism in female rat, mouse and human liver microsomes. Carcinogenesis 15:589–593

51. Moorthy B, Sriram P, Pathak DN et al (1996) Tamoxifen metabolic activation: comparison of DNA adducts formed by microsomal and chemical activation of tamoxifen and 4-hydroxytamoxifen with DNA adducts formed in vivo. Cancer Res 56:53–57

52. Pongracz K, Pathak DN, Nakamura T et al (1995) Activation of the tamoxifen derivative metabolite E to form DNA adducts: comparison with the adducts formed by microsomal activation of tamoxifen. Cancer Res 55:3012–3015

53. Potter GA, McCague R, Jarman M (1994) A mechanistic hypothesis for DNA adduct formation by tamoxifen following hepatic oxidative metabolism. Carcinogenesis 15:439–442

54. Phillips DH, Carmichael PL, Hewer A et al (1994) alpha-Hydroxytamoxifen, a metabolite of tamoxifen with exceptionally high DNA-binding activity in rat hepatocytes. Cancer Res 54:5518–5522

55. Phillips DH, Potter GA, Horton MN et al (1994) Reduced genotoxicity of [D5-ethyl]-tamoxifen implicates alpha-hydroxylation of the ethyl group as a major pathway of tamoxifen activation to a liver carcinogen. Carcinogenesis 15:1487–1492

56. Osborne MR, Hewer A, Hardcastle IR et al (1996) Identification of the major tamoxifen-deoxyguanosine adduct formed in the liver DNA of rats treated with tamoxifen. Cancer Res 56:66–71

57. Phillips DH, Carmichael PL, Hewer A et al (1996) Activation of tamoxifen and its metabolite alpha-hydroxytamoxifen to DNA-binding products: comparisons between human, rat and mouse hepatocytes. Carcinogenesis 17:89–94

58. Osborne MR, Hewer A, Phillips DH (2001) Resolution of alpha-hydroxytamoxifen; R-isomer forms more DNA adducts in rat liver cells. Chem Res Toxicol 14:888–893

59. Osborne MR, Hewer A, Phillips DH (2004) Stereoselective metabolic activation of alpha-hydroxy-N-desmethyltamoxifen: the R-isomer forms more DNA adducts in rat liver cells. Chem Res Toxicol 17:697–701

60. Phillips DH (2001) Understanding the genotoxicity of tamoxifen? Carcinogenesis 22:839–849

61. Jordan VC (1995) What if tamoxifen (ICI 46,474) had been found to produce rat liver tumors in 1973? A personal perspective. Ann Oncol 6:29–34

62. Jordan VC, Gradishar WJ (1997) Molecular mechanisms and future uses of antiestrogens. Mol Aspects Med 18:167–247

63. Jordan VC (1984) Biochemical pharmacology of antiestrogen action. Pharmacol Rev 36:245–276

64. Jordan VC (1988) Chemosuppression of breast cancer with tamoxifen: laboratory evidence and future clinical investigations. Cancer Invest 6:589–595

65. Lerner LJ, Jordan VC (1990) Development of antiestrogens and their use in breast cancer: eighth Cain memorial award lecture. Cancer Res 50:4177–4189

66. Jordan VC (2001) Selective estrogen receptor modulation: a personal perspective. Cancer Res 61:5683–5687

67. Jordan VC (2003) Antiestrogens and selective estrogen receptor modulators as multifunctional medicines. 2. Clinical considerations and new agents. J Med Chem 46:1081–1111
68. Ariazi EA, Ariazi JL, Cordera F, Jordan VC et al (2006) Estrogen receptors as therapeutic targets in breast cancer. Curr Top Med Chem 6:195–216
69. Buzdar AU, Marcus C, Holmes F et al (1988) Phase II evaluation of Ly156758 in metastatic breast cancer. Oncology 45:344–345
70. Snyder KR, Sparano N, Malinowski JM (2000) Raloxifene hydrochloride. Am J Health Syst Pharm 57:1669–1675, quiz 76–8
71. Kemp DC, Fan PW, Stevens JC (2002) Characterization of raloxifene glucuronidation in vitro: contribution of intestinal metabolism to presystemic clearance. Drug Metab Dispos 30:694–700
72. Jeong EJ, Liu Y, Lin H, Hu M (2005) Species- and disposition model-dependent metabolism of raloxifene in gut and liver: role of UGT1A10. Drug Metab Dispos 33:785–794
73. Suh N, Lamph WW, Glasebrook AL et al (2002) Prevention and treatment of experimental breast cancer with the combination of a new selective estrogen receptor modulator, arzoxifene, and a new rexinoid, LG 100268. Clin Cancer Res 8:3270–3275
74. Baselga J, Llombart-Cussac A, Bellet M et al (2003) Randomized, double-blind, multicenter trial comparing two doses of arzoxifene (LY353381) in hormone-sensitive advanced or metastatic breast cancer patients. Ann Oncol 14:1383–1390
75. Buzdar A, O'Shaughnessy JA, Booser DJ et al (2003) Phase II, randomized, double-blind study of two dose levels of arzoxifene in patients with locally advanced or metastatic breast cancer. J Clin Oncol 21:1007–1014
76. Bolognese M, Krege JH, Utian WH et al (2009) Effects of arzoxifene on bone mineral density and endometrium in postmenopausal women with normal or low bone mass. J Clin Endocrinol Metab 94:2284–2289
77. Downs RW Jr, Moffett AM, Ghosh A et al (2010) Effects of arzoxifene on bone, lipid markers, and safety parameters in postmenopausal women with low bone mass. Osteoporos Int 21:1215–1226
78. Kendler DL, Palacios S, Cox DA et al (2012) Arzoxifene versus raloxifene: effect on bone and safety parameters in postmenopausal women with osteoporosis. Osteoporos Int 23:1091–1101
79. Falany JL, Pilloff DE, Leyh TS, Falany CN (2006) Sulfation of raloxifene and 4-hydroxytamoxifen by human cytosolic sulfotransferases. Drug Metab Dispos 34:361–368
80. Rosati RL, Da Silva JP, Cameron KO et al (1998) Discovery and preclinical pharmacology of a novel, potent, nonsteroidal estrogen receptor agonist/antagonist, CP-336156, a diaryltetrahydronaphthalene. J Med Chem 41:2928–2931
81. Ke HZ, Paralkar VM, Grasser WA et al (1998) Effects of CP-336,156, a new, nonsteroidal estrogen agonist/antagonist, on bone, serum cholesterol, uterus and body composition in rat models. Endocrinology 139:2068–2076
82. Ke HZ, Qi H, Crawford DT et al (2000) Lasofoxifene (CP-336,156), a selective estrogen receptor modulator, prevents bone loss induced by aging and orchidectomy in the adult rat. Endocrinology 141:1338–1344
83. Tatee T, Carlson KE, Katzenellenbogen JA et al (1979) Antiestrogens and antiestrogen metabolites: preparation of tritium-labeled (+/−)-cis-3-[p-(1,2,3,4-tetrahydro-6-methoxy-2-phenyl-1-naphthyl)phenoxyl]-1,2-propanediol (U-23469) and characterization and synthesis of a biologically important metabolite. J Med Chem 22:1509–1517
84. Legha SS, Slavik M, Carter SK (1976) Nafoxidine–an antiestrogen for the treatment of breast cancer. Cancer 38:1535–1541
85. Cohen LA, Pittman B, Wang CX et al (2001) LAS, a novel selective estrogen receptor modulator with chemopreventive and therapeutic activity in the N-nitroso-N-methylurea-induced rat mammary tumor model. Cancer Res 61:8683–8688
86. Robertson DW, Katzenellenbogen JA, Hayes JR, Katzenellenbogen BS (1982) Antiestrogen basicity–activity relationships: a comparison of the estrogen receptor binding and

antiuterotrophic potencies of several analogues of (Z)-1,2-diphenyl-1-[4-[2-(dimethylamino) ethoxy]phenyl]-1-butene (tamoxifen, Nolvadex) having altered basicity. J Med Chem 25:167–171

87. Hellmann-Blumberg U, Taras TL, Wurz GT, DeGregorio MW et al (2000) Genotoxic effects of the novel mixed antiestrogen FC-1271a in comparison to tamoxifen and toremifene. Breast Cancer Res Treat 60:63–70

88. Qu Q, Zheng H, Dahllund J et al (2000) Selective estrogenic effects of a novel triphenylethylene compound, FC1271a, on bone, cholesterol level, and reproductive tissues in intact and ovariectomized rats. Endocrinology 141:809–820

89. DeGregorio MW, Wurz GT, Taras TL et al (2000) Pharmacokinetics of (deaminohydroxy) toremifene in humans: a new, selective estrogen-receptor modulator. Eur J Clin Pharmacol 56:469–475

90. Rutanen EM, Heikkinen J, Halonen K et al (2003) Effects of ospemifene, a novel SERM, on hormones, genital tract, climacteric symptoms, and quality of life in postmenopausal women: a double-blind, randomized trial. Menopause 10:433–439

91. Komi J, Lankinen KS, Harkonen P et al (2005) Effects of ospemifene and raloxifene on hormonal status, lipids, genital tract, and tolerability in postmenopausal women. Menopause 12:202–209

92. Namba R, Young LJ, Maglione JE et al (2005) Selective estrogen receptor modulators inhibit growth and progression of premalignant lesions in a mouse model of ductal carcinoma in situ. Breast Cancer Res 7:R881–R889

93. Wurz GT, Read KC, Marchisano-Karpman C et al (2005) Ospemifene inhibits the growth of dimethylbenzanthracene-induced mammary tumors in Sencar mice. J Steroid Biochem Mol Biol 97:230–240

94. Dehal SS, Kupfer D (1997) CYP2D6 catalyzes tamoxifen 4-hydroxylation in human liver. Cancer Res 57:3402–3406

95. Beverage JN, Sissung TM, Sion AM et al (2007) CYP2D6 polymorphisms and the impact on tamoxifen therapy. J Pharm Sci 96:2224–2231

96. Bradford LD (2002) CYP2D6 allele frequency in European Caucasians, Asians, Africans and their descendants. Pharmacogenomics 3:229–243

97. Raimundo S, Toscano C, Klein K et al (2004) A novel intronic mutation, 2988G>A, with high predictivity for impaired function of cytochrome P450 2D6 in white subjects. Clin Pharmacol Ther 76:128–138

98. Hanioka N, Kimura S, Meyer UA, Gonzalez FJ (1990) The human CYP2D locus associated with a common genetic defect in drug oxidation: a G1934—A base change in intron 3 of a mutant CYP2D6 allele results in an aberrant 3′ splice recognition site. Am J Hum Genet 47:994–1001

99. Bernard S, Neville KA, Nguyen AT, Flockhart DA (2006) Interethnic differences in genetic polymorphisms of CYP2D6 in the U.S. population: clinical implications. Oncologist 11:126–135

100. Lim YC, Desta Z, Flockhart DA, Skaar TC (2005) Endoxifen (4-hydroxy-N-desmethyl-tamoxifen) has anti-estrogenic effects in breast cancer cells with potency similar to 4-hydroxy-tamoxifen. Cancer Chemother Pharmacol 55:471–478

101. Lim YC, Li L, Desta Z et al (2006) Endoxifen, a secondary metabolite of tamoxifen, and 4-OH-tamoxifen induce similar changes in global gene expression patterns in MCF-7 breast cancer cells. J Pharmacol Exp Ther 318:503–512

102. Stearns V, Johnson MD, Rae JM et al (2003) Active tamoxifen metabolite plasma concentrations after coadministration of tamoxifen and the selective serotonin reuptake inhibitor paroxetine. J Natl Cancer Inst 95:1758–1764

103. Jin Y, Desta Z, Stearns V et al (2005) CYP2D6 genotype, antidepressant use, and tamoxifen metabolism during adjuvant breast cancer treatment. J Natl Cancer Inst 97:30–39

104. Fisher B, Costantino J, Redmond C et al (1989) A randomized clinical trial evaluating tamoxifen in the treatment of patients with node-negative breast cancer who have estrogen-receptor-positive tumors. N Engl J Med 320:479–484

105. Fisher B, Dignam J, Wolmark N et al (1999) Tamoxifen in treatment of intraductal breast cancer: National Surgical Adjuvant Breast and Bowel Project B-24 randomised controlled trial. Lancet 353:1993–2000
106. Fisher B, Costantino JP, Wickerham DL et al (1998) Tamoxifen for prevention of breast cancer: report of the National Surgical Adjuvant Breast and Bowel Project P-1 Study. J Natl Cancer Inst 90:1371–1388
107. Loprinzi CL, Kugler JW, Sloan JA et al (2000) Venlafaxine in management of hot flashes in survivors of breast cancer: a randomised controlled trial. Lancet 356:2059–2063
108. Loprinzi CL, Sloan JA, Perez EA et al (2002) Phase III evaluation of fluoxetine for treatment of hot flashes. J Clin Oncol 20:1578–1583
109. Stearns V, Beebe KL, Iyengar M, Dube E (2003) Paroxetine controlled release in the treatment of menopausal hot flashes: a randomized controlled trial. JAMA 289:2827–2834
110. Crewe HK, Ellis SW, Lennard MS, Tucker GT (1997) Variable contribution of cytochromes P450 2D6, 2C9 and 3A4 to the 4-hydroxylation of tamoxifen by human liver microsomes. Biochem Pharmacol 53:171–178
111. Coller JK, Krebsfaenger N, Klein K et al (2002) The influence of CYP2B6, CYP2C9 and CYP2D6 genotypes on the formation of the potent antioestrogen Z-4-hydroxy-tamoxifen in human liver. Br J Clin Pharmacol 54:157–167
112. Lessard E, Yessine MA, Hamelin BA et al (2001) Diphenhydramine alters the disposition of venlafaxine through inhibition of CYP2D6 activity in humans. J Clin Psychopharmacol 21:175–184
113. Albers LJ, Reist C, Vu RL et al (2000) Effect of venlafaxine on imipramine metabolism. Psychiatry Res 96:235–243
114. Yoon YR, Cha IJ, Shon JH et al (2000) Relationship of paroxetine disposition to metoprolol metabolic ratio and CYP2D6*10 genotype of Korean subjects. Clin Pharmacol Ther 67:567–576
115. Jeppesen U, Gram LF, Vistisen K et al (1996) Dose-dependent inhibition of CYP1A2, CYP2C19 and CYP2D6 by citalopram, fluoxetine, fluvoxamine and paroxetine. Eur J Clin Pharmacol 51:73–78
116. Andersson T, Flockhart DA, Goldstein DB et al (2005) Drug-metabolizing enzymes: evidence for clinical utility of pharmacogenomic tests. Clin Pharmacol Ther 78:559–581
117. Borges S, Desta Z, Li L et al (2006) Quantitative effect of CYP2D6 genotype and inhibitors on tamoxifen metabolism: implication for optimization of breast cancer treatment. Clin Pharmacol Ther 80:61–74
118. Dieudonne AS, Lambrechts D, Claes B et al (2009) Prevalent breast cancer patients with a homozygous mutant status for CYP2D6*4: response and biomarkers in tamoxifen users. Breast Cancer Res Treat 118:531–538
119. Schroth W, Goetz MP, Hamann U et al (2009) Association between CYP2D6 polymorphisms and outcomes among women with early stage breast cancer treated with tamoxifen. JAMA 302:1429–1436
120. Kiyotani K, Mushiroda T, Imamura CK et al (2010) Significant effect of polymorphisms in CYP2D6 and ABCC2 on clinical outcomes of adjuvant tamoxifen therapy for breast cancer patients. J Clin Oncol 28:1287–1293
121. Lammers LA, Mathijssen RH, van Gelder T et al (2010) The impact of CYP2D6-predicted phenotype on tamoxifen treatment outcome in patients with metastatic breast cancer. Br J Cancer 103:765–771
122. Madlensky L, Natarajan L, Tchu S et al (2011) Tamoxifen metabolite concentrations, CYP2D6 genotype, and breast cancer outcomes. Clin Pharmacol Ther 89:718–725
123. Lash TL, Cronin-Fenton D, Ahern TP et al (2011) CYP2D6 inhibition and breast cancer recurrence in a population-based study in Denmark. J Natl Cancer Inst 103:489–500
124. Regan MM, Leyland-Jones B, Bouzyk M et al (2012) CYP2D6 genotype and tamoxifen response in postmenopausal women with endocrine-responsive breast cancer: the breast international group 1–98 trial. J Natl Cancer Inst 104:441–451

125. Rae JM, Drury S, Hayes DF et al (2012) CYP2D6 and UGT2B7 genotype and risk of recurrence in tamoxifen-treated breast cancer patients. J Natl Cancer Inst 104:452–460

126. Brauch H, Schroth W, Goetz MP et al (2013) Tamoxifen use in postmenopausal breast cancer: CYP2D6 matters. J Clin Oncol 31(2):176–180

127. Lim JS, Chen XA, Singh O et al (2011) Impact of CYP2D6, CYP3A5, CYP2C9 and CYP2C19 polymorphisms on tamoxifen pharmacokinetics in Asian breast cancer patients. Br J Clin Pharmacol 71:737–750

128. Murdter TE, Schroth W, Bacchus-Gerybadze L et al (2011) Activity levels of tamoxifen metabolites at the estrogen receptor and the impact of genetic polymorphisms of phase I and II enzymes on their concentration levels in plasma. Clin Pharmacol Ther 89:708–717

129. Jordan VC, Fritz NF, Tormey DC (1987) Endocrine effects of adjuvant chemotherapy and long-term tamoxifen administration on node-positive patients with breast cancer. Cancer Res 47:624–630

130. Ravdin PM, Fritz NF, Tormey DC, Jordan VC (1988) Endocrine status of premenopausal node-positive breast cancer patients following adjuvant chemotherapy and long-term tamoxifen. Cancer Res 48:1026–1029

131. Irvin WJ Jr, Walko CM, Weck KE et al (2011) Genotype-guided tamoxifen dosing increases active metabolite exposure in women with reduced CYP2D6 metabolism: a multicenter study. J Clin Oncol 29:3232–3239

132. Barginear MF, Jaremko M, Peter I et al (2011) Increasing tamoxifen dose in breast cancer patients based on CYP2D6 genotypes and endoxifen levels: effect on active metabolite isomers and the antiestrogenic activity score. Clin Pharmacol Ther 90:605–611

133. Kiyotani K, Mushiroda T, Imamura CK et al (2012) Dose-adjustment study of tamoxifen based on CYP2D6 genotypes in Japanese breast cancer patients. Breast Cancer Res Treat 131:137–145

134. Jordan VC (1976) Antiestrogenic and antitumor properties of tamoxifen in laboratory animals. Cancer Treat Rep 60:1409–1419

135. Jordan VC, Allen KE (1980) Evaluation of the antitumour activity of the non-steroidal antioestrogen monohydroxytamoxifen in the DMBA-induced rat mammary carcinoma model. Eur J Cancer 16:239–251

136. Rouanet P, Linares-Cruz G, Dravet F et al (2005) Neoadjuvant percutaneous 4-hydroxytamoxifen decreases breast tumoral cell proliferation: a prospective controlled randomized study comparing three doses of 4-hydroxytamoxifen gel to oral tamoxifen. J Clin Oncol 23:2980–2987

137. Jordan VC, Fenuik L, Allen KE et al (1981) Structural derivatives of tamoxifen and oestradiol 3-methyl ether as potential alkylating antioestrogens. Eur J Cancer 17:193–200

138. Wakeling AE, Dukes M, Bowler J (1991) A potent specific pure antiestrogen with clinical potential. Cancer Res 51:3867–3873

Chapter 4
Adjuvant Therapy: The Breakthrough

Abstract The finding that long-term tamoxifen therapy of rats previously treated with a chemical carcinogen 7,12-dimethylbenzanthracene (DMBA) had a suppression of mammary tumorigenesis as long as treatment was continued, created a new strategy to save lives. These pivotal laboratory studies changed clinical practice. The initiation of numerous international randomized clinical trials of extended adjuvant tamoxifen therapy for patients with ER-positive tumors demonstrated longer was better to save lives. Recurrences were controlled by tamoxifen and mortality decreased by at least 30 %. Current indications are that 10 years of adjuvant tamoxifen is superior to 5 years of adjuvant tamoxifen.

Introduction

The initial success of adjuvant monotherapy with L-phenylalanine mustard [1] or combination chemotherapy [2] to delay the recurrence of node-positive breast cancer encouraged the investigation of other, perhaps less toxic, therapies. Most of the beneficial effects of adjuvant chemotherapy were noted in premenopausal women. In retrospect, this result was almost certainly a "chemical oophorectomy" produced by the cancer treatment. During the 1970s and 1980s, numerous reports [3, 4] described the changes in women's endocrinology as ovarian function is destroyed. Indeed, in the premenopausal women with breast cancer, combination cytotoxic chemotherapy can be considered to be endocrine therapy [5]. The low reported incidence of side effects noted with tamoxifen [6, 7] with modest efficacy naturally caused clinicians to consider adjuvant antiestrogen therapy. But the question to be addressed was "How long is long enough for adjuvant tamoxifen therapy?"

During the 1970's, at the time when tamoxifen was only available in the United Kingdom for the treatment of metastatic breast cancer in postmenopausal women, this was also true in the United States until approval by the FDA in December 1977 for the treatment of metastatic breast cancer. The laboratory studies in the 1970s

P.Y. Maximov et al., *Tamoxifen*, Milestones in Drug Therapy,   69
DOI 10.1007/978-3-0348-0664-0_4, © Springer Basel 2013

would encourage the testing of long-term adjuvant treatment, but the change in conservative clinical philosophy about using a "palliative" treatment of low efficacy would take a decade [8].

Laboratory studies using the DMBA-induced rat mammary carcinoma model were first used to explore whether tamoxifen would be an effective adjuvant therapy and whether the drug produces a tumoristatic or tumoricidal effect in vivo. Studies with estrogen receptor (ER) in positive MCF-7 breast cancer cells in vitro had previously indicated that tamoxifen could be a tumoricidal drug [9], but the results from the DMBA studies in vivo (first reported at a breast cancer symposium at King's College, Cambridge, England, in September 1977) (Fig. 4.1) demonstrated that a short course of tamoxifen therapy (1 month) given 1 month after the carcinogenic insult only delayed the appearance of mammary tumors; continuous therapy (for 6 months) resulted in 90 % of the animals remaining tumor free (Fig. 4.2) [12, 13]. Indeed if tamoxifen therapy is stopped, tumors appear [14]. Thus, tamoxifen was shown to have a tumoristatic component to its mode of action, and the laboratory results indicated that long-term (up to 5 years) or indefinite therapy might be the best clinical strategy for adjuvant treatment. Subsequent laboratory studies using DMBA- or N-nitrosomethylurea (NMU)-induced rat mammary tumors [15–17] or human breast cancer cell lines inoculated into athymic mice [18–20] have all supported the initial observation. However, most attention has naturally focused on the clinical evaluation of adjuvant tamoxifen therapy.

Adjuvant Therapy with Tamoxifen

Several trials of tamoxifen monotherapy as an adjuvant to mastectomy were initiated toward the end of the 1970s. The majority of clinical trial organizations selected a conservative course of 1 year of adjuvant tamoxifen [21–27]. This decision was, however, based on a number of reasonable concerns. Patients with advanced disease usually respond to tamoxifen for 1 year, and it was expected that ER-negative disease would be encouraged to grow prematurely during adjuvant therapy. If this growth was to occur, then the physician would have already used a valuable palliative drug and would have only combination chemotherapy to slow the relentless growth of recurrent disease. A related argument involved the changing strategy for the application of adjuvant combination chemotherapy. Recurrent treatment cycles (2 years) of cytotoxic chemotherapy were found to be of no long-term benefit for the patient. An aggressive course of short-term treatment (6 months) with the most active cytotoxic drugs could have the best chance to kill tumor cells before the premature development of drug resistance. The same argument provided an intuitive reluctance to use long-term tamoxifen therapy because it would lead to premature drug resistance: longer might not be better.

Finally, there were sincere concerns about the side effects of adjuvant therapy and the ethical issues of treating patients who might never have recurrent disease.

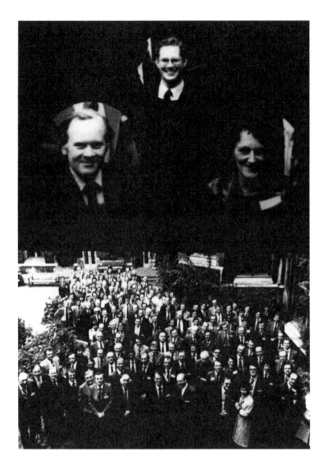

Fig. 4.1 Breast cancer symposium at King's College, Cambridge, England, in September 1977. The concept of extended adjuvant tamoxifen treatment was first proposed at this meeting. Clinical studies of 1-year adjuvant tamoxifen were in place; regrettably, a decade later, this approach was shown to produce little survival benefit for patients. In the inserts, (*top*) V. Craig Jordan, who presented the new concept, (*bottom left*) Mr. Michael Baum who planned to use 2 years of adjuvant tamoxifen and (*bottom right*) Dr. Helen Stewart, who was a participant at the conference. She would initiate a pilot trial in 1978 and, led by Sir Patrick Forest, would later guide the full randomized Scottish trial of the 5-year adjuvant tamoxifen treatment versus control in the 1980s. Both clinical trials were later proven to produce survival advantages for patients. The concept of longer tamoxifen treatment producing more survival benefits for patients was eventually established indirectly by the Oxford Overview Analysis in 1992 [10] and directly by the Swedish group led by Dr. Lars Rutqvist [11]

Although this argument primarily focused on chemotherapy and node-negative patients, it is fair to say that few women in the mid-1970s had received extended therapy with tamoxifen, so that long-term side effects were largely unknown. The majority of tamoxifen-treated patients had received only about 2 years of treatment for advanced disease before drug resistance occurred. Potential side effects of thrombosis, osteoporosis, and so on were only of secondary importance. The use of tamoxifen in the disease-free patient would change that perspective.

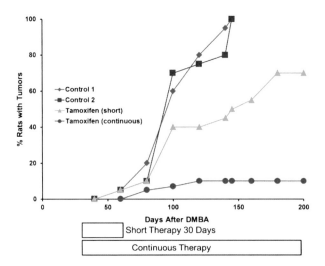

Fig. 4.2 The effectiveness of long-term tamoxifen treatment in the dimethylbenzanthracene (DMBA)-induced rat mammary carcinoma model. The administration of 20-mg DMBA by gavage to 50-day-old female Sprague-Dawley rats results in all animals developing mammary tumors 160 days later. The short-term (30 days) administration of different daily doses (12.5–800 µg) of tamoxifen between days 30 and 60 after DMBA results in a delay of tumor formation. However, not all animals are protected from the carcinogen. In contrast, the daily administration of a clinically relevant dose (50 µg daily = 0.25 mg/kg in rats or 20 mg daily to a 70 kg woman) of tamoxifen continuously, starting 30 days after DMBA, results in 90 % of animals remaining tumor free

In 1977, Dr. Douglass C. Tormey organized the first evaluation of long-term tamoxifen therapy in node-positive patients treated with combination chemotherapy plus tamoxifen [28, 29]. This pilot study was initiated to determine whether patients could tolerate 5 years of adjuvant tamoxifen therapy and whether metabolic tolerance would occur during long-term tamoxifen therapy. No unusual side effects of tamoxifen therapy were noted, and blood levels of tamoxifen and its metabolites N-desmethyltamoxifen and metabolite Y remained stable throughout the 5 years of treatment. Although this study was not a randomized trial, those patients who received long-term tamoxifen therapy continued to make excellent progress, and many patients took the drug for more than 14 years. We reported [30] that tamoxifen does not produce metabolic tolerance during 10 years of administration. Serum levels of tamoxifen and its metabolites are maintained.

The metabolic stability data and the DMBA-induced rat mammary carcinoma data [31] were used to support randomized Eastern Cooperative Oncology Group (ECOG) trials EST 4181 and 5181. An early analysis of EST 4181, which compares short-term tamoxifen with long-term tamoxifen (both with combination chemotherapy), demonstrated an increase in disease-free survival with long-term tamoxifen therapy [32]. In fact, the 5-year tamoxifen arm went through a second randomization either to stop the tamoxifen or to continue the antiestrogen indefinitely. The National Surgical Adjuvant Breast and Bowel Project (NSABP) clinical trial organization conducted a registration study of 2 years of combination chemotherapy (L-PAM, 5-FU) plus tamoxifen with an additional year of tamoxifen alone [33] to build on the successes of the earlier trials that demonstrated the efficacy of tamoxifen in receptor-positive postmenopausal patients [34–36]. Overall, these investigators conclude that 3 years of tamoxifen confers a significant advantage for patients over 2 years of tamoxifen.

Although the 2-year adjuvant tamoxifen study that was conducted by the Nolvadex Adjuvant Trial Organization (NATO) was the first to demonstrate a survival advantage for women [37], subsequent clinical trials all evaluated a longer duration of tamoxifen therapy. A small, randomized clinical trial of 3 years of tamoxifen versus no treatment demonstrated a survival advantage for ER-positive patients who receive tamoxifen [38]. Similarly, the Scottish trial that evaluated 5 years of tamoxifen versus no treatment demonstrated a survival advantage for patients who take tamoxifen [39]. The Scottish trial is particularly interesting because it addressed the question of whether to administer tamoxifen early as an adjuvant or to save the drug until recurrence. This comparison was possible because most patients in the control arm received tamoxifen at recurrence. Early concerns that long-term adjuvant tamoxifen would result in premature drug resistance were unjustified, because the patients have a survival advantage on the adjuvant tamoxifen arm. Indeed, an analysis of non-cancer-related deaths in the Scottish trial demonstrated a significant decrease in fatal myocardial infarction for patients receiving adjuvant tamoxifen for 5 years [40]. A number of other studies also demonstrate a decrease in coronary heart disease with tamoxifen [41, 42] but there is no overall consensus on this point and the overview analysis of clinical trials does not support enhanced survival by reduced coronary heart disease in women taking tamoxifen.

Studies in Premenopausal Women

Tamoxifen was initially used in premenopausal women to treat menometrorrhagia [43] and to induce ovulation in infertile women [44, 45]. Subsequent evaluation of the endocrine effects of tamoxifen by Groom and Griffiths [46] revealed an increase in ovarian estrogen production.

Although concerns have been expressed about the potential for the reversal of tamoxifen's action in a high-estrogen environment, tamoxifen can effectively control the growth of advanced breast cancer in premenopausal patients [47–51], and small clinical trials have demonstrated that tamoxifen and oophorectomy [52, 53] have similar efficacy. Adjuvant monotherapy with tamoxifen has shown efficacy in node-positive premenopausal patients [54], but most experience has been derived from the study B_{14} of node-negative ER-positive premenopausal patients conducted by the NSABP [56]. Tamoxifen increases the disease-free survival and, perhaps most importantly, the antiestrogen is active in premenopausal women. The protocol used an initial treatment period of 5 years of adjuvant tamoxifen, and then stop or continue tamoxifen for an additional 5-year period. No advantages were found for longer adjuvant therapy but there were more reported side effects [55, 56]. However, this is a very small trial and the issue of extending tamoxifen therapy in the ATLAS (Adjuvant Tamoxifen: Longer Against Shorter) trial from 5 to 10 years is currently being addressed. The following questions have now been asked: (1) What are the advantages and disadvantages of 5 versus 10 years of adjuvant tamoxifen? (2) What are the improvements in mortality during and after 10 years of adjuvant tamoxifen? The initial results of the ATLAS trial with 12,984 women who have completed 5 years of adjuvant tamoxifen are randomized to stop or continue for a further 5 years. The report of 6,846 women with ER-positive disease is reported [57] and compared with the earlier analysis of no treatment versus 5 years of adjuvant tamoxifen [58]. These enormous data sets confirm that endometrial cancer is the only side effect of concern in postmenopausal women, but deaths from endometrial cancer do not offset the benefits of adjuvant tamoxifen with an enhanced 50 % decrease in mortality in the decade after 10 years of tamoxifen.

These data [57] will be compared with aTTom (adjuvant Tamoxifen Treatment—offer more?) in 2013 and regular follow-ups will occur with reporting over the next 2 years.

Tamoxifen is currently available to treat select patients at each stage of breast cancer, but the overview analysis of randomized clinical trials has precisely described the worth of antiestrogen therapy. By way of an introduction, the overview analysis wonderfully demonstrated that "longer is better" for the effectiveness of different durations of adjuvant tamoxifen alone used to treat premenopausal women with ER-positive breast cancer. One year of adjuvant therapy is completely ineffective in improving either recurrence or survival (Fig. 4.3). Five years of tamoxifen produces 30 % decrease in mortality and a 50 % decrease in recurrence.

Overview of Clinical Trials

The first overview analysis of adjuvant therapy for breast cancer was conducted in 1984 by Richard Peto, Rory Collins, and Richard Gray leading the team for the Clinical Trials Unit of Oxford University. Analysis of clinical trials' results pertaining to tamoxifen demonstrated not only a decrease in recurrence-free survival for postmenopausal women receiving tamoxifen but also increase in overall survival. These data were refined, checked, and presented again at the National Cancer Institute Consensus Conference in Bethesda, Maryland, in 1985, where the panel concluded that adjuvant tamoxifen should be the standard of care for all postmenopausal women with ER-positive primary tumor and positive nodes [59].

As an aside, this was the year that ICI Pharmaceutical Division (Zeneca) was awarded the start of their "use patent" for tamoxifen as a treatment for breast cancer originally submitted and denied from 1965 onward (25 years!) (see Chap. 2). The patent would now extend into the twenty-first century creating the resources to advance chemoprevention and tamoxifen in the United States and the major clinical

Fig. 4.3 The antitumorigenic action of tamoxifen in postmenopausal women. The results from the overview analysis have proven "the longer the better" concept for treatment with tamoxifen

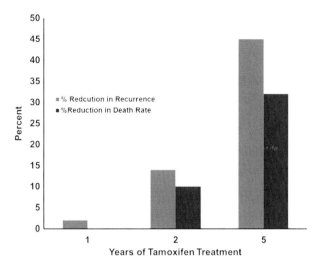

trial of anastrozole, their aromatase inhibitor. The Anastrazole versus Tamoxifen and the combination (ATAC) trial, then the single largest adjuvant endocrine clinical trial which became pivotal to lead progress with breast cancer therapy [60].

The overview of the clinical trials with tamoxifen was published in 1998 and 2005 [61, 62]. The 1998 and 2005 reports had three major therapeutic conclusions:

1. Tamoxifen was only effective as an adjuvant therapy in patients with an ER-positive breast tumor.
2. Longer was better than short adjuvant therapy in the treatment of ER-positive breast cancer. The power of this principle was best illustrated (Fig. 4.3) in premenopausal women receiving tamoxifen monotherapy: 1 year of adjuvant tamoxifen was completely ineffective at improving either recurrence rates or mortality but 5 years decreased recurrence by 50 % and mortality by 30 %. The scientific principles [8], published before any of the trials had started to recruit patients, were proven to have veracity.
3. The concern that the increased incidence of endometrial cancer during long-term adjuvant tamoxifen therapy might significantly reduce the value of tamoxifen as a cheap and effective life-saving medicine was calculated to be incorrect [61, 62].

We will now summarize the 2011 report of the relevance of breast cancer hormone receptors to the efficacy of adjuvant tamoxifen [58]. The meta-analysis of data was derived from 20 randomized clinical trials (n = 21,457) of adjuvant tamoxifen employing a 5-year treatment duration (80 % compliance). Again the continuing evaluation of adjuvant tamoxifen demonstrates the veracity of science in "the real world":

1. In ER positive disease (n = 10,645), tamoxifen reduced recurrence rates during the first 10 years but thereafter, there was no gain or loss out to 15 years.

2. Marginal ER-positive disease (10–19 femtomoles/mg cytosol protein—from assays no longer used or quantitation employed) recurrence rates were substantial and significant.
3. Progesterone receptor was of no value to predict responsiveness to tamoxifen.
4. Breast cancer mortality was reduced by a third for the first 15 years.
5. All-cause mortality was substantially reduced despite small increases in thromboembolic and uterine cancer deaths (only women over 55 years of age) in women taking tamoxifen.

However, with the shift of the use of tamoxifen to aromatase inhibitors in postmenopausal patients, we felt it is appropriate to summarize the clinical trial to clarify the state of knowledge with the use of aromatase inhibitors versus tamoxifen.

Arrival of Aromatase Inhibitors as Adjuvant Therapy

The meta-analysis of the data from different trials (the Austrian Breast and Colorectal Cancer Study Group (ABCSG) XII trial, the Breast International Group (BIG) I-98/International Breast Cancer Study Group (IBCSG) 18–98 trial, and the ATAC trial) submitted to the Early Breast Cancer Trialists' Collaborative Group (EBCTCG) was published in 2010 and described the comparison of the third-generation aromatase inhibitors (AI) against tamoxifen in breast cancer patients [63]. The patients were divided into two cohorts: cohort one comprised 9,856 patients that underwent treatment with AI immediately after surgery for 5 years and were compared to patients treated with tamoxifen; cohort two comprised 9,015 patients to assess the AI treatment with AI after 2–3 years of tamoxifen. The results of this analysis have shown that the administration of AI immediately after surgery for 5 years in the first cohort of patients has significantly reduced the recurrence of breast cancer by 23 % comparing to 5 years of tamoxifen. In the other cohort of patients, the efficacy of the switch to AI after 2–3 years of tamoxifen treatment was analyzed and it was shown that there was a 40 % reduction in risk of recurrence during the 3 following years after tamoxifen treatment. The authors of that study suggest that tamoxifen treatment after 3 years has sensitized the cancer cells to AI treatment; however, there is no experimental data supporting that. Also patients in both cohorts had follow-ups (5.8 years in cohort one and 3.9 years in cohort two) to assess the recurrence of the disease. The reduction of recurrence of breast cancer in both cohorts at 5 years after diagnosis was approximately 3 % and highly significant (2.9 %, SE = 0.7 % in cohort 1; and 3.1 %, SE = 0.6 % in cohort 2). The mortality rates in both cohorts were analogous at 5 years after diagnosis; however, there was a further decrease of mortality from breast cancers in the second cohort (AI after 2–3 years of tamoxifen). The authors concluded that AIs achieve "modest" improvements in breast cancer end points with significant reductions in recurrence in both cohorts of patients and specifically reduced mortality from breast cancer in

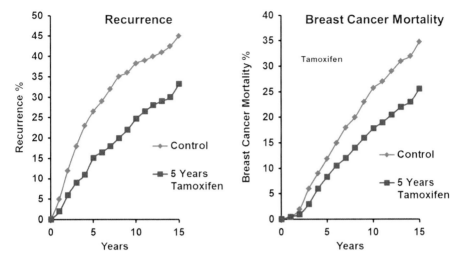

Fig. 4.4 The therapeutic action of tamoxifen after the treatment termination. The decrease of recurrence and mortality from breast cancer continues even 15 years after the treatment with tamoxifen stopped

the second cohort. However, it should be noted that AIs also have different side effects versus tamoxifen. AIs are associated with fewer endometrial cancers and thromboembolic events than tamoxifen but with increased incidence of arthralgia and bone fractures [64, 65].

Increasing Survivorship Following 5 Years of Adjuvant Tamoxifen

A significant mystery is why mortality continues to decrease following 5 years of adjuvant tamoxifen, i.e., after tamoxifen treatment has stopped [58, 62] (Fig. 4.4). Tamoxifen is a competitive inhibitor of estrogen action at the tumor ER, so no drug would imply estrogen would bind to the unoccupied ER to cause tumor regrowth and increase mortality. But it does not!

However, a possible explanation occurred more by accident than design, through a study of acquired drug resistance to tamoxifen (Chap. 9). With the acceptance that long-term adjuvant tamoxifen was the appropriate strategy for the treatment of node-positive/node-negative breast cancer, in the late 1980s, it was imperative to develop a realistic model of acquired drug resistance to tamoxifen in the laboratory to determine mechanisms and diverse strategies for second-line therapy. The first transplantable model of acquired resistance was propagated in athymic mice. The ER-positive MCF-7 breast cancer cell line was used to develop the model [20]. Acquired resistance to tamoxifen developed within 2 years and once resistance was acquired either tamoxifen or physiologic estradiol utilizing the tumor ER to cause growth [66]. However, the tumors could only be propagated in mice, and no successful transfer from tumor to tissue culture occurred. The model did not seem to replicate adjuvant therapy but rather metastatic breast cancer that fails tamoxifen treatments within 2 years. This seemed to be bad news but this became the good news as the unique tumor model could only be retained for study by routine propagation to tamoxifen-treated mice over years.

The finding that, following 5 years of retransplantation of tumors with acquired tamoxifen resistance into successive generations of tamoxifen-treated athymic mice, physiologic estrogen causes tumors to melt away was both mystifying and exciting. We will expand on this exciting new biology of estrogen-induced apoptosis in Chap. 9, but suffice to say it raised the possibility that acquired drug resistance to tamoxifen evolves and that the act of stopping tamoxifen after 5 years of adjuvant therapy causes the woman's own estrogen to seek out the appropriately reconfigured and sensitized breast cancer cells and triggers apoptosis. These data were first reported at the St. Gallen Breast Cancer Meeting with the hypothesis that the women's own estrogen caused the decrease in the patient mortality by killing appropriately sensitive microscopic foci of breast cancer cells [67].

In closing this chapter, it is important to stress that the hypothesis was not well received by the clinical community or the idea that physiologic estrogen administration might be of therapeutic significance. Despite the fact that no peer-reviewed funding was forthcoming, our research was sustained through philanthropy by the Lynn Sage Breast Cancer Foundation and the Robert H. Lurie Comprehensive Cancer Center at Northwestern University in Chicago, IL. Almost by chance, talented surgeons (Drs. Yao, Lee, England, and Bentrem) were looking for a project to exploit and this was it. They reproduced the Wolf data [67] over a 5-year period and it became clear that by year 5 of tamoxifen treatment, physiologic estrogen administration killed breast cancer cells with acquired resistance to tamoxifen. Estradiol killed the resistant cells but the remaining cells were again sensitive to antihormone therapy [68]. The process was cyclical (Fig. 4.5) and would eventually be tested in clinical trial and the molecular biology of estradiol-induced apoptosis clarified (Chap. 9). The concept was extended to the SERM raloxifene in an exceptionally long 10-year transplantation study of an MCF-7 study of acquired raloxifene resistance in athymic mice [69]. The original Wolf study and Balaburski study some 20 years apart are illustrated in Fig. 4.5.

Postscript. Perhaps the most important continuing support that ICI Pharmaceutical Division made to the development of tamoxifen (Nolvadex) was the hundreds of rats they chauffeured from Alderley Park to Leeds University Medical School. Over the years (1974–1978), this strategy, instituted and paid for by Dr. Roy Cotton in the clinical department, was visionary. He was investing in a young enthusiastic pharmacologist who wanted to develop drugs to treat cancer. To a young faculty member in the Department of Pharmacology at Leeds University, armed with additional grants from the Yorkshire Cancer Research Campaign to purchase expensive ultracentrifuges (they were happy to invest in a BTA, Been to America), and ultimately an ICI/University of Leeds Joint Research Scheme

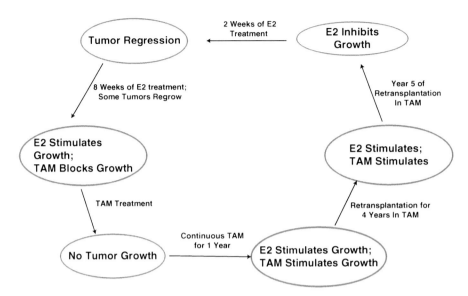

Fig. 4.5 The cyclical sensitivity and resistance of breast cancer cells to tamoxifen and estradiol. Estradiol is able to induce apoptosis in resistant cells; however, the remaining cells were again sensitive to tamoxifen treatment

co-headed by Walpole for ICI and I for Leeds to create 6,7-substituted alkylating estrogens (Chap. 9), the unlimited animals were more valuable than gold. What did the investment yield? We did extensive studies on the mechanism of action of tamoxifen [70–76]; we were the first to discover the pharmacological properties of 4-hydroxytamoxifen [15, 17, 77–82], discovered the metabolic activation of tamoxifen, and most importantly created the strategy with animal models, to employ long-term adjuvant tamoxifen treatment for patients with ER-positive breast cancer [83–87]. Oh, and chemoprevention (Chap. 7).

We had two strategic goals with the studies of Karen Allen, an extremely talented technician who had trained in my group when she was an undergraduate in the Department of Pharmacology, and Clive Dix, an exceptional PhD student funded with an ICI Graduate Student Fellowship. Our first goal was to establish whether short-term high-dose tamoxifen administered to rats 30 days after the DMBA to induce mammary cancer for a short period of time (4 weeks which we considered to be equivalent to 1 year in a woman's life) would "cure the animals." It did not, but we realized that suppression of tumor development by tamoxifen was dose related, i.e., once the accumulated and slowly excreted tamoxifen was gone from the body, the tumors appeared. Clive demonstrated that continuous tamoxifen treatment was necessary to prevent tumorigenesis, almost completely, and was superior to oophorectomy [15]. Thus, long-term adjuvant therapy was going to be better to control the recurrence of ER-positive disease effectively after primary surgery.

Our second goal was to determine whether 4-hydroxytamoxifen, a more potent antiestrogen than tamoxifen, was a more potent antitumor agent in the rat. It was not, although continuous therapy was effective at controlling tumor development [17]. We concluded that rapidly excreted hydroxylated antiestrogens were poor antitumor agents, a principle that was to recur with polyhydroxylated raloxifene [16] when used for the prevention of breast cancer [88] and proven over the next 30 years!

The opportunity to present our new concept for the adjuvant use of tamoxifen occurred in September 1977 at an ICI Pharmaceutical Division Breast Cancer Symposium at King's College, Cambridge, England. Michael Baum was the chair of my session and it was clear that plans were in place to increase the duration of adjuvant tamoxifen therapy from the standard 1 year to 2 years with the NATO trial (the acronym was based on the belief the Americans would read their subsequent papers and refer to them in their publications if they believed it was an American sponsored trial. The acronym actually stands for "Nolvadex Adjuvant Trial Organization") and the proposed 5 years for the Scottish trial. Each of the trialists considered their choice of trial design was arbitrary, but we already had the scientific basis published that would prove to be successful in their clinical trials.

The week following the King's College meeting I began a 3-month sabbatical at the University of Wisconsin Clinical Cancer Center, Madison, Wisconsin. There I proposed the "tamoxifen forever" clinical strategy as a forward thinking goal to accelerate tamoxifen's development and prevent disease recurrence. I should restate that tamoxifen at that time was not FDA approved in the United States even for the treatment of metastatic breast cancer. This would occur on 29 December 1977. Presentation of the strategy with compelling laboratory data to create potential survival advantages for patients with ER-positive breast cancer caught on with both the Eastern Cooperative Oncologic Group (ECOG) and the National Adjuvant Breast and Bowel Project (NSABP) as they advanced their adjuvant therapy trials from 2 to 5 years. This was a critical decision that saved hundreds of thousands of women's lives worldwide.

The good news for my career was that this 3-month sabbatical time in the Wisconsin Clinical Cancer Center in Madison resulted in a job offer because by this time I had lots of publications and Eliahu Caspi's lesson had been learned! (See Chap. 2.) After a year setting up the Ludwig Institute in Bern, Switzerland (1979–1980), and forging friendships that would last a career, I moved to Wisconsin to learn and recreate my Tamoxifen Team in America (Chap. 5).

References

1. Fisher B, Carbone P, Economou SG et al (1975) 1-Phenylalanine mustard (L-PAM) in the management of primary breast cancer. A report of early findings. N Engl J Med 292:117–122
2. Bonadonna G, Brusamolino E, Valagussa P et al (1976) Combination chemotherapy as an adjuvant treatment in operable breast cancer. N Engl J Med 294:405–410

3. Jordan VC, Fritz NF, Tormey DC (1987) Endocrine effects of adjuvant chemotherapy and long-term tamoxifen administration on node-positive patients with breast cancer. Cancer Res 47:624–630

4. Rose DP, Davis TE (1980) Effects of adjuvant chemohormonal therapy on the ovarian and adrenal function of breast cancer patients. Cancer Res 40:4043–4047

5. Jordan VC (1998) Chemotherapy is antihormonal therapy–how much proof do oncologists need? Eur J Cancer 34:606–608

6. Cole MP, Jones CT, Todd ID (1971) A new anti-oestrogenic agent in late breast cancer. An early clinical appraisal of ICI46474. Br J Cancer 25:270–275

7. Ward HW (1973) Anti-oestrogen therapy for breast cancer: a trial of tamoxifen at two dose levels. Br Med J 1:13–14

8. Jordan VC (2008) Tamoxifen: catalyst for the change to targeted therapy. Eur J Cancer 44:30–38

9. Lippman ME, Bolan G (1975) Oestrogen-responsive human breast cancer in long term tissue culture. Nature 256:592–593

10. Early Breast Cancer Trialists' Collaborative Group (1992) Systemic treatment of early breast cancer by hormonal, cytotoxic, or immune therapy. 133 randomised trials involving 31,000 recurrences and 24,000 deaths among 75,000 women. Lancet 339:1–15

11. Swedish Breast Cancer Cooperative Group (1996) Randomized trial of two versus five years of adjuvant tamoxifen for postmenopausal early stage breast cancer. J Natl Cancer Inst 88:1543–1549

12. Jordan VC (1978) Use of the DMBA-induced rat mammary carcinoma system for the evaluation of tamoxifen as a potential adjuvant therapy. Rev Endocr Relat Cancer:49–55

13. Jordan VC, Dix CJ, Allen KE (1979) The effectiveness of long-term treatment in a laboratory model for adjuvant hormone therapy of breast cancer. In: Salmon SE, Jones SE (eds) Adjuvant therapy of cancer II. Greene and Stratton, New York, pp 19–26

14. Robinson SP, Mauel DA, Jordan VC (1989) Antitumor actions of toremifene in the 7,12-dimethylbenzanthracene (DMBA)-induced rat mammary tumor model. Eur J Cancer Clin Oncol 24:1817–1821

15. Jordan VC, Allen KE, Dix CJ (1980) Pharmacology of tamoxifen in laboratory animals. Cancer Treat Rep 64:745–759

16. Gottardis MM, Jordan VC (1987) Antitumor actions of keoxifene and tamoxifen in the N-nitrosomethylurea-induced rat mammary carcinoma model. Cancer Res 47:4020–4024

17. Jordan VC, Allen KE (1980) Evaluation of the antitumour activity of the non-steroidal antioestrogen monohydroxytamoxifen in the DMBA-induced rat mammary carcinoma model. Eur J Cancer 16:239–251

18. Osborne CK, Hobbs K, Clark GM (1985) Effect of estrogens and antiestrogens on growth of human breast cancer cells in athymic nude mice. Cancer Res 45:584–590

19. Osborne CK, Coronado EB, Robinson JP (1987) Human breast cancer in the athymic nude mouse: cytostatic effects of long-term antiestrogen therapy. Eur J Cancer Clin Oncol 23:1189–1196

20. Gottardis MM, Robinson SP, Jordan VC (1988) Estradiol-stimulated growth of MCF-7 tumors implanted in athymic mice: a model to study the tumoristatic action of tamoxifen. J Steroid Biochem 30:311–314

21. Ribeiro G, Palmer MK (1983) Adjuvant tamoxifen for operable carcinoma of the breast: report of clinical trial by the Christie Hospital and Holt Radium Institute. Br Med J (Clin Res Ed) 286:827–830

22. Rose C, Thorpe SM, Andersen KW et al (1985) Beneficial effect of adjuvant tamoxifen therapy in primary breast cancer patients with high oestrogen receptor values. Lancet 1:16–19

23. Ribeiro G, Swindell R (1985) The Christie Hospital tamoxifen (Nolvadex) adjuvant trial for operable breast carcinoma–7-yr results. Eur J Cancer Clin Oncol 21:897–900

24. Cummings FJ, Gray R, Davis TE et al (1985) Adjuvant tamoxifen treatment of elderly women with stage II breast cancer. A double-blind comparison with placebo. Ann Intern Med 103:324–329

25. Baum M, and other members of the Nolvadex Adjuvant Trial Organization (1985) Controlled trial of tamoxifen as single adjuvant agent in management of early breast cancer. Lancet 1:836–840
26. Pritchard KI, Meakin JW, Boyd NF, Ambus K, DeBoer G, Paterson AHG, Sutherland DJA, Wilkinson RH, Bassett AA, Evans WK, Beale FA, Clark RM, Keane TJ (1984) A randomized trial of adjuvant tamoxifen in postmenopausal women with axillary node positive breast cancer. In: Jones SE, Salmon SE (eds) Adjuvant therapy of breast cancer. Grune and Stratton, New York, pp 339–348
27. Wallgren A, Baral E, Castensen J, Friberg S, Glas U, Hjalmar JL, Kargas M, Nordenskjold B, Skoog L, There N-O, Wilking N (1984) Should adjuvant tamoxifen be given for several years in breast cancer. In: Jones SE, Salmon SE (eds) Adjuvant therapy of breast cancer. Grune and Stratton, New York, pp 331–338
28. Tormey DC, Jordan VC (1984) Long-term tamoxifen adjuvant therapy in node-positive breast cancer: a metabolic and pilot clinical study. Breast Cancer Res Treat 4:297–302
29. Tormey DC, Rasmussen P, Jordan VC (1987) Long-term adjuvant tamoxifen study: clinical update. Breast Cancer Res Treat 9:157–158
30. Langan-Fahey SM, Tormey DC, Jordan VC (1990) Tamoxifen metabolites in patients on long-term adjuvant therapy for breast cancer. Eur J Cancer 26:883–888
31. Jordan VC (1983) Laboratory studies to develop general principles for the adjuvant treatment of breast cancer with antiestrogens: problems and potential for future clinical applications. Breast Cancer Res Treat 3(Suppl):S73–S86
32. Falkson HC, Gray R, Wolberg WH et al (1990) Adjuvant trial of 12 cycles of CMFPT followed by observation or continuous tamoxifen versus four cycles of CMFPT in postmenopausal women with breast cancer: an Eastern Cooperative Oncology Group phase III study. J Clin Oncol 8:599–607
33. Fisher B, Brown A, Wolmark N et al (1987) Prolonging tamoxifen therapy for primary breast cancer. Findings from the National Surgical Adjuvant Breast and Bowel Project clinical trial. Ann Intern Med 106:649–654
34. Fisher B, Redmond C, Brown A et al (1981) Treatment of primary breast cancer with chemotherapy and tamoxifen. N Engl J Med 305:1–6
35. Fisher B, Redmond C, Brown A et al (1983) Influence of tumor estrogen and progesterone receptor levels on the response to tamoxifen and chemotherapy in primary breast cancer. J Clin Oncol 1:227–241
36. Fisher B, Redmond C, Brown A et al (1986) Adjuvant chemotherapy with and without tamoxifen in the treatment of primary breast cancer: 5-year results from the National Surgical Adjuvant Breast and Bowel Project Trial. J Clin Oncol 4:459–471
37. Nolvadex Adjuvant Trailb Organisation (1983) Controlled trial of tamoxifen as adjuvant agent in management of Early Breast Cancer. Interim analysis at four years by the Nolvadex Adjuvant Trial Orginisation. Lancet 321:257–261
38. Delozier T, Julien JP, Juret P et al (1986) Adjuvant tamoxifen in postmenopausal breast cancer: preliminary results of a randomized trial. Breast Cancer Res Treat 7:105–109
39. Scottish Cancer Trials Office (MRC) (1987) Adjuvant tamoxifen in the management of operable breast cancer: the Scottish Trial. Report from the Breast Cancer Trials Committee. Lancet 2:171–175
40. McDonald CC, Stewart HJ (1991) Fatal myocardial infarction in the Scottish adjuvant tamoxifen trial. The Scottish Breast Cancer Committee. BMJ 303:435–437
41. Rutqvist LE, Mattsson A (1993) Cardiac and thromboembolic morbidity among postmeno-pausal women with early-stage breast cancer in a randomized trial of adjuvant tamoxifen. The Stockholm Breast Cancer Study Group. J Natl Cancer Inst 85:1398–1406
42. Hackshaw A, Roughton M, Forsyth S et al (2011) Long-term benefits of 5 years of tamoxifen: 10-year follow-up of a large randomized trial in women at least 50 years of age with early breast cancer. J Clin Oncol 29:1657–1663
43. el Sheikha Z, Klopper A, Beck JS (1972) Treatment of menometrorrhagia with an anti-oestrogen. Clin Endocrinol (Oxf) 1:275–282

44. Klopper A, Hall M (1971) New synthetic agent for the induction of ovulation: preliminary trials in women. Br Med J 1:152–154
45. Williamson JG, Ellis JD (1973) The induction of ovulation by tamoxifen. J Obstet Gynaecol Br Commonw 80:844–847
46. Groom GV, Griffiths K (1976) Effect of the anti-oestrogen tamoxifen on plasma levels of luteinizing hormone, follicle-stimulating hormone, prolactin, oestradiol and progesterone in normal pre-menopausal women. J Endocrinol 70:421–428
47. Manni A, Trujillo JE, Marshall JS et al (1979) Antihormone treatment of stage IV breast cancer. Cancer 43:444–450
48. Pritchard KI, Thomson DB, Myers RE et al (1980) Tamoxifen therapy in premenopausal patients with metastatic breast cancer. Cancer Treat Rep 64:787–796
49. Kalman AM, Thompson T, Vogel CL (1982) Response to oophorectomy after tamoxifen failure in a premenopausal patient. Cancer Treat Rep 66:1867–1868
50. Planting AS, Alexieva-Figusch J, Blonk-vdWijst J, van Putten WL (1985) Tamoxifen therapy in premenopausal women with metastatic breast cancer. Cancer Treat Rep 69:363–368
51. Sawka CA, Pritchard KI, Paterson AH et al (1986) Role and mechanism of action of tamoxifen in premenopausal women with metastatic breast carcinoma. Cancer Res 46:3152–3156
52. Ingle JN, Krook JE, Green SJ et al (1986) Randomized trial of bilateral oophorectomy versus tamoxifen in premenopausal women with metastatic breast cancer. J Clin Oncol 4:178–185
53. Buchanan RB, Blamey RW, Durrant KR et al (1986) A randomized comparison of tamoxifen with surgical oophorectomy in premenopausal patients with advanced breast cancer. J Clin Oncol 4:1326–1330
54. CRC Adjuvant Breast Trial Working Party (1988) Cyclophosphamide and tamoxifen as adjuvant therapies in the management of breast cancer. Br J Cancer 57:604–607
55. Fisher B, Dignam J, Bryant J et al (1996) Five versus more than five years of tamoxifen therapy for breast cancer patients with negative lymph nodes and estrogen receptor-positive tumors. J Natl Cancer Inst 88(21):1529–1542
56. Fisher B, Costantino J, Redmond C et al (1989) A randomized clinical trial evaluating tamoxifen in the treatment of patients with node-negative breast cancer who have estrogen-receptor-positive tumors. N Engl J Med 320:479–484
57. Davies C, Hongchao P, Godwin J et al (2012) Long-term effects of continuing adjuvant tamoxifen to 10 years versus stopping at 5 years after diagnosis of oestrogen receptor-positive breast cancer: ATLAS, a randomized trial. Lancet
58. Davies C, Godwin J, Gray R et al (2011) Relevance of breast cancer hormone receptors and other factors to the efficacy of adjuvant tamoxifen: patient-level meta-analysis of randomised trials. Lancet 378:771–784
59. Consensus Conference (1985) Adjuvant chemotherapy for breast cancer. JAMA 254:3461–3463
60. Howell A, Cuzick J, Baum M et al (2005) Results of the ATAC (arimidex, tamoxifen, alone or in combination) trial after completion of 5 years' adjuvant treatment for breast cancer. Lancet 365:60–62
61. EBCTCG (1998) Tamoxifen for early breast cancer: an overview of the randomised trials. Lancet 351:1451–1467
62. EBCTCG (2005) Effects of chemotherapy and hormonal therapy for early breast cancer on recurrence and 15-year survival: an overview of the randomised trials. Lancet 365:1687–1717
63. Dowsett M, Cuzick J, Ingle J et al (2010) Meta-analysis of breast cancer outcomes in adjuvant trials of aromatase inhibitors versus tamoxifen. J Clin Oncol 28:509–518
64. Lin NU, Winer EP (2008) Advances in adjuvant endocrine therapy for postmenopausal women. J Clin Oncol 26:798–805
65. Lonning PE, Geisler J (2008) Indications and limitations of third-generation aromatase inhibitors. Expert Opin Investig Drugs 17:723–739
66. Gottardis MM, Jordan VC (1988) Development of tamoxifen-stimulated growth of MCF-7 tumors in athymic mice after long-term antiestrogen administration. Cancer Res 48:5183–5187

67. Wolf DM, Jordan VC (1993) A laboratory model to explain the survival advantage observed in patients taking adjuvant tamoxifen therapy. Recent Results Cancer Res 127:23–33
68. Yao K, Lee ES, Bentrem DJ et al (2000) Antitumor action of physiological estradiol on tamoxifen-stimulated breast tumors grown in athymic mice. Clin Cancer Res 6:2028–2036
69. Balaburski GM, Dardes RC, Johnson M et al (2010) Raloxifene-stimulated experimental breast cancer with the paradoxical actions of estrogen to promote or prevent tumor growth: a unifying concept in anti-hormone resistance. Int J Oncol 37:387–398
70. Abbott AC, Clark ER, Jordan VC (1976) Inhibition of oestradiol binding to oestrogen receptor proteins by a methyl-substituted analogue of tamoxifen. J Endocrinol 69:445–446
71. Jordan VC (1976) Antiestrogenic and antitumor properties of tamoxifen in laboratory animals. Cancer Treat Rep 60:1409–1419
72. Jordan VC, Prestwich G (1977) Binding of [3H]tamoxifen in rat uterine cytosols: a comparison of swinging bucket and vertical tube rotor sucrose density gradient analysis. Mol Cell Endocrinol 8:179–188
73. Jordan VC, Dix CJ, Rowsby L, Prestwich G (1977) Studies on the mechanism of action of the nonsteroidal antioestrogen tamoxifen (I.C.I. 46,474) in the rat. Mol Cell Endocrinol 7:177–192
74. Jordan VC, Naylor KE (1979) The binding of [3H]-oestradiol-17 beta in the immature rat uterus during the sequential administration of non-steroidal anti-oestrogens. Br J Pharmacol 65:167–173
75. Jordan VC, Prestwich G (1978) Effect of non-steroidal anti-oestrogens on the concentration of rat uterine progesterone receptors. J Endocrinol 76:363–364
76. Jordan VC, Rowsby L, Dix CJ, Prestwich G (1978) Dose-related effects of non-steroidal antioestrogens and oestrogens on the measurement of cytoplasmic oestrogen receptors in the rat and mouse uterus. J Endocrinol 78:71–81
77. Jordan VC, Collins MM, Rowsby L, Prestwich G (1977) A monohydroxylated metabolite of tamoxifen with potent antioestrogenic activity. J Endocrinol 75:305–316
78. Jordan VC, Dix CJ, Naylor KE et al (1978) Nonsteroidal antiestrogens: their biological effects and potential mechanisms of action. J Toxicol Environ Health 4:363–390
79. Jordan VC, Dix CJ (1979) Effect of oestradiol benzoate, tamoxifen and monohydroxy-tamoxifen on immature rat uterine progesterone receptor synthesis and endometrial cell division. J Steroid Biochem 11:285–291
80. Dix CJ, Jordan VC (1980) Subcellular effects of monohydroxytamoxifen in the rat uterus: steroid receptors and mitosis. J Endocrinol 85:393–404
81. Allen KE, Clark ER, Jordan VC (1980) Evidence for the metabolic activation of non-steroidal antioestrogens: a study of structure-activity relationships. Br J Pharmacol 71:83–91
82. Dix CJ, Jordan VC (1980) Modulation of rat uterine steroid hormone receptors by estrogen and antiestrogen. Endocrinology 107:2011–2020
83. Jordan VC, Dowse LJ (1976) Tamoxifen as an anti-tumour agent: effect on oestrogen binding. J Endocrinol 68:297–303
84. Jordan VC, Jaspan T (1976) Tamoxifen as an anti-tumour agent: oestrogen binding as a predictive test for tumour response. J Endocrinol 68:453–460
85. Jordan VC, Jaspan T (1976) Oestrogen binding as a predictive test for DMBA-induced tumour response to tamoxifen therapy. In: Hellman K, Conors TA (eds) Chemotherapy. Plenum, New York, pp 89–94
86. Jordan VC (1978) Use of the DMBA-induced rat mammary carcinoma system for the evaluation of tamoxifen as a potential adjuvant therapy. Rev Endocr Relat Cancer:49–55 (October supplement)
87. Jordan VC, Dix CJ, Allen KE (1979) The effectiveness of long term tamoxifen treatment in a laboratory model for adjuvant hormone therapy of breast cancer. In: Salmon SE, Jones SE (eds) Adjuvant therapy of cancer II. Grune and Strattin, New York, pp 19–26
88. Vogel VG, Costantino JP, Wickerham DL et al (2010) Update of the National Surgical Adjuvant Breast and Bowel Project study of tamoxifen and raloxifene (STAR) P-2 trial: preventing breast cancer. Cancer Prev Res (Phila) 3:696–706

Chapter 5
The Wisconsin Story in the 1980s: Discovery of Target Site-Specific Estrogen Action

Abstract The idea that tamoxifen could potentially be employed to prevent breast cancer in populations of women with high risk, naturally mandated an extensive laboratory and clinical investigation of potential toxicological concerns. It was reasoned that if estrogen was necessary to maintain bone density and protect women from coronary heart disease, then an "antiestrogen" might prevent breast cancer but increase the risks of osteoporosis and coronary heart disease. Laboratory results and translation to clinical trial proved the reverse was true, and the new drug group, selective estrogen receptor modulators (SERMs), was discovered. Tamoxifen (and raloxifene) paradoxically prevented bone loss in ovariectomized rats (estrogen-like) but prevented rat mammary carcinogenesis (antiestrogen-like). The same was true in patients with tamoxifen (and raloxifene) maintaining bone density but preventing breast cancer. Additionally, circulating cholesterol decreased (an estrogen-like effect) in patients. However, an estrogen-like effect of tamoxifen that became a concern was the discovery that in the laboratory, tamoxifen prevented breast cancer growth but enhanced the growth of endometrial cancer.

Introduction

In the early 1980s, Professor Trevor Powles, the head of the Breast Cancer Unit at the Royal Marsden hospital, took the bold step to initiate a pilot clinical trial of tamoxifen to treat healthy women with a high risk of breast cancer. The goals were to determine whether healthy women without disease would take tamoxifen for years, monitor side effects, and use the experience gained as a vanguard for a large placebo-controlled chemotherapeutics study of tamoxifen. The scientific rationale was based on two dominant facts: (1) In the laboratory, tamoxifen was known to prevent the initiation and promotion of mammary cancer by estrogen in the DMBA-induced rat mammary carcinoma model [1, 2]. (2) Tamoxifen, used as an adjuvant

P.Y. Maximov et al., *Tamoxifen*, Milestones in Drug Therapy,
DOI 10.1007/978-3-0348-0664-0_5, © Springer Basel 2013

therapy, was noted in a letter to the Lancet [3] to reduce the incidence of contralateral breast cancer.

In other words, tamoxifen inhibited rat mammary carcinogenesis in the standard laboratory model used in breast cancer research at the time, and tamoxifen actually inhibited the incidence of primary breast cancer.

At this time in the 1980s, tamoxifen was classified as a nonsteroidal antiestrogen [4] and clinical trials with long-term adjuvant therapy were reporting a good safety profile for the drug administered between 2 years and potentially indefinite therapy [5–7]. However, the idea of treating healthy women with an "antiestrogen" raised some important issues that had to be addressed. If estrogen was important to maintain bone density and, at the time, there was the conviction that estrogen protected women from coronary heart disease, then the administration of an "antiestrogen" might well prevent half a dozen breast cancers per year in a 1,000 high-risk women, but the antiestrogenic interaction would expose the majority of women to crushing osteoporosis and an increased risk of dying from coronary heart disease. The target site pharmacology needed to be investigated in the laboratory, and steps had to be taken to translate the findings to clinical practice.

Two approaches were addressed that were ultimately to change clinical perceptions about "nonsteroidal antiestrogens" and, more importantly, to change the application of these drugs in medicine. We will describe the developing set of laboratory studies that would result in a new understanding of the pharmacology of tamoxifen and raloxifene (then called keoxifene) and then describe the clinical studies that occurred simultaneously that opened the door to the descriptions of a new drug group—the selective estrogen receptive modulators or SERMs. This program was unique to the Wisconsin Comprehensive Cancer Center, so we will describe the associated information from others that confirmed or supported our research strategy during the 1980s.

Laboratory Studies on the Target Site-Specific Pharmacology of "Nonsteroidal Antiestrogens"

The early studies in the literature concerning ICI 46,474 (later tamoxifen) described its antifertility and antiestrogenic properties in the immature rat uterus and in ovariectomized rat Allen-Doisy tests [8, 9]. Paradoxically, tamoxifen was estrogenic in the mouse uterus [10–12]. Tamoxifen was also known to lower circulating cholesterol in the rat with no significant increase in circulating desmosterol [8]. In contrast, LY156758 (keoxifene to become raloxifene) and LY117018 were both antiestrogens in the rat and mouse uterus and blocked estrogen and tamoxifen induced increase in uterine weight [13–17]. There was initially no information about circulating cholesterol in animals, as all interest was then focused upon the use of keoxifene as a treatment for breast cancer, an indication for which it was eventually to fail, and work was discontinued at Eli Lilly in the late 1980s.

There was interest in comparing and contrasting the actions of tamoxifen and keoxifene on the rodent uterus, rat bone density, and carcinogen-induced rat mammary cancers and human tumors (breast and endometrial) grown in athymic mice. The differential effects of tamoxifen in the athymic mouse uterus transplanted with a growing estrogen-stimulated ER-positive MCF-7 tumor was particularly interesting. Administration of estradiol caused an increase in uterine weight and the growth of the MCF-7 tumor. However, tamoxifen caused an increase in mouse uterine weight but did not cause MCF-7 tumor growth. In fact, tamoxifen blocked estrogen-stimulated growth. We analyzed the tamoxifen metabolites in both estrogen target organs and found they were comparable, so we concluded "that the drug can selectively stimulate or inhibit events in the target tissues of different species without metabolic intervention" [18]. It was realized, however, that the target site specificity had clinical relevance to the application of tamoxifen as a long-term adjuvant therapy and as a potential chemopreventive.

Dr. Satyaswaroop at Penn State Medical School in Hershey, Pennsylvania, had dedicated considerable efforts to establish human endometrial cancer that grew in athymic mice [19]. He also noted that tamoxifen would increase the growth of human endometrial cancers [20] but had not stated that these data could be translated to clinical practice. In a pioneering experiment that hereafter changed clinical practice, human endometrial cancer and an MCF-7 tumor were transplanted into athymic mice and treated with both physiologic estrogen and tamoxifen. The goal was to establish whether tamoxifen would stop the estrogen-stimulated growth of both human tumors in the same mouse. The results (Fig. 5.1) demonstrated that tamoxifen inhibited estrogen-stimulated tumor growth but enhanced the growth of the human endometrial tumor. It was concluded that "these findings suggest that the disparate pharmacology of TAM is a tissue-specific phenomenon" [21] and suggested that "Until the influence of TAM and other antiestrogens on endometrial cancers has been fully investigated, vigilance by physicians treating patients with these agents is needed to establish the clinical relevance (if any) of these observations." In other words, it was possible that tamoxifen could prevent the growth of breast cancer but enhance the growth of endometrial cancer. The clinical community was quick to replicate the same target tissue concept in patients treated with long-term adjuvant tamoxifen therapy [22] with tamoxifen decreasing contralateral breast cancer but increasing the incidence of endometrial cancer in postmenopausal women. It was clear that tamoxifen was enhancing the growth of some target tissues but blocking the growth of others, so tamoxifen may not be appropriate in postmenopausal women at high risk of breast cancer.

A new dimension was necessary. Chemoprevention was to be a reality with antiestrogens and that new dimension would be keoxifene (raloxifene). Raloxifene was compared with tamoxifen in rats to prevent mammary carcinogenesis [23] and endometrial cancer [24]. Tamoxifen was better than raloxifene at preventing mammary cancer, but raloxifene blocked endometrial cancer growth.

There was a concern about "nonsteroidal antiestrogens" inhibiting bone regeneration and causing osteoporosis during long-term adjuvant tamoxifen treatment or

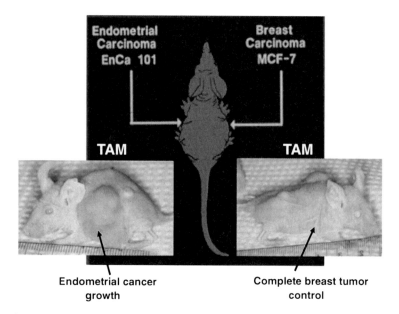

Fig. 5.1 The pioneering bitransplantation study by Gottardis [21] with an ER-positive breast tumor (MCF-7) implanted in one axilla and an ER-positive endometrial tumor (EnCa 101) in the other axilla. Tamoxifen blocks estrogen-stimulated growth of the breast tumor, but tamoxifen encourages the growth of the endometrial tumor

during the use of tamoxifen as a chemopreventive, so there was a focus on measurements of rat bone following ovariectomy and antiestrogen treatment. Earlier, Beall and coworkers [25] had reported that clomiphene (a mixture of estrogenic and antiestrogenic geometric isomers) maintained bone density in ovariectomized retired breeder rats. However, since the administered drug was an impure mixture and not an antiestrogenic drug specifically, there was no proof that the estrogenic isomer (Chap. 1) had not caused an increase in bone density.

In contrast, the same model was used in the rat to determine the effect of the pure antiestrogenic isomer tamoxifen, and the results were compared with raloxifene, an antiestrogen with less estrogen-like actions than tamoxifen in the rat uterus and a fixed ring structures. Both antiestrogens maintained bone density, and in fact a combination of antiestrogens and estrogen was additive [26]. A study of tamoxifen and raloxifene to prevent rat mammary carcinogenesis demonstrated efficacy for both antiestrogens, but tamoxifen was shown to be superior and raloxifenes' effectiveness was found to be not long lasting [23]. More than 20 years later, these data were to be relevant in the STAR trial (Chap. 8) with tamoxifen having long-term and lasting actions to prevent breast tumor incidence, but raloxifene was not able to sustain the antitumor effect after treatment was stopped [27].

Finally, raloxifene was less effective at stimulating the growth of human endometrial cancer in laboratory models [24] and less effective at stimulating the growth of rodent uteri in vivo [15]. Taken together, these data generated in the same laboratory over a period of 2–3 years, described the target site-specific actions of nonsteroidal antiestrogens to switch on and switch off estrogen target sites around the body. Those data lead to the proposal first stated at the First International Chemoprevention Conference in New York [28].

> …an extensive clinical investigation of available antioestrogens. Could analogs be developed to treat osteoporosis or even retard the development of atherosclerosis? Should the agent also retain anti-breast tumour actions then it might be expected to act as a chemosuppressive on all developing breast cancers.
>   …….a bold commitment to drug discovery and clinical pharmacology will potentially place us in a key position to prevent the development of breast cancer by the end of this century.

This vision became a reality and it led to the further clinical evaluation of tamoxifen in bone and then raloxifene as a selective estrogen/antiestrogen in target sites around a human's body. Tamoxifen was the drug of choice to study because it was approved clinically. The agent of choice by the clinical community to study chemoprevention in high-risk women was tamoxifen as raloxifene (aka keoxifene) that was unavailable for clinical testing at that time; but that would change.

The Wisconsin Tamoxifen Study

A preliminary study of bone mineral density in women treated with adjuvant tamoxifen showed no detrimental effects at 2 years, i.e., the antiestrogenic actions of tamoxifen did not decrease bone density [29]. These data encouraged the establishment of a double-blind placebo-controlled trial of node-negative postmenopausal (no menses for 12 months) breast cancer patients with a diagnosis up to 10 years previously. The Principal Investigator was Dr. Richard R. Love.

It is important to emphasize that in the late 1980s, adjuvant tamoxifen treatment was not the standard of care for the node-negative patient. Women were randomized to either tamoxifen or placebo for 2 years (Fig. 5.2) with evaluations for bone density, symptoms, and cardiovascular risk factors at baseline, 3, 6, 12, 18, and 24 months later.

The main results were reported in a series of publications in the early 1990s [30–32]. The changes in cardiovascular risk factors during tamoxifen treatment were encouraging for long-term safety of adjuvant tamoxifen and as a potential chemopreventive agent in high-risk women. Total cholesterol decreased by 12 % during the 2-year period and this remained statistically significant ($P < 0.001$). The main effect was driven by a specific decrease of 20 % in low-density lipoprotein (LDL) cholesterol ($P < 0.0001$) with stable high-density lipoprotein (HDL) cholesterol. Fibrinogen rapidly decreased by 20 % at 6 months ($P < 0.0003$) and a 7 % decrease in platelets with a significant decrease in antithrombin III was observed in tamoxifen-treated women.

The bone parameters were highly significant and established the idea that tamoxifen could maintain or build bone translated from the laboratory [26, 33–35] to clinical practice. The placebo group had a decrease in radius of

Fig. 5.2 The design of the Wisconsin Tamoxifen Study recruited 140 node-negative breast cancer patients to be randomized to either tamoxifen (20 mg/daily) or placebo. Bone mineral density was measured by dual-photon absorptiometry at regular intervals, and bloods were drawn to determine circulating lipids and clotting factors

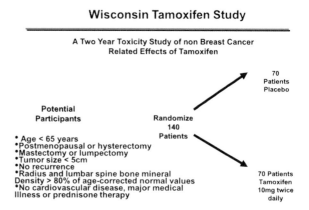

1–1.292 % per year (P < 0.0001) and spine of −0.9967 % per year (P < 0.0008). Tamoxifen-treated women lost bone in the radius from baseline of −0.878 % per year (P < 0.0002) and lumbar spine a gain of 0.611 % per year (P < 0.04). A comparison of both lumbar spine linear rates was highly significant by 2 years (P < 0.0001). Symptoms were consistent with prior reports with only a modest rise in hot flashes compared with placebo. Gynecological symptoms increased modestly when vaginal discharge, vaginal dryness, bleeding, and genital pruritus were identified. Interestingly, there were fewer headaches.

In general, these data from the Wisconsin Tamoxifen Study were confirmed by other publications around this time [36–40].

Translational Research

The results with tamoxifen and raloxifene in the ovariectomized rat in the mid-1980s were subsequently confirmed by others, first for tamoxifen [33–35] and then eventually raloxifene [41–43]. The clinical research on tamoxifen was set to demonstrate that circulating cholesterol was reduced and postmenopausal bone density was maintained in contrast to placebo-treated controls. The links between tamoxifen and endometrial cancer (Chap. 6) and rat liver carcinogenesis were naturally of concern for the testing of tamoxifen as a chemopreventive (Chap. 6), but a new strategy was in place in the refereed literature when Leonard Lerner and I were awarded the Bruce F. Cain Award by the American Association for Cancer Research for laboratory research that resulted in a successful strategy to treat cancer [44]. Simply stated, the roadmap for pharmaceutical industry to follow was as follows:

> Is this the end of the possible applications for antioestrogens? Certainly not. We have obtained valuable clinical information about this group of drugs that can be applied in other disease states. Research does not travel in straight lines and observations in one field of science often become major discoveries in another. Important clues have been garnered

about the effects of tamoxifen on bone and lipids so it is possible that derivatives could find targeted applications to retard osteoporosis or atherosclerosis. The ubiquitous application of novel compounds to prevent diseases associated with the progressive changes after menopause may, as a side effect, significantly retard the development of breast cancer. The target population would be post-menopausal women in general, thereby avoiding the requirement to select a high risk group to prevent breast cancer.

Numerous companies followed the roadmap but not before keoxifene was renamed raloxifene and became the first SERM to treat and prevent osteoporosis and prevent breast cancer in postmenopausal women.

Postscript. During the 1980s, the nascent Breast Cancer Program led by Dr. Douglass Tormey, former head of the Breast Cancer Program at the National Cancer Institute, was building rapidly to create a multidisciplinary group able to conduct important translational research with the potential to "export" ideas to the Eastern Cooperative Oncology Group. Tormey had been the chief of the Breast Committee throughout the 1970s and was instrumental in recruiting me to Wisconsin. Lois Trench was also key, as the drug monitor for tamoxifen, and was the one to "get me started" at the Worcester Foundation for Experimental Biology (1972–1974). I was ICI America's first scientific consultant to use my laboratory results to facilitate clinical trials in America. I arrived in Madison, Wisconsin, in 1980 following a period establishing a breast cancer center for the Ludwig Institute for Cancer Research in Bern, Switzerland (1979–1980). My brief in Madison was to establish a major center for tamoxifen research and act as a link between basic science at the University of Wisconsin and clinical trials. Remember, tamoxifen was only approved to treat metastatic breast cancer by the FDA at the end of 1977, but we had plans! To achieve this, all my students had Dr. Jack Gorski on their Ph. D. thesis committee, and I recruited (with Jack's encouragement) numerous of his trainees to my laboratory at the Comprehensive Cancer Center. The late Mara Lieberman, Wade Welshons, and Mike Fritsch were all outstanding.

Another important scientist of note at the cancer center was Dr. David Rose who introduced me to a range of new antiestrogens (LY117018, trioxifene, LY156758) from Eli Lilly. David left Madison in the early 1980s, and it was decided that I should assume the responsibility for his staff, his laboratory space, and the ER clinical laboratory that served the hospitals in Southern Wisconsin. This was a frightening turn of events, so I called my mentor Bill McGuire in San Antonio to explain that I did not feel prepared for the task. He replied that I was looking at this incorrectly—"it's an opportunity" and so it was. In 1988, I was appointed as the director of the Breast Cancer Research and Treatment Program for the cancer center.

Wisconsin created the optimal environment to advance exciting translational science and create new careers. There we created an outstanding Tamoxifen Team in the Department of Human Oncology for 14 years; everyone was excellent, played their part, and contributed important skills and publications that changed medicine. It was a superb cancer center where young ambitions could be realized in a nurturing environment of an outstanding community focused on science. But from the many in my Tamoxifen Team, several must be mentioned because they either changed medical practice, created new knowledge in tamoxifen pharmacology that would change the way we perceived mechanisms, or created new models that would be critical for future advances.

Anna Riegel (née Tate) demonstrated outstanding skills as an undergraduate student at Leeds University Department of Pharmacology where I was her tutor, and she received a first-class honors degree in pharmacology, a distinction in her master's degree in steroid endocrinology, and was awarded a Fulbright Hays Scholarship to study for a Ph.D. with me at the McArdle Laboratory for Cancer Research at the University of Wisconsin-Madison. She published a pivotal paper in cancer research with myself, Elwood Jensen, and Geoffrey Greene, on the shape of the estrogen and 4-hydroxytamoxifen ER complex conceived through a study of antibodies to the human ER [45]. This model complemented studies I was conducting with Jack Gorski [46] that presaged (rather accurately) the subsequent crystallization of the ligand-binding domain of the ER with estrogens and antiestrogens some 15 years later [47, 48]. Anna was also an important part of our team that contributed to the debate in the early 1980s about the localization of the ER within the cells of estrogen target tissues. The two-step hypothesis stated that estrogen diffuses into the cell, binds with high affinity to the cytoplasmic ER, and is translocated to the nucleus where it is transformed (activated) to initiate estrogen-specific gene transcription (protein synthesis and growth) [49]. However, McGuire's group in San Antonio and others had suggested that unoccupied ER was actually in the nucleus [50]. Two pieces of evidence swayed scientific opinion to create a new model of estrogen action: monoclonal antibodies demonstrated nuclear ER in breast cancer cells in an estrogen-free environment [51] and the Gorski group used cytochalasin B with GH3 rat pituitary cells to create nucleoplasts and cytoplasts to show ER only on the nucleoplasts [52]. It was strange to recall I had worked as a summer student with Steven Carter, at ICI Pharmaceuticals Division in the summer of 1967, who discovered the cell enucleation property of the natural product cytochalasin B [53].

In 1983, we reported to the Endocrine Society in San Antonio that tamoxifen analogs that could not be metabolically activated to 4-hydroxytamoxifen switched on growth of the immature rat uterus and induced progesterone synthesis but apparently without translocating the ER complex from the cytoplasm to the nucleus. The person responsible for these studies was the late Barbara Gosden whom Anna recommended for a job in my laboratory for 2 years. Anna and Barbara were students of the master's course in steroid endocrinology at Leeds in 1979. When Barbara completed her studies in vivo, she was concerned that she had the wrong answer-but she has made a discovery, this was exploited and confirmed using triphenylethylene estrogens that only weakly bound to the ER in the rat uterus. The uterus grew and progesterone receptors were made, but the ER "appeared" to remain in the cytosolic fraction (or cytoplasmic) and not in the nuclear fraction. We got the same result as the metabolically resistant tamoxifen analogs and proposed, using this example of tamoxifen structural pharmacology, to suggest that it was the technique of uterine cell disruption that caused the abnormal result inconsistent with the 2-step model—but nobody cared [54]!

Marco M. Gottardis was a superb experimentalist with animal models. I inherited him from David Rose in 1983, and he accepted my invitation to become a Ph.D. student on the Human Oncology Ph.D. Training Program in 1984. The publications from his Ph.D. changed medicine. Marco demonstrated the chemopreventive actions of tamoxifen and raloxifene in carcinogen-induced rat mammary carcinoma model [23]. He concluded that raloxifene in the long term would not be superior to tamoxifen. The update of the STAR trial (Chap. 8) was to prove his data correct some 20 years later [27]. In the mid-1980s, at a time when long-term adjuvant tamoxifen treatment was being tested, there was no knowledge about acquired drug resistance to tamoxifen. Marco established the first laboratory model of acquired tamoxifen resistance in athymic mice [55]. Tamoxifen resistance is unique in the transplantable model as it takes the form of tamoxifen-stimulated growth. He showed that both estrogen withdrawal (a decade later this was equivalent to aromatase inhibitor treatment) and he used the first pure antiestrogen [56] to demonstrate that these strategies were appropriate second-line therapies to be used in clinic following tamoxifen failure.

Perhaps of greatest significance clinically was the superb experimental model of bitransplantation of a human endometrial and breast tumor in athymic mice. The tumors were both ER positive, but tamoxifen only blocked estrogen-stimulated growth of the breast tumor but enhanced the growth of the endometrial tumor. The clinical significance was clear. Women taking long-term tamoxifen needed to be checked for endometrial cancer growth. I presented a pivotal lecture in Italy during a celebration of the 900th anniversary of the University of Bologna, and this was noted by clinicians in the audience. Dr. Hardell from Sweden immediately reported about our laboratory finding in a letter to the Lancet and described several anecdotal cases he had observed of endometrial cancer in tamoxifen-treated patients. I replied [57] that we needed a placebo-controlled clinical evaluation to settle the matter once and for all. Fornander and colleagues [22] showed that 5 years of adjuvant tamoxifen would increase the detection of endometrial cancer by fivefold in postmenopausal women compared to placebo-treated women. The standard of care changed for women treated with tamoxifen with the introduction of routine gynecological examinations. This saved lives and is an excellent example of the potential for improvements in women's health with rapid clinical translation. The process from conceiving the laboratory study to publicizing and publishing the results in Cancer Research, followed by correspondence to the Lancet and the fast clinical publications in the Lancet, was 2–3 years.

Shun Yen Jiang came to my laboratory on a 4-year scholarship from Taiwan to learn molecular biology. However, she gave my Tamoxifen Team far more with a succession of firsts. She created two estrogen deprivation-resistant breast cancer cell lines from MCF-7 cells. These are MCF7:5C [58] that was to be so critical for our understanding of estrogen-induced apoptosis. These cells were waiting for Joan Lewis to "discover" in the deep freeze a decade later (Chap. 9). Shun Yen also created the MCF7:2A cells, the only breast cancer cells with a high molecular weight ER protein completely characterized by John Pink and found to be 6 and 7 exon repeats in the ligand-binding domain [59, 60]. John also documented the two different systems regulating ER synthesis in breast cancer [61] and with Cathy Murphy the first ER-positive to ER-negative transition in breast cancer cell lines during estrogen deprivation [62, 63]. Shun Yen Jiang subsequently reversed the process by creating the first stable transfectant of the ER gene into an ER-negative breast cancer cell line MDA-MB-231 [64]. This advance in cell biology was passed on to Bill Catherino who created a stable transfectant of a natural mutant ER asp351tyr (BC2) [65] from a tamoxifen-stimulated tumor developed by Doug Wolf [66] who discovered the mutant ER in one particular tumor cell line [66].

All my students start with multiple projects in the expectation that one would bear fruit. With Doug, all bore fruit but this was not clear at the time. But this is what good (and reliable) results in the laboratory really are. I gave Doug another couple of projects to address and to discover the mechanism of tamoxifen-stimulated growth. One hypothesis at the time in the early 1990s was that metabolic activation of tamoxifen to the 4-hydroxytamoxifen metabolite would also produce an estrogenic *cis* isomer to cause growth (Cathy Murphy demonstrated that this was not true as not all isomers were antiestrogenic [67]). Doug used a fixed ring tamoxifen analog that could not isomerize to prove that it was the actual drug not an isomer that caused growth [68]. All of this closely interconnected research passed from generations of students to the next as the optimal model for progress. Progress and knowledge to aid patients was achieved in the nested environment at UW-Madison. A big breakthrough for us at the UW-Madison was yet to come. In the early 1990s, growth factor pathways were the answer to cancer. I set Doug Wolf the problem of characterizing estrogen and tamoxifen-stimulated tumor growth through their growth factor pathways in Marco's model of tamoxifen resistance. However, when Doug addressed the question, all the physiologic estrogen-stimulated tumors derived from acquired tamoxifen-resistant tumors disappeared. He was embarrassed and very apologetic that he had repeated the experiment several times—tamoxifen-stimulated tumors grew just as Marco described 5 years earlier, but estrogen caused tumors to melt away. He believed he had failed to deliver the expected result from Marco's work, but he had made a discovery— estrogen-induced apoptosis [69]. This was confirmed at a new institution, the Robert Lurie Comprehensive Cancer Center at North Western University [70], and ultimately changed medicine through first providing us with data to be funded by the Department of Defense to study mechanisms that would be used to develop treatment for antihormone-resistant breast cancer [71] and the results of the WHI estrogen-alone study where there is a significant decrease in breast cancers and mortality [72].

But it did not end there with innovation of discovery by students. Mei Wei Jeng was a student from Taiwan, who had obtained a master's degree in Iowa. She made several important advances in cellular pharmacology. Using Shun Yen Jiang's stable transfectants of wild-type ER in MDA-MB-231 cells (S-10s, all my students named their own cell lines!), Mei Wei Jeng addressed what seemed the obvious hypothesis that the cause of estrogen action to stop growth of the S-10 cells was because it blocked TGF-α (a growth-stimulating hormone) production but increased TGF-β (a growth inhibitor) production. This was not true [73], it was the other way around, but new knowledge gave the Tamoxifen Team standard estrogen target gene TGF-α for all our subsequent work. Mei Wei Jeng was also very keen to discover the role of the progestogens in the modulation of TGF-β. Instead, she discovered that 19-nortestosterone derivatives of the oral contraceptives were estrogens on MCF-7 cell growth [74], as was the antiprogestin RU486 at high doses [75].

So why did we ever do a bone study? Dr. Urban Lindgren, from the Karolinska Institute in Stockholm, was doing a sabbatical at the UW-Madison. He approached me to consider creating a rapidly developing osteoporosis model in ovariectomized rats. Nothing was really known about the effect of individual nonsteroidal antiestrogens on rat bone, so it seemed fairly simple as an experiment: antiestrogens would create bone loss in the ovariectomized rat. I obviously selected tamoxifen as there was really nothing known clinically about the action on bone, and it might aid the move to clinical testing of tamoxifen as a preventive for breast cancer. After Eli Lilly abandoned their anticancer program to create a rival to tamoxifen with keoxifene for breast cancer treatment, I was left with a large quantity of the nonsteroidal antiestrogen in the laboratory. I selected keoxifene as a competitor to tamoxifen. The reason was because keoxifene was less estrogenic in the uterus than tamoxifen [15]; this would probably make bone loss much worse. Lindgren taught Eric Phelps, an undergraduate student at UW-Madison, how to do the ash density study and then to our surprise another discovery! Tamoxifen was estrogen-like in bone as was keoxifene, and the combination with estradiol benzoate was additive [26]. These data were repeatedly rejected in "Bone" journals, so I wrote our results up for the refereed journal Breast Cancer Research and Treatment as I guessed correctly that the medical community would be interested in our findings. The results with tamoxifen were confirmed by others, and the Wisconsin Tamoxifen Study was propelled forward with other clinicians committed to the idea that tamoxifen would built bone [40]. Keoxifene became raloxifene, and funnily enough, the target site specificity of a combination of estrogen and a nonsteroidal antiestrogen being clinically valuable has now evolved into bazedoxifene and conjugated equine estrogen being used to control menopausal symptoms but with uterine and breast safety (Chap. 10)! A lot was initiated in Wisconsin that would change medical science with selective estrogen receptor modulators (SERMs).

All of this decade of discovery at the Wisconsin Comprehensive Cancer Center would provide a foundation for the subsequent interrogation of the modulation of the ER by selective ER modulator by AnaitLevenson, Jennifer MacGregor-Schafer [76, 77] and Hong Liu [78, 79] at the Robert H. Lurie Cancer Center, Northwestern University, Chicago. The Wisconsin scientists would pass the baton of estrogen-induced apoptosis to the Northwestern Medical Scientists Kathy Yao, Dave Bentrem [70, 80], Clodio Osipo [81], Hong Liu [82], and Joan Lewis [83] (Chap. 9). It has always been a Tamoxifen Team effort from generation to generation.

References

1. Jordan VC (1976) Effect of tamoxifen (ICI 46,474) on initiation and growth of DMBA- 409 induced rat mammary carcinomata. Eur J Cancer 12:419–424.
2. Jordan VC, Allen KE (1980) Evaluation of the antitumor activity of the nonsteroidal antiestrogen monohydroxytamoxifen in the DMBA-induced rat mammary carcinoma model. Eur J Cancer 16:239–251.
3. Cuzick J, Baum M (1985) Tamoxifen and contralateral breast cancer. Lancet 2:282
4. Jordan VC (1984) Biochemical pharmacology of antiestrogen action. Pharmacol Rev 36:245–276
5. Nolvadex Adjuvant Trail Organisation (1983) Controlled trial of tamoxifen as adjuvant agent in management of early breast cancer. Lancet 1:257–261
6. Tormey DC, Jordan VC (1984) Long-term tamoxifen adjuvant therapy in node-positive breast cancer: a metabolic and pilot clinical study. Breast Cancer Res Treat 4:297–302
7. Scottish Cancer Trials Office (MRC) (1987) Adjuvant tamoxifen in the management of operable breast cancer: the Scottish Trial. Report from the Breast Cancer Trials Committee. Lancet 2:171–175
8. Harper MJ, Walpole AL (1967) A new derivative of triphenylethylene: effect on implantation and mode of action in rats. J Reprod Fertil 13:101–119
9. Harper MJ, Walpole AL (1967) Mode of action of I.C.I. 46,474 in preventing implantation in rats. J Endocrinol 37:83–92
10. Harper MJ, Walpole AL (1966) Contrasting endocrine activities of cis and trans isomers in a series of substituted triphenylethylenes. Nature 212:87
11. Terenius L (1970) Two modes of interaction between oestrogen and anti-oestrogen. Acta Endocrinol (Copenh) 64:47–58
12. Terenius L (1971) Structure-activity relationships of anti-oestrogens with regard to interaction with 17-beta-oestradiol in the mouse uterus and vagina. Acta Endocrinol (Copenh) 66:431–447
13. Black LJ, Goode RL (1980) Uterine bioassay of tamoxifen, trioxifene and a new estrogen antagonist (LY117018) in rats and mice. Life Sci 26:1453–1458
14. Black LJ, Goode RL (1981) Evidence for biological action of the antiestrogens LY117018 and tamoxifen by different mechanisms. Endocrinology 109:987–989
15. Black LJ, Jones CD, Falcone JF (1983) Antagonism of estrogen action with a new benzothiophene derived antiestrogen. Life Sci 32:1031–1036
16. Jordan VC, Gosden B (1983) Inhibition of the uterotropic activity of estrogens and antiestrogens by the short acting antiestrogen LY117018. Endocrinology 113:463–468
17. Jordan VC, Gosden B (1983) Differential antiestrogen action in the immature rat uterus: a comparison of hydroxylated antiestrogens with high affinity for the estrogen receptor. J Steroid Biochem 19:1249–1258
18. Jordan VC, Robinson SP (1987) Species-specific pharmacology of antiestrogens: role of metabolism. Fed Proc 46:1870–1874
19. Satyaswaroop PG, Zaino RJ, Mortel R (1983) Human endometrial adenocarcinoma transplanted into nude mice: growth regulation by estradiol. Science 219:58–60
20. Satyaswaroop PG, Zaino RJ, Mortel R (1984) Estrogen-like effects of tamoxifen on human endometrial carcinoma transplanted into nude mice. Cancer Res 44:4006–4010
21. Gottardis MM, Robinson SP, Satyaswaroop PG, Jordan VC (1988) Contrasting actions of tamoxifen on endometrial and breast tumor growth in the athymic mouse. Cancer Res 48:812–815
22. Fornander T, Rutqvist LE, Cedermark B et al (1989) Adjuvant tamoxifen in early breast cancer: occurrence of new primary cancers. Lancet 1:117–120
23. Gottardis MM, Jordan VC (1987) Antitumor actions of keoxifene and tamoxifen in the N-nitrosomethylurea-induced rat mammary carcinoma model. Cancer Res 47:4020–4024

24. Gottardis MM, Ricchio ME, Satyaswaroop PG, Jordan VC (1990) Effect of steroidal and nonsteroidal antiestrogens on the growth of a tamoxifen-stimulated human endometrial carcinoma (EnCa101) in athymic mice. Cancer Res 50:3189–3192

25. Beall PT, Misra LK, Young RL et al (1984) Clomiphene protects against osteoporosis in the mature ovariectomized rat. Calcif Tissue Int 36:123–125

26. Jordan VC, Phelps E, Lindgren JU (1987) Effects of anti-estrogens on bone in castrated and intact female rats. Breast Cancer Res Treat 10:31–35

27. Vogel VG, Costantino JP, Wickerham DL et al (2010) Update of the National Surgical Adjuvant Breast and Bowel Project study of tamoxifen and raloxifene (STAR) P-2 trial: preventing breast cancer. Cancer Prev Res (Phila) 3:696–706

28. Jordan VC (1988) Chemosuppression of breast cancer with tamoxifen: laboratory evidence and future clinical investigations. Cancer Invest 6:589–595

29. Love RR, Mazess RB, Tormey DC et al (1988) Bone mineral density in women with breast cancer treated with adjuvant tamoxifen for at least two years. Breast Cancer Res Treat 12:297–302

30. Love RR, Newcomb PA, Wiebe DA et al (1990) Effects of tamoxifen therapy on lipid and lipoprotein levels in postmenopausal patients with node-negative breast cancer. J Natl Cancer Inst 82:1327–1332

31. Love RR, Wiebe DA, Newcomb PA et al (1991) Effects of tamoxifen on cardiovascular risk factors in postmenopausal women. Ann Intern Med 115:860–864

32. Love RR, Mazess RB, Barden HS et al (1992) Effects of tamoxifen on bone mineral density in postmenopausal women with breast cancer. N Engl J Med 326:852–856

33. Turner RT, Wakley GK, Hannon KS, Bell NH (1987) Tamoxifen prevents the skeletal effects of ovarian hormone deficiency in rats. J Bone Miner Res 2:449–456

34. Turner RT, Wakley GK, Hannon KS, Bell NH (1988) Tamoxifen inhibits osteoclast-mediated resorption of trabecular bone in ovarian hormone-deficient rats. Endocrinology 122:1146–1150

35. Turner RT, Evans GL, Wakley GK (1993) Mechanism of action of estrogen on cancellous bone balance in tibiae of ovariectomized growing rats: inhibition of indices of formation and resorption. J Bone Miner Res 8:359–366

36. Jones AL, Powles TJ, Treleaven JG et al (1992) Haemostatic changes and thromboembolic risk during tamoxifen therapy in normal women. Br J Cancer 66:744–747

37. Kedar RP, Bourne TH, Powles TJ et al (1994) Effects of tamoxifen on uterus and ovaries of postmenopausal women in a randomised breast cancer prevention trial. Lancet 343:1318–1321

38. Powles TJ, Jones AL, Ashley SE et al (1994) The Royal Marsden Hospital pilot tamoxifen chemoprevention trial. Breast Cancer Res Treat 31:73–82

39. Powles TJ, Hickish T, Kanis JA et al (1996) Effect of tamoxifen on bone mineral density measured by dual-energy x-ray absorptiometry in healthy premenopausal and postmenopausal women. J Clin Oncol 14:78–84

40. Turken S, Siris E, Seldin D et al (1989) Effects of tamoxifen on spinal bone density in women with breast cancer. J Natl Cancer Inst 81:1086–1088

41. Black LJ, Sato M, Rowley ER et al (1994) Raloxifene (LY139481 HCI) prevents bone loss and reduces serum cholesterol without causing uterine hypertrophy in ovariectomized rats. J Clin Invest 93:63–69

42. Evans G, Bryant HU, Magee D et al (1994) The effects of raloxifene on tibia histomorphometry in ovariectomized rats. Endocrinology 134:2283–2288

43. Evans GL, Bryant HU, Magee DE, Turner RT (1996) Raloxifene inhibits bone turnover and prevents further cancellous bone loss in adult ovariectomized rats with established osteopenia. Endocrinology 137:4139–4144

44. Lerner LJ, Jordan VC (1990) Development of antiestrogens and their use in breast cancer: eighth Cain memorial award lecture. Cancer Res 50:4177–4189

45. Tate AC, Greene GL, DeSombre ER et al (1984) Differences between estrogen- and antiestrogen-estrogen receptor complexes from human breast tumors identified with an antibody raised against the estrogen receptor. Cancer Res 44:1012–1018
46. Lieberman ME, Gorski J, Jordan VC (1983) An estrogen receptor model to describe the regulation of prolactin synthesis by antiestrogens in vitro. J Biol Chem 258:4741–4745
47. Brzozowski AM, Pike AC, Dauter Z et al (1997) Molecular basis of agonism and antagonism in the oestrogen receptor. Nature 389:753–758
48. Shiau AK, Barstad D, Loria PM et al (1998) The structural basis of estrogen receptor/coactivator recognition and the antagonism of this interaction by tamoxifen. Cell 95:927–937
49. Jensen EV, DeSombre ER (1973) Estrogen-receptor interaction. Science 182:126–134
50. Zava DT, McGuire WL (1977) Estrogen receptor. Unoccupied sites in nuclei of a breast tumor cell line. J Biol Chem 252:3703–3708
51. King WJ, Greene GL (1984) Monoclonal antibodies localize oestrogen receptor in the nuclei of target cells. Nature 307:745–747
52. Welshons WV, Lieberman ME, Gorski J (1984) Nuclear localization of unoccupied oestrogen receptors. Nature 307:747–749
53. Carter SB (1967) Effects of cytochalasins on mammalian cells. Nature 213:261–264
54. Jordan VC, Tate AC, Lyman SD et al (1985) Rat uterine growth and induction of progesterone receptor without estrogen receptor translocation. Endocrinology 116:1845–1857
55. Gottardis MM, Jordan VC (1988) Development of tamoxifen-stimulated growth of MCF-7 tumors in athymic mice after long-term antiestrogen administration. Cancer Res 48:5183–5187
56. Gottardis MM, Jiang SY, Jeng MH, Jordan VC (1989) Inhibition of tamoxifen-stimulated growth of an MCF-7 tumor variant in athymic mice by novel steroidal antiestrogens. Cancer Res 49:4090–4093
57. Jordan VC (1989) Tamoxifen and endometrial cancer. Lancet 1:733–734
58. Jiang SY, Wolf DM, Yingling JM et al (1992) An estrogen receptor positive MCF-7 clone that is resistant to antiestrogens and estradiol. Mol Cell Endocrinol 90:77–86
59. Pink JJ, Jiang SY, Fritsch M, Jordan VC (1995) An estrogen-independent MCF-7 breast cancer cell line which contains a novel 80-kilodalton estrogen receptor-related protein. Cancer Res 55:2583–2590
60. Pink JJ, Wu SQ, Wolf DM et al (1996) A novel 80 kDa human estrogen receptor containing a duplication of exons 6 and 7. Nucleic Acids Res 24:962–969
61. Pink JJ, Jordan VC (1996) Models of estrogen receptor regulation by estrogens and antiestrogens in breast cancer cell lines. Cancer Res 56:2321–2330
62. Murphy CS, Meisner LF, Wu SQ, Jordan VC (1989) Short- and long-term estrogen deprivation of T47D human breast cancer cells in culture. Eur J Cancer Clin Oncol 25:1777–1788
63. Pink JJ, Bilimoria MM, Assikis J, Jordan VC (1996) Irreversible loss of the oestrogen receptor in T47D breast cancer cells following prolonged oestrogen deprivation. Br J Cancer 74:1227–1236
64. Jiang SY, Jordan VC (1992) Growth regulation of estrogen receptor-negative breast cancer cells transfected with complementary DNAs for estrogen receptor. J Natl Cancer Inst 84:580–591
65. Catherino WH, Wolf DM, Jordan VC (1995) A naturally occurring estrogen receptor mutation results in increased estrogenicity of a tamoxifen analog. Mol Endocrinol 9:1053–1063
66. Wolf DM, Jordan VC (1994) The estrogen receptor from a tamoxifen stimulated MCF-7 tumor variant contains a point mutation in the ligand binding domain. Breast Cancer Res Treat 31:129–138
67. Murphy CS, Langan-Fahey SM, McCague R, Jordan VC (1990) Structure-function relationships of hydroxylated metabolites of tamoxifen that control the proliferation of estrogen-responsive T47D breast cancer cells in vitro. Mol Pharmacol 38:737–743

68. Wolf DM, Langan-Fahey SM, Parker CJ et al (1993) Investigation of the mechanism of tamoxifen-stimulated breast tumor growth with nonisomerizable analogues of tamoxifen and metabolites. J Natl Cancer Inst 85:806–812

69. Wolf DM, Jordan VC (1993) A laboratory model to explain the survival advantage observed in patients taking adjuvant tamoxifen therapy. Recent Results Cancer Res 127:23–33

70. Yao K, Lee ES, Bentrem DJ et al (2000) Antitumor action of physiological estradiol on tamoxifen-stimulated breast tumors grown in athymic mice. Clin Cancer Res 6:2028–2036

71. Ellis MJ, Gao F, Dehdashti F et al (2009) Lower-dose vs high-dose oral estradiol therapy of hormone receptor-positive, aromatase inhibitor-resistant advanced breast cancer: a phase 2 randomized study. JAMA 302:774–780

72. Anderson GL, Chlebowski RT, Aragaki AK et al (2012) Conjugated equine oestrogen and breast cancer incidence and mortality in postmenopausal women with hysterectomy: extended follow-up of the Women's Health Initiative randomised placebo-controlled trial. Lancet Oncol 13:476–486

73. Jeng MH, Jiang SY, Jordan VC (1994) Paradoxical regulation of estrogen-dependent growth factor gene expression in estrogen receptor (ER)-negative human breast cancer cells stably expressing ER. Cancer Lett 82:123–128

74. Jeng MH, Parker CJ, Jordan VC (1992) Estrogenic potential of progestins in oral contraceptives to stimulate human breast cancer cell proliferation. Cancer Res 52:6539–6546

75. Jeng MH, Langan-Fahey SM, Jordan VC (1993) Estrogenic actions of RU486 in hormone-responsive MCF-7 human breast cancer cells. Endocrinology 132:2622–2630

76. MacGregor Schafer J, Liu H, Bentrem DJ et al (2000) Allosteric silencing of activating function 1 in the 4-hydroxytamoxifen estrogen receptor complex is induced by substituting glycine for aspartate at amino acid 351. Cancer Res 60:5097–5105

77. Schafer JI, Liu H, Tonetti DA, Jordan VC (1999) The interaction of raloxifene and the active metabolite of the antiestrogen EM-800 (SC 5705) with the human estrogen receptor. Cancer Res 59:4308–4313

78. Liu H, Lee ES, Deb Los Reyes A et al (2001) Silencing and reactivation of the selective estrogen receptor modulator-estrogen receptor alpha complex. Cancer Res 61:3632–3639

79. Liu H, Park WC, Bentrem DJ et al (2002) Structure-function relationships of the raloxifene-estrogen receptor-alpha complex for regulating transforming growth factor-alpha expression in breast cancer cells. J Biol Chem 277:9189–9198

80. Bentrem D, Fox JE, Pearce ST et al (2003) Distinct molecular conformations of the estrogen receptor alpha complex exploited by environmental estrogens. Cancer Res 63:7490–7496

81. Osipo C, Gajdos C, Liu H et al (2003) Paradoxical action of fulvestrant in estradiol-induced regression of tamoxifen-stimulated breast cancer. J Natl Cancer Inst 95:1597–1608

82. Liu H, Lee ES, Gajdos C et al (2003) Apoptotic action of 17beta-estradiol in raloxifene-resistant MCF-7 cells in vitro and in vivo. J Natl Cancer Inst 95:1586–1597

83. Lewis JS, Meeke K, Osipo C et al (2005) Intrinsic mechanism of estradiol-induced apoptosis in breast cancer cells resistant to estrogen deprivation. J Natl Cancer Inst 97:1746–1759

Chapter 6
Carcinogenesis and Tamoxifen

Abstract The laboratory study to show that tamoxifen was likely to increase the risk of endometrial cancer in women was initially rapidly confirmed by examination of an adjuvant clinical trials database. However, there was a concern raised that tamoxifen was producing high-grade endometrial cancer, but this claim turned out to be unsubstantiated. In general, the NSABP (P-1) study showed low-grade good prognosis disease with no deaths from endometrial cancer. In contrast, the laboratory finding in the early 1990s that select strains of rats were vulnerable to hepatocarcinoma following lifetime exposure to high daily doses of tamoxifen was of concern and caused labeling changes for tamoxifen. The concerns that there would be significant increases in fatal hepatocellular carcinomas were unfounded on examination of clinical trials data and subsequently ongoing monitoring of epidemiology databases.

Introduction

The toxicological requirements to develop a drug as a breast cancer therapy contrast dramatically from the requirements necessary for approval for a drug to be used in well women. Metastatic breast cancer is fatal, so a small therapeutic index between toxicity and clinical benefit is appropriate. In contrast, drugs must be rigorously tested and demonstrate no toxicological issues in tests of mutagenesis and carcinogenesis in preclinical models prior to FDA approval for use in humans without disease.

Tamoxifen was launched as a treatment for metastatic breast cancer in postmenopausal women in the United Kingdom in 1973, and similar approvals occurred in the United States in December 1977. Toxicology was based on short-term tests in two species, and clinical data showed efficiency with a remarkable lack of side effects [1, 2]. However, the successful use of tamoxifen as an adjuvant therapy in node-positive breast cancer and the expanded use of tamoxifen as an adjuvant therapy in node-negative breast cancer, where the majority of patients are cured

P.Y. Maximov et al., *Tamoxifen*, Milestones in Drug Therapy,

DOI 10.1007/978-3-0348-0664-0_6, © Springer Basel 2013

by early surgery and radiation, enhanced enthusiasm to use tamoxifen to prevent breast cancer in high-risk populations of well women. The laboratory data supported the development of prospective clinical trials [3, 4], and it was already known that tamoxifen, used as an adjuvant therapy, reduced the incidence of contralateral breast cancer by 50 % [5]. The idea that tamoxifen would be used in well women therefore mandated a renewed evaluation of the toxicology of tamoxifen despite the fact that the drug had been successfully used ubiquitously in breast cancer therapy for 20 years.

A surprise was in store. Firstly was the finding that tamoxifen was target site specific and enhanced endometrial cancer growth but, at the same time, prevented estrogen-stimulated breast tumor growth [6] (Fig. 5.1, Chap. 5). Secondly was the findings of long-term carcinogenesis studies in the rat; tamoxifen was a liver carcinogen.

Tamoxifen and the Endometrial Carcinoma

The association between tamoxifen and endometrial carcinoma in humans is based upon clinical observations during the period 1988–1994. There is believed to be an increased incidence of endometrial carcinoma associated with breast cancer; therefore, physicians need to take extra precautions for the routine care of their patients. Tamoxifen is known to have estrogen-like properties in the uterus of some patients [7–9], so treatment would be expected to encourage the growth of preexisting disease, a principle which was first illustrated in the laboratory (Fig. 5.1, Chap. 5). When a breast tumor and endometrial carcinoma are co-transplanted into athymic mice, tamoxifen will block the estrogen-stimulated growth of the breast tumor while stimulating the endometrial carcinoma to grow [6, 10]. This is a demonstration of tamoxifen's target site specificity.

When evaluating reports of tamoxifen-induced endometrial carcinoma, it is important to appreciate that the incidence of occult endometrial tumors found in autopsy specimens is approximately five times the reported incidence in the general population [11]. The estrogen-like properties of tamoxifen can cause uterine hyperplasia and proliferation, facilitating the growth of occult disease and leading to symptoms such as spotting and bleeding. Deaths from endometrial carcinoma occurred during tamoxifen therapy for breast cancer, initially raising the possibility that an aggressive form of the disease could be caused by tamoxifen. However, it should be remembered that only one-third of metastatic endometrial cancer is hormonally responsive, so tamoxifen would not be expected to control the majority of advanced endometrial cancer.

Deaths from Endometrial Carcinoma

Magriples and coworkers [12] completed a computer search of the Yale New Haven Hospital tumor registry for the decade 1980–1990 and identified 53 patients with a history of breast cancer who subsequently developed endometrial cancer. Fifteen of these patients received tamoxifen and 38 did not. A total of 3,457 women were initially identified with breast cancer, but the proportion receiving tamoxifen was not stated. Interestingly enough, all of the tamoxifen-treated patients received 40-mg tamoxifen daily rather than the standard 20 mg daily. Five patients died of endometrial carcinoma during tamoxifen therapy, and the tumors from tamoxifen-treated patients were in general (67 %) poorly differentiated endometrial carcinomata (Table 6.1). The authors concluded "it appears that women receiving tamoxifen as treatment for breast cancer who subsequently develop uterine cancer are at risk for high-grade endometrial cancers that have a poor prognosis." Examination of the duration of tamoxifen therapy received by women before detection and subsequent death from endometrial carcinoma shows that three patients received tamoxifen for 12 months or less.

Deaths in women taking tamoxifen for relatively short time periods were also reported in the Stockholm study [13] (Table 6.2) and the NSABP study B14 [14] (Table 6.3). In the Stockholm study, 931 patients were randomized to receive either 2 or 5 years of tamoxifen 40 mg daily. Seventeen patients have been diagnosed with endometrial carcinoma; however, examination of patient records shows that each of the women received tamoxifen for less than 2 years, and the reported tumors were grades 1 and 2. One of the major conclusions of the study was that the probability of developing endometrial carcinoma was increased with duration of tamoxifen therapy [15]. However, examination of the 17 cases of endometrial carcinoma detected in the nearly 1,000 patients shows that 13 of the women who developed endometrial carcinoma received less than 2 years of tamoxifen treatment [13].

In the NSABP study [14], 1,419 patients were randomized to receive 20-mg tamoxifen daily for 5 years, and 1,220 patients were recruited and registered to receive at least 5 years of tamoxifen. Twenty-three women developed endometrial carcinoma with an average time of evaluation of 8 years and 5 years for randomized and registered patients, respectively. Six patients in the tamoxifen-treated arms died after a diagnosis of endometrial carcinoma (Table 6.3). Three of the six women took tamoxifen for less than 2 years, and one woman never took tamoxifen, although she was included in the analysis based on intention to treat. Overall, eight of the total of 23 women taking tamoxifen received the drug for less than 2 years.

Based on an analysis of clinical trials data available in the 1990s, it was possible to address the question [12] of whether an aggressive high-grade disease develops during tamoxifen therapy.

Table 6.1 Clinical and pathological features of tamoxifen-treated breast cancer patients who died of endometrial carcinoma in the Yale Haven Cancer Survey [12]

Patient	Age	Months on tamoxifen	Endometrial histology	FIGO stage
1	71	120	Adenosquamous FG3	NS
2	85	96	Endometrial	IIIC
3	60	12	Endometrioid FG3	NS
4	71	12	MMT	IVB
5	87	3	Papillary serous	NS

NS not stated, MMT mixed Mullerian tumor

Table 6.2 Clinical and pathological features of tamoxifen-treated patients who died of endometrial carcinoma in the Stockholm trial [13]

Age	Months on tamoxifen	Patient	Endometrial histology	FIGO stage
68	24	1	NS grade I	I
69	13	2	NS grade II	I
70	11	3	NS grade II	IV

Table 6.3 Characteristics and pathological feature of tamoxifen-treated breast cancer patients who died of endometrial carcinoma (EC) in the NSABP B14 trial [14]

Patient	Age	Months on tamoxifen	Off tamoxifen to diagnosis (months)	Histology	FIGO stage	Cause of death
1	68	65	0	Papillary	IVG1	PE
2	54	42	23	Carcinosarcoma	11BG3	EC
3	58	22	73	Papillary	1BG3	EC
4	68	5	0	Endometrioid	1A	CV disease
5	63	9	0	Endometrioid	1BG2	EC
6	66	0	0	Endometrioid	1BG1	EC

CV cardiovascular, PE pulmonary embolus

Tamoxifen and the Stage of Endometrial Carcinoma

The discovery that high doses of tamoxifen will cause adduct formation in rat liver DNA [16] occurred at the same time that Magriples and coworkers [12] reported tamoxifen was associated with high-grade endometrial carcinoma. This naturally lead to the possibility that tamoxifen may be causing progression of preexisting disease. However, randomized clinical trial [14] and an epidemiology study [17] did not support this proposition, although, in each case, the authors state that the numbers are too low to draw any definite conclusions. Fisher and coworkers [14] compared the stages of endometrial carcinoma and tumor grades found in their study and in the Yale Tumor Registry Study and the Swedish Trail. An epidemiology study from the Netherlands Cancer Institute is included for comparison [17] (Table 6.4). It is difficult to make absolute comparisons of these data, but several points can be made. The studies all found that the majority of tumors reported were stage 1 endometrial carcinoma. The percentage of low-grade tumors was variable with 78 %, 33 %, 53 %, and 52 % for the NSABP, Yale, Swedish, and Netherlands studies, respectively. Additionally, for comparison purposes, a Gynecologic Oncology Group Study [18] of 222 patients found the distribution of cases to be 82 % low-grade cases (FIGO I and 2) and 18 % high-grade cases (FIGO 3). Overall, the Yale group stood alone having the largest proportion of high-grade tumors, with 67 %. However, the fact that the events were so low, and patients with already advanced endometrial carcinoma were being given tamoxifen to treat breast cancer, made this fact not unexpected. Based on this analysis of available data, there was insufficient evidence to support the statement that "women receiving tamoxifen as treatment for breast cancer who subsequently develop uterine cancer are at high risk for high-grade endometrial cancers that have a poor prognosis [12]." Nevertheless, the fact that there was an increase in the incidence of endometrial cancer was a major clue with the use of tamoxifen for both treatment and prevention in the 1990s. How bad was the fear of tamoxifen for some patients? In the mid-1990s, one patient said to me: "Thank God! I have been diagnosed with ER-negative breast cancer and I don't have to take tamoxifen."

Incidence of Endometrial Cancer with Tamoxifen

It is now possible to give a precise rate for the incidence of endometrial carcinoma in tamoxifen-treated patients. The results from the Early Breast Cancer Trialists' Collaborative Group (EBCTCG) [19] have shown that tamoxifen increases the incidence of endometrial cancer and was strongly correlated with age. The risk of incidence or death from endometrial cancer was very little in the younger age group (<45, or 45–54 years) with only one death and 11 incidents of endometrial cancer in the <45 years group with ER-positive breast cancer and seven deaths and 71 incident cases of endometrial cancer in the 55–69 years group with ER-positive breast cancer (incidence 3.8 % in the tamoxifen group vs. 1.1 % in the control group; absolute increase 2.6 %, 95 % CI) [19].

Most importantly, the new knowledge about the small but significant increase in endometrial cancer in postmenopausal patients treated with long-term adjuvant tamoxifen therapy acted as a forewarning for the NCI NSABP P-1 prevention trial to remain vigilant for signs of spotting and bleeding on protocol. Accurate results for the detection of endometrial cancer in pre- and postmenopausal women at risk for breast cancer are documented. There is a significant increase in endometrial cancer in postmenopausal population, but not in premenopausal women at risk for breast cancer [20, 21]. It is important to note that no patient died from endometrial cancer in the NCI/NSABP P-1 study, probably because of the meticulous surveillance practices during the study.

Finally, another clinical trial Study of Tamoxifen and Raloxifene (STAR), also known as NSABP P-2 trial, concluded, as well, that tamoxifen treatment increases the incidence of invasive uterine cancer in comparison to women with high risk of breast cancer treated with raloxifene [22]. Increase by 45 % (RR, 0.55; 95 % CI,

Table 6.4 Comparison of the uterine cancers in tamoxifen-treated and control patients [12–14, 17]

	NSABP		Yale tumor registry				Swedish trial				Netherlands cancer institute			
	Tamoxifen n = 25		Tamoxifen n = 15		No tamoxifen n = 38		Tamoxifen n = 17		No tamoxifen n = 5		Tamoxifen n = 23		No tamoxifen n = 75	
	Events	%	Events	%	Events	%	Events	%	Events	%	Events	%	Events	%
Stage														
I	21	88	7	78	23	88	14	82	4	100	17	85	62	87
II–IV	3	12	2	22	3	12	3	18	0	0	3	15	9	13
Total no. staged	24		9		26		17		4		20		71	
Histological grade														
Low (good)	18	78	5	33	26	74	8	53	4	100	12	52[a]	24	32[a]
High (poor)	5	22	10	67	9	26	7	47	0	0	11	48	51	68
Total no. graded	23		15		35		15		4		23		75	

[a]Calculated from a statement made by the authors in the discussion of the paper [17]. No breakdown of histological grade was presented in the results, although the morphological classification for users and nonusers of tamoxifen was in the same proportions. The proportion of well-differentiated tumors in the no tamoxifen group of this study is very low in comparison to all the studies and the survey in [18]

0.36–0.83) for invasive uterine cancer, and 80 % higher incidence of endometrial cancer in tamoxifen-treated group than in raloxifene treated (RR, 0.19; 95 %CI, 0.12–0.29).

Tamoxifen and Rat Liver Carcinogenesis

It is now clear that if I had pursued the idea of giving high doses of tamoxifen to prevent rat mammary carcinogenesis [4], then rat liver carcinogenesis would have been discovered in 1973 [23], and there would have been no tamoxifen, and hundreds of thousands of women would now be dead of breast cancer. There would probably be no aromatase inhibitors or SERMs. The pharmacological indus-try would not have advanced a known carcinogen for long-term therapy (adjuvant therapy) or chemoprevention, so the "gold standard" would not have existed for others to beat.

High daily doses of tamoxifen will produce hepatocellular carcinoma in the rat (Table 6.5) if administered for up to half the animal's lifetime. This is particularly true at a 45.2 mg/kg dose, when tumors are formed within 6 months in 29 % of the animals [24]. There is general agreement that high daily doses of tamoxifen result in the premature death of rats. In the study by Greaves and coworkers [25], 50 % of control female rats were alive and well at about 104 weeks (2 years), but treatment with 35 mg/kg tamoxifen daily produced 50 % deaths by 42 weeks. Interestingly, the low dose of 5 mg/kg/day increases the survival of male and female rats at 2 years (males, 30 % deaths in treated vs. 70 % deaths in controls; females, 25 % deaths in treated vs. 50 % deaths in controls). The authors note [25] that their low tamoxifen dose (5 mg/kg/day) completely inhibited the incidence of adenomas in the pituitary gland and adenocarcinomas of the mammary gland in female rats and almost completely inhibited adenomas of the pituitary gland and parathyroid gland in male rats.

The published studies indicate that there is a threshold level for liver carcinoge-nicity, which is approximately 3 mg/kg/day [24]. However, the study by Dragan and coworkers [27], using a different rat strain and experimental design, observed no hepatocellular carcinomata after 15 months of treatment. The design of the study divided carcinogenesis into initiation and promotion. Carcinogenesis was initiated with diethylnitrosamine (DEN 10 mg/kg oral) in partially hepatectomized Fischer F344 rats, and promotion to carcinogenesis was completed with tamoxifen in the feed at 250 ppm. Blood levels of tamoxifen were 230 ± 30 ng/ml (i.e., in the range of clinical experience [27]). It can be estimated that a 200-g rat consumes 10 g of food containing 2.5 mg tamoxifen per day, so a rat received a daily dose of 12.5 mg/ kg, which is within the 10–30 mg/kg/day dosing regimens of other studies [24]. No hepatocellular carcinomata were observed if DEN, the initiator, was omitted, but tumors were seen if DEN was given with tamoxifen, leading the authors to conclude that tamoxifen is a promoter of hepatocellular carcinoma in the Fischer rat. How-ever, all the other studies, mainly using Sprague-Dawley strains of rats and bolus administration of drug by lavage, suggest that tamoxifen is a complete carcinogen at high doses.

Table 6.5 The occurrence of hepatocellular carcinoma in various rat strains during long-term tamoxifen treatment

Strain of rat	Daily dose (mg/kg)	n	Duration (months)	Hepatocellular carcinoma %	(n)	Reference
1. Sprague-Dawley	2.8	57	15	0	(22)	[24]
(Crl:CD(BR))	11.3	57	15	45	(11)	
	45.2	57	12	75	(4)	
2. Wistar (Alpk: ApfSD)	5	52	24	16	(51)	[25]
	20	52	24	64	(51)	
	35	52	24	64	(51)	
3. Sprague-Dawley	11.3	84	12	44	(36)	[26]
(Crl:CD(BR))	22.6	75	12	100	(24)	
4. Fischer F344	12.5[a]	20	15	0	(8)	[27]

[a]Based on estimate of daily food intake of 10 g per day of 250-mg tamoxifen/kg feed

Tamoxifen and DNA Adduct Formation

Carcinogenesis requires genotoxicity, so it is important to correlate the formation of DNA adducts with the formation of tumors in a particular organ for a sensitive species. Mani and Kupfer [28] first showed that in human and rat liver microsome systems in vitro [^{14}C], tamoxifen was metabolized by an NADPH-dependent cytochrome P450-mediated activation system to intermediate(s) which covalently bound to microsomal proteins. Han and Liehr [16] subsequently showed that the administration intraperitoneally (i.p.) of tamoxifen (20 mg/kg/day) to Sprague-Dawley rats resulted in two DNA adducts after only 1 day and up to six adducts after 6 consecutive days of treatment. A similar result was observed by Hard and associates [26] using 48 mg/kg/day tamoxifen for 7 days in Sprague-Dawley rats.

It is clear that large doses of tamoxifen can produce DNA adducts, but White and coworkers [29] have investigated the dose adduct relationship in rats. Seven days of dosing with between 5 and 45 mg tamoxifen/kg/day produced an almost linear dose-dependent increase in DNA adducts in the Fischer 344 rat. At doses of less than 5 mg/kg/day, tamoxifen did not alter the chromatograph from ^{32}P post-labeled DNA from treated rats. It would appear, therefore, that there is a threshold for the appearance of adducts with tamoxifen and the induction of liver tumors. The metabolite α-hydroxytamoxifen was subsequently found to be responsible for DNA adducts in rats (see Chap. 3).

White and colleagues [29] also examined whether adduct formation occurs in the mouse, which does not produce liver tumors in response to tamoxifen. There is DNA adduct formation in both C57Bl/6 and DBA/2 mice; however, this is approximately 30 % of that observed with a similar dosing schedule in the Fischer rats [29], raising questions about the correlation between adduct formation and clinically evident tumors.

In humans, DNA adducts were not observed in the livers of tamoxifen-treated women; however, only limited samples were screened [30]. A study in vitro [31] demonstrated the ability to form DNA adducts with human and rat liver microsomes using 100-μM tamoxifen. Although the levels of DNA adducts are low and in the range of the studies in vivo with mice, the human liver was two to three times more effective at producing DNA adducts than the rat. The Sprague-Dawley rat livers used in the studies in vitro [31] are from a strain that is extremely sensitive to the carcinogenic actions of tamoxifen in vivo. Adduct formation in vitro can be dramatically altered by adding different cofactors [31], and the level of DNA adduct formation that is required for carcinogenesis may be dose related, as in the rat in vivo [29]. The level of adducts, $1-3 \times 10^8$ nucleotides, observed in the study of rat liver microsomes in vitro [31] is not in the carcinogenic range in vivo [29], although caution must be used when comparing in vivo and in vitro studies.

Overall, these data demonstrated that DNA adducts could be formed in vitro and in vivo, but the level of adduct formation seems critical for carcinogenesis. Adduct formation using human microsomes is very low, but this can be enhanced into the mouse range using cumene hydroperoxide as a cofactor [31]. However, mice do not produce liver tumors after long-term treatment. Thus, the most important issues in the 1990s were the species differences, the correlation between liver carcinogenesis and DNA adduct formation, the effect of the rate of repair of DNA in different species, and the relative doses used to demonstrate the carcinogenic effects of tamoxifen. However, the epidemiology of human liver cancer did not support patient risk evaluations in women taking tamoxifen. No correlation has been noted to this day, but in the 1990s, the concern was justified with the move to prevention and the possibility that the liver carcinogenesis could occur decades after taking the drug.

Doses of Tamoxifen in Animals and Man

A key argument made regarding rat liver carcinogenesis studies was that since the serum concentrations of tamoxifen obtained in the rat (Table 6.6) were within the range of serum concentrations achieved during the treatment of breast cancer, then the results are clinically relevant. It is generally believed that toxicology testing should be conducted to mimic human pharmacokinetics. However, the rat and mouse clear tamoxifen from the body at a much faster rate than the human so that higher doses must be administered to maintain the blood level in the human range used for treatment. Examination of the relative dosage regimens in different species and the resulting serum levels of tamoxifen illustrate the point. Serum levels of tamoxifen during the treatment of breast cancer with 10 mg twice daily (approximately 285 μg/kg daily for a 70-kg postmenopausal woman) are usually between 100 and 200 ng/ml [32]. In contrast, the administration of 50- or 100-μg tamoxifen daily to ovariectomized mature mice (approximately 2.5 mg/kg for a 20-g mouse) or immature rats (approximately 3 mg/kg for a 35-g rat) for 7–10 days results in pharmacological effects but produces serum levels of tamoxifen often below the level of detection by high performance liquid chromatography [33]. Only by giving high doses of tamoxifen (200 mg/kg) to animals can one adequately study circulating levels of drug [33]. We studied the circulating levels of tamoxifen in patients receiving high daily doses of tamoxifen. Increasing the daily dose to the limits of toxicity (10 mg/kg) [35] in humans reaches the dose range (5–35 mg/kg) used to treat rats in the liver carcinogenesis studies (Table 6.6). However, the blood levels are tenfold higher in the human. Comparable serum levels in the rat and human during tamoxifen treatment can only be produced by treating rats with high doses of tamoxifen. The schedules that are used to demonstrate liver carcinogenesis in the rat (5–40 mg/kg) are 20 times greater than the standard treatment regimen in women (20 mg daily or 285 µg/kg).

Testing at Comparable Therapeutic Levels

Tamoxifen, at a daily dose of 50 µg (250 µg/kg), inhibits the growth and development of dimethylbenzanthracene-induced rat mammary tumors [36]. This is equivalent to the therapeutic dose used to treat metastatic breast cancer and as an adjuvant therapy in node-positive and node-negative disease. The duration of therapy for the treatment of breast cancer can be indefinite in some clinical trials [37, 38], but most treatment plans use 5 years of adjuvant tamoxifen at a dose of 20 mg daily. With the life expectancy of most women being 80 years of age, this translates into about 6 % of a woman's lifetime, and most women are treated during their postmenopausal years. In contrast, studies of rat liver carcinogenesis employ a test system that starts at 6 weeks of age (just post-puberty) and treats daily with approximately 20 times the human dose for the rest of the animals' life. At a dose of 11.3 mg/kg, approximately half the rats develop liver tumors within a year [26] (Table 6.7).

It is important to state that the general need for carcinogenic testing is to establish whether an agent is carcinogenic per se not just at the level of therapeutic value. To achieve this, animals are tested with a high dose, with lower doses approaching the therapeutic range. A positive result in the animal test does not mean that human therapeutic levels will be carcinogenic but provides a warning of such a possibility. A treatment regimen of tamoxifen, 0.25 mg/kg daily, for 2–3 months during the second year of the rats' life would be an equivalent bioassay. This approach would give a realistic view of the toxicological risks observed in patients. Since the doses to be used are far below the level that causes adduct formation [29] and repair mechanisms occur after the cessation of therapy, there is little probability that animals will develop liver tumors, thus duplicating clinical experience.

Table 6.6 Circulating serum levels obtained with different dosage regimens in the rat, mouse, and human (70-kg postmenopausal women)

Species	Dosage per day (mg/kg)	Duration	Tamoxifen concentration (ng/ml)	Reference
Human	0.28	>2 years	148	[32]
Rat	3	7 days	<1	[33]
Rat	200	7 days	1,000	[33]
Mouse	2.5	7 days	<10	[33]
Mouse	200	10 days	300	[33]
Human	4.9	1 year	1,300	[33, 34]
Human	Approx. 10	11 days	1,855	[35]

Table 6.7 The levels of circulating tamoxifen achieved with the dosing regimens used in rats during carcinogenesis experiments

Rats	Dosage regimen (mg/kg)	Tamoxifen concentration (ng/ml)	Liver tumors	Reference
1. Mature Wistar	5	166	Yes	[24]
	20	644		
	35	636		
2. Mature Sprague-Dawley	11.3	138 ± 41	Yes	[25]
	22.6	172 ± 103		
3. Mature Fischer	12.5[a]	230 ± 30	Yes	[27]

[a]Based on estimate of daily food intake of 10 g per day of 250-mg tamoxifen/kg feed

Toxicological testing of new drugs in development to reduce the risks to patients is crucial, but tamoxifen has received extensive clinical testing over the past 40 years without producing major toxicities. Although it is argued that a decade is required for iatrogenic carcinogenesis in patients [39], there is currently little or no information to demonstrate that tamoxifen is a significant liver carcinogen in the human, as has been demonstrated for the rat [24]. The divergence of effects in rats and women is because of differences in the dose, duration and timing of tamoxifen treatment, differential metabolism, rapid repair responses in humans, and the susceptibility of some inbred strains of rat to hepatocellular carcinogens.

Conclusion

Overall, the effective translational research on the link between tamoxifen and the growth of endometrial cancer with the important step of taking our laboratory finding [6] to the clinical community [15], resulted in lives saved and put in place new gynecologic procedures that remain to this day. It was specifically stated: "Until the influence of TAM and other antiestrogens on endometrial cancers has been fully investigated, vigilance by physicians treating patients with these agents is needed to establish the clinical relevance (if any) of these observations."

However, the other toxicological issue, rat liver carcinogenesis was not to evaporate so easily and is a lasting example of those observations in laboratory that do not necessarily translate to the clinic. However, Zeneca (originally ICI pharmaceuticals division) formally required a "black box" designation to comply with the toxicological findings. A lesson learned, but not unlike the fact the tamoxifen was a superb antifertility agent in the laboratory but did exactly the opposite in clinical practice!

Postscript. The results of the pioneering experiment by my Ph.D. student Marco Gottardis [6] on the target site specificity in breast cancer, and endometrial cancer was used by us to appeal to the clinical community to monitor their adjuvant clinical trials. This story is told in the Postscript to Chap. 5. Marco and I traveled to ICI pharmaceutical division in 1987, and he presented his work at Alderley Park for their staff. The staff at ICI took immediate action and contacted the Stockholm adjuvant clinical trial group to look at their database with different durations of tamoxifen [15, 40]. The results of their data collection process replicated our laboratory study, fewer contralateral breast cancers and more endometrial cancers with tamoxifen. It is interesting to observe that an examination of their paper published in 1989 shows that the axis for the duration of patient monitoring of their adjuvant tamoxifen trial for endometrial cancer extends for 10.5 years. In other words, they already had the data by the year 1987 when we first talked about our animal studies of human disease in 1987. The NSABP followed up with their evaluation of tamoxifen and endometrial cancer in 1991 [41]. All of these translational research successes were essential to prepare the clinical trials community for monitoring the proposed chemoprevention trials in women without breast cancer for endometrial cancer.

Wisconsin with its two cancer centers: the Wisconsin Comprehensive Cancer Center and McArdle Laboratory for Cancer Research had significant researchers in carcinogenesis. Henry Pitot, a former director of the McArdle Laboratory, was a world authority on hepatocarcinogenesis. Here was a superb opportunity to join forces on a "hot topic" in toxicology—rat carcinogenesis with nonsteroidal antiestrogens. Henry had a talented, keen, and enthusiastic postdoc Yvonne Dragon, who successfully wrote up our proposal, and Henry generously insisted that I was the principal investigator as this was a "topical tamoxifen issue," and I was better positioned to be successful. He was correct and numerous publications subsequently followed. This is what cancer centers are all about—collaboration to aid and understanding of topics that will affect the well-being of patients, in this case the concern was about liver cancer with tamoxifen use. It also provided me with the opportunity to participate in the debate about the safety of tamoxifen at the national level and especially at hearings in the state of California. All through the development of tamoxifen, I had a philosophy of looking at "the good, the bad, and the ugly" of tamoxifen. Patient safety and patient mortality was always the goal.

References

1. Cole MP, Jones CT, Todd ID (1971) A new anti-oestrogenic agent in late breast cancer. An early clinical appraisal of ICI46474. Br J Cancer 25:270–275
2. EBCTCG (1988) Effects of adjuvant tamoxifen and of cytotoxic therapy on mortality in early breast cancer. An overview of 61 randomized trials among 28,896 women. N Engl J Med 319:1681–1692
3. Jordan VC (1974) Antitumour activity of the antiestrogen ICI 46,474 (Tamoxifen) in the dimethylbenzanthracene (DMBA)-induced rat mammary carcinoma model. J Steroid Biochem 5:354
4. Jordan VC (1976) Effect of tamoxifen (ICI 46,474) on initiation and growth of DMBA-induced rat mammary carcinomata. Eur J Cancer 12:419–424
5. Cuzick J, Baum M (1985) Tamoxifen and contralateral breast cancer. Lancet 2:282
6. Gottardis MM, Robinson SP, Satyaswaroop PG, Jordan VC (1988) Contrasting actions of tamoxifen on endometrial and breast tumor growth in the athymic mouse. Cancer Res 48:812–815
7. Cross SS, Ismail SM (1990) Endometrial hyperplasia in an oophorectomized woman receiving tamoxifen therapy. Case report. Br J Obstet Gynaecol 97:190–192
8. Gal D, Kopel S, Bashevkin M et al (1991) Oncogenic potential of tamoxifen on endometria of postmenopausal women with breast cancer–preliminary report. Gynecol Oncol 42:120–123
9. De Muylder X, Neven P, De Somer M et al (1991) Endometrial lesions in patients undergoing tamoxifen therapy. Int J Gynaecol Obstet 36:127–130
10. Satyaswaroop PG, Zaino RJ, Mortel R (1984) Estrogen-like effects of tamoxifen on human endometrial carcinoma transplanted into nude mice. Cancer Res 44:4006–4010
11. Horwitz RI, Feinstein AR (1986) Estrogens and endometrial cancer. Responses to arguments and current status of an epidemiologic controversy. Am J Med 81:503–507
12. Magriples U, Naftolin F, Schwartz PE, Carcangiu ML (1993) High-grade endometrial carcinoma in tamoxifen-treated breast cancer patients. J Clin Oncol 11:485–490
13. Fornander T, Hellstrom AC, Moberger B (1993) Descriptive clinicopathologic study of 17 patients with endometrial cancer during or after adjuvant tamoxifen in early breast cancer. J Natl Cancer Inst 85:1850–1855
14. Fisher B, Costantino JP, Redmond CK et al (1994) Endometrial cancer in tamoxifen-treated breast cancer patients: findings from the National Surgical Adjuvant Breast and Bowel Project (NSABP) B-14. J Natl Cancer Inst 86:527–537
15. Fornander T, Rutqvist LE, Cedermark B et al (1989) Adjuvant tamoxifen in early breast cancer: occurrence of new primary cancers. Lancet 1:117–120
16. Han XL, Liehr JG (1992) Induction of covalent DNA adducts in rodents by tamoxifen. Cancer Res 52:1360–1363
17. van Leeuwen FE, Benraadt J, Coebergh JW et al (1994) Risk of endometrial cancer after tamoxifen treatment of breast cancer. Lancet 343:448–452
18. Boronow RC, Morrow CP, Creasman WT et al (1984) Surgical staging in endometrial cancer: clinical-pathologic findings of a prospective study. Obstet Gynecol 63:825–832
19. Davies C, Godwin J, Gray R et al (2011) Relevance of breast cancer hormone receptors and other factors to the efficacy of adjuvant tamoxifen: patient-level meta-analysis of randomised trials. Lancet 378:771–784
20. Fisher B, Costantino JP, Wickerham DL et al (2005) Tamoxifen for the prevention of breast cancer: current status of the National Surgical Adjuvant Breast and Bowel Project P-1 study. J Natl Cancer Inst 97:1652–1662
21. Fisher B, Costantino JP, Wickerham DL et al (1998) Tamoxifen for prevention of breast cancer: report of the National Surgical Adjuvant Breast and Bowel Project P-1 Study. J Natl Cancer Inst 90:1371–1388

22. Runowicz CD, Costantino JP, Wickerham DL et al (2011) Gynecologic conditions in participants in the NSABP breast cancer prevention study of tamoxifen and raloxifene (STAR). Am J Obstet Gynecol 205:535 e1–535 e5
23. Jordan VC (1995) What if tamoxifen (ICI 46,474) had been found to produce rat liver tumors in 1973? A personal perspective. Ann Oncol 6:29–34
24. Williams GM, Iatropoulos MJ, Djordjevic MV, Kaltenberg OP (1993) The triphenylethylene drug tamoxifen is a strong liver carcinogen in the rat. Carcinogenesis 14:315–317
25. Greaves P, Goonetilleke R, Nunn G et al (1993) Two-year carcinogenicity study of tamoxifen in Alderley Park Wistar-derived rats. Cancer Res 53:3919–3924
26. Hard GC, Iatropoulos MJ, Jordan K et al (1993) Major difference in the hepatocarcinogenicity and DNA adduct forming ability between toremifene and tamoxifen in female Crl:CD(BR) rats. Cancer Res 53:4534–4541
27. Dragan YP, Fahey S, Street K et al (1994) Studies of tamoxifen as a promoter of hepatocarcinogenesis in female Fischer F344 rats. Breast Cancer Res Treat 31:11–25
28. Mani C, Kupfer D (1991) Cytochrome P-450-mediated activation and irreversible binding of the antiestrogen tamoxifen to proteins in rat and human liver: possible involvement of flavin-containing monooxygenases in tamoxifen activation. Cancer Res 51:6052–6058
29. White IN, de Matteis F, Davies A et al (1992) Genotoxic potential of tamoxifen and analogues in female Fischer F344/n rats, DBA/2 and C57BL/6 mice and in human MCL-5 cells. Carcinogenesis 13:2197–2203
30. Martin EA, Rich KJ, White IN et al (1995) 32P-postlabelled DNA adducts in liver obtained from women treated with tamoxifen. Carcinogenesis 16:1651–1654
31. Pathak DN, Bodell WJ (1994) DNA adduct formation by tamoxifen with rat and human liver microsomal activation systems. Carcinogenesis 15:529–532
32. Langan-Fahey SM, Tormey DC, Jordan VC (1990) Tamoxifen metabolites in patients on long-term adjuvant therapy for breast cancer. Eur J Cancer 26:883–888
33. Robinson SP, Langan-Fahey SM, Johnson DA, Jordan VC (1991) Metabolites, pharmacodynamics, and pharmacokinetics of tamoxifen in rats and mice compared to the breast cancer patient. Drug Metab Dispos 19:36–43
34. Jordan VC, Bain RR, Brown RR et al (1983) Determination and pharmacology of a new hydroxylated metabolite of tamoxifen observed in patient sera during therapy for advanced breast cancer. Cancer Res 43:1446–1450
35. Trump DL, Smith DC, Ellis PG et al (1992) High-dose oral tamoxifen, a potential multidrug-resistance-reversal agent: phase I trial in combination with vinblastine. J Natl Cancer Inst 84:1811–1816
36. Jordan VC (1983) Laboratory studies to develop general principles for the adjuvant treatment of breast cancer with antiestrogens: problems and potential for future clinical applications. Breast Cancer Res Treat 3(Suppl):S73–S86
37. Falkson HC, Gray R, Wolberg WH et al (1990) Adjuvant trial of 12 cycles of CMFPT followed by observation or continuous tamoxifen versus four cycles of CMFPT in postmenopausal women with breast cancer: an Eastern Cooperative Oncology Group phase III study. J Clin Oncol 8:599–607
38. Tormey DC, Gray R, Abeloff MD et al (1992) Adjuvant therapy with a doxorubicin regimen and long-term tamoxifen in premenopausal breast cancer patients: an Eastern Cooperative Oncology Group trial. J Clin Oncol 10:1848–1856
39. Jordan VC, Lababidi MK, Mirecki DM (1990) Anti-oestrogenic and anti-tumour properties of prolonged tamoxifen therapy in C3H/OUJ mice. Eur J Cancer 26:718–721
40. Fornander T, Rutqvist LE (1989) Adjuvant tamoxifen and second cancers. Lancet 1:616
41. Fisher B, Redmond C (1991) New perspective on cancer of the contralateral breast: a marker for assessing tamoxifen as a preventive agent. J Natl Cancer Inst 83:1278–1280

Chapter 7
Chemoprevention: Cinderella Waiting for the Ball

Abstract Tamoxifen was first shown to prevent the initiation and promotion of rat mammary carcinogenesis in the 1970s. During the 1990s, numerous trials were initiated to test the worth of tamoxifen to decrease the incidence of breast cancer in otherwise healthy women. The Royal Marsden study was first with a vanguard study in the 1980s followed by the National Surgical Adjuvant Breast and Bowel Project (NSABP) P-1 trial, the Italian Study of women not at risk, and the International Breast Cancer Study Group (IBIS). Multiple subsequent analyses all showed some efficacy to reduce breast cancer incidence, but the NSABP study was the strongest powered clinical trial uniformly demonstrating a 50 % decrease in incidence for both pre- and postmenopausal women at risk. As predicted, endometrial cancer was the most troublesome side effect, but only in postmenopausal women taking tamoxifen.

Introduction

The idea of the prevention of breast cancer is not new, but significant practical progress has been made, through translational research, to make the idea feasible in some women. It is now possible to reduce the incidence of breast cancer through the inhibition of estrogen action.

Professor Antoine Lacassagne [1] stated a vision for the prevention of breast cancer at the annual meeting of the American Association of Cancer Research in Boston in 1936.

> If one accepts the consideration of adenocarcinoma of the breast as the consequence of a special hereditary sensibility to the proliferative actions of estrone, one is led to imagine a therapeutic preventative for subjects predisposed by their heredity to this cancer. It would consist – perhaps in the very near future when the knowledge and use of hormones will be better understood – in the suitable use of a hormone antagonistic or excretory, to prevent the stagnation of estrone in the ducts of the breast.

But no agent that was "antagonistic to prevent the stagnation of oestrone in the breast" was available to the clinician for clinical trial until tamoxifen [2, 3].

Tamoxifen became the "antiestrogen" of choice because of the following (a) there was a large body of basic biological evidence that this was a valid hypothesis to test, (b) tamoxifen was noted to reduce the incidence of contralateral breast cancer when used as an adjuvant therapy to treat micrometastases from the original primary tumor, (c) there was a huge and expanding clinical experience with tamoxifen as a long-term treatment for node-positive and node-negative breast cancer. The later point was important as the majority of patients with estrogen receptor (ER)-positive node-negative breast cancers are cured by surgery (plus radiation) alone, so 5 years of adjuvant tamoxifen was essentially already being used in the majority of these cured "well women" [4, 5].

In this chapter, the changing fashions in endocrine chemoprevention will be described. The change in fashion occurred because of significant advances in our understanding of the pharmacology of the drug group called the "nonsteroidal antiestrogens" [6] that underwent a metamorphosis in the mid-1980s [7] to become the new drug group called the selective ER modulators (SERMs) [8, 9]. See Chap. 5.

The Link Between Estrogen and Breast Cancer

The topic has recently been reviewed [10] in the refereed research literature so only essential facts will be considered here. The link between estrogen action for breast cancer growth of the original tumor, ER, and 5 years of adjuvant tamoxifen therapy to block tumor growth is compelling and proven in randomized clinical trials [11]. The findings can be simply summarized: breast tumors that are ER negative do not respond to tamoxifen treatment, tamoxifen dramatically reduces recurrence and mortality during 5 years of treatment for patients with ER-positive breast cancer, and this is maintained for at least 15 years following completion of therapy (see Chap. 4). Tamoxifen reduces the incidence of contralateral breast cancer by 50 % and this is sustained, but tamoxifen also increases the incidence of endometrial cancer in postmenopausal women (and mortality). The negative actions of adjuvant tamoxifen, such as deaths from endometrial cancer or thromboembolic disease, do not affect the overall benefit of treatment [11], but do impact on the use of tamoxifen for chemoprevention. Profound target site-specific actions of tamoxifen on the uterus in the recent overview [11] recapitulate and confirm the translational research with tamoxifen completed in the 1980s [12, 13] with the recognition of a small but significant increase in the incidence of endometrial cancer in postmenopausal women treated with tamoxifen. This finding eventually resulted in the paradigm shift away from tamoxifen to new opportunities, but this advances our story too quickly. In the 1980s, tamoxifen was the only medicine available for testing therapeutic and chemopreventive strategies with SERMs in the 1990s. The clinical community advanced with a responsibility to weigh risks and benefits in clinical trials to ensure the safety and long-term health of women at risk for breast cancer.

The treatment trials database and translational research were essential to address the hypothesis that tamoxifen, a nonsteroidal antiestrogen, could effectively block

Selective Action of Tamoxifen

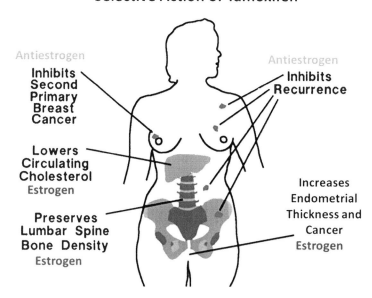

Fig. 7.1 Selective action of tamoxifen in target tissues. Tamoxifen is a SERM and has antiestrogenic action in the breast, but estrogenic properties in the bone, endometrium

the genesis and growth of ER-positive breast cancer but would be ineffective against the growth of ER-negative disease. Nevertheless in the 1980s, estrogen was also considered to be an essential component of women's health by maintaining bone density and preventing coronary heart disease. Thus, if tamoxifen, an antiestrogen, prevented the development and growth of ER-positive breast cancer in half a dozen high-risk women per year per thousand [14], hundreds of other women in the selected population might subsequently develop osteoporosis and coronary heart disease. The intervention with tamoxifen would be detrimental to public health. The good news was tamoxifen was not an antiestrogen everywhere; it was the lead compound of the drug group that selectively modulated ER target tissues around the body (Fig. 7.1). The original work (described in Chap. 5) to investigate the target site pharmacology of tamoxifen in the laboratory was to provide a database with which to predict clinical outcomes and safety for future chemoprevention trials. This discovery ultimately facilitated the development of a new strategy for the utilization of new SERMs as chemopreventives in breast cancer.

Prevention of Mammary Cancer in Rodents

The expanding literature on the prevention of rodent mammary cancer was used to support the clinical use of tamoxifen to prevent breast cancer. As mentioned earlier, Lacassagne predicted that a therapeutic intervention could be developed that would "prevent or antagonize the congestion of estrone in the breast." Unfortunately, no therapeutic agent was available and all his predictions were based upon the known effect of early oophorectomy on the development of mammary cancer in high-incidence strains of mice [1]. Clearly, the indiscriminate oophorectomy of young women would be an inappropriate intervention. The animal studies with tamoxifen were undertaken for two reasons: first, to establish the efficacy of tamoxifen in well-described models of carcinogenesis and, second, to discover whether tamoxifen would always be an inhibitor or whether the drug would ever exacerbate tumorigenesis. Two animal model systems were used extensively: the carcinogen-induced rat mammary carcinoma model and mouse mammary tumor virus (MMTV)-infected strains of mice.

The mammary carcinogens 7,12-dimethylbenz[α]anthracene (DMBA) [15] and N-nitrosomethylurea (NMU) [16] induce tumors in young female rats. The timing of the carcinogenic insult is very important, because as the animals age they become resistant to the mammary carcinogens. Tumorigenesis does not occur in oophorectomized animals, and the sooner oophorectomy is performed after the carcinogenic insult, the more effective it is in preventing the development of tumors [17].

The administration of tamoxifen to carcinogen-treated rats prevents the initiation of carcinogenesis, and animals remain tumor-free [18, 19]. The short-term administration of tamoxifen at different times after the carcinogenic insult is effective in reducing the number of tumors that develop [20, 21], although most animals develop at least one tumor after therapy is stopped.

Continuous tamoxifen therapy that is started at 1 month after the administration of carcinogens completely inhibits the appearance of mammary tumors [22, 23]. Under these circumstances, tamoxifen is preventing promotion and suppressing the appearance of occult disease. In fact, if treatment is stopped prematurely (i.e., a 3–4-month duration of therapy), the microfoci of transformed cells grow into palpable tumors. Because the timing of initiation in human breast cancer is unknown, and unlike the laboratory model not all women will develop tumors, tamoxifen will be given to target populations to suppress, and there is expectation that this will reverse the promotional effects of estrogen during carcinogenesis. Lacassagne performed his pioneering mammary tumor experiments linking estrogen with carcinogens in the high-risk mouse [24], so this was another model to use.

Until 1989, there was a paucity of information about the efficacy of tamoxifen to inhibit mouse mammary tumorigenesis. This was true in part because tamoxifen is estrogenic in short-term tests in oophorectomized [25] and immature mice [26]. However, the finding that long-term tamoxifen therapy renders the oophorectomized mouse vagina [27] and athymic mouse uterus [12] refractory to estrogenic stimuli prompted a reconsideration of the value of tamoxifen as a preventive in mouse mammary tumor models.

High-incidence strains of mice that develop mammary tumors are infected with MMTV, which is transferred to the offspring in the mothers' milk [28]. Tumorigenesis appears to be ovarian dependent, because the highest incidence of tumors appears in females, and tumorigenesis can be delayed or prevented depending upon the age at oophorectomy [29]. Steroid hormones activate the pro-viral MMTV [30], which in turn can initiate an increase in growth factors from the viral integration site Int. 2 [31]. Promotion of the initiated cells with steroid hormones and prolactin then completes tumorigenesis.

Long-term tamoxifen therapy, after an early cycle of pregnancy and weaning to facilitate early tumorigenesis, is equivalent to an ovariectomy performed at 4 months in reducing tumorigenesis to 50 % at 14 months of age. However, tamoxifen is superior to oophorectomy, even after therapy is stopped, because ovariectomized animals continue to develop tumors, whereas animals previously treated with tamoxifen do not develop any more tumors [32].

We followed up on initial observations with an investigation of tumorigenesis in virgin mice. In this study design, mice develop mammary tumors during their second year of life. Again, long-term tamoxifen therapy started at 3 months of age is superior to oophorectomy at 3 months. Fifty percent of the oophorectomized animals develop tumors by the third year of life, whereas 90 % of tamoxifen-treated mice remain tumor-free [33]. These studies are illustrated in Fig. 7.2.

Overall, the results of the studies in the mouse model are particularly interesting because they changed our view of the interspecies pharmacology of tamoxifen. Long-term treatment with tamoxifen results in an initial classification of tamoxifen as an estrogen, but within a few weeks the pharmacology changes and tamoxifen becomes an antiestrogen. An understanding of this process was seen to have important implications for the long-term use of tamoxifen as an adjuvant therapy and a preventive.

Tamoxifen: The First SERM for the Prevention of Breast Cancer in High-Risk Populations

Forty years ago, tamoxifen was shown to prevent the induction [18] and promotion [20] of carcinogen-induced mammary cancer in rats. Similarly, tamoxifen was also shown to prevent the development of mammary cancer induced by ionizing radiation in rats [34]. These laboratory observations, coupled with the emerging preliminary clinical observation that adjuvant tamoxifen could prevent contralateral breast cancer in women [35], provided a rationale for Dr. Trevor Powles, who, in 1986, established the vanguard study at the Royal Marsden Hospital in England to test whether tamoxifen could prevent breast cancer in high-risk women [36].

During the 1990s, much progress was achieved to answer the question: "Does tamoxifen have worth in the prevention of breast cancer in select high-risk women?" The results of four international trials that address this question—the Royal Marsden study, the NSABP/NCI study, the Italian study, and the IBIS trial—have been reported. These data will be presented in detail as well as their subsequent updates in the past decade. A summary of trial characteristics and findings are presented in Table 7.1.

Fig. 7.2 The ability of long-term tamoxifen treatment or ovariectomy on the development of the mammary tumors in virgin C3H/OUJ mice. Long-term tamoxifen therapy is more effective as a chemopreventive than ovariectomy

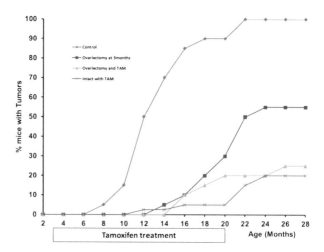

Table 7.1 Comparison of the characteristics of various breast cancer treatment trials

Characteristic	NSABP	Royal Marsden	Italian	IBIS
Sample size	13,388	2,471	5,408	7,152
Women years of follow-up	46,858	12,355	5,408	29,800
Participants <50	40 %	62 %	36 %	52 %
Breast cancer incidence per 1,000				
Placebo	6.7	5.5	2.3	6.7
Tamoxifen	3.4	4.7	2.1	4.7

Royal Marsden Study

Powles and coworkers recruited 2,484 women aged 30–70 to a placebo-controlled trial using 20 mg of tamoxifen daily for up to 8 years. Women were eligible if their risk of breast cancer was increased due to family history. Each participant had at least one first-degree relative with breast cancer under age 50; or a first-degree relative affected at any age, plus an additional affected first- or second-degree relative; or a first-degree relative with bilateral breast cancer. Women with a history of benign breast biopsy and an affected first-degree relative of any age were also eligible. Women with a history of venous thrombosis, any previous malignancy, or an estimated life expectancy of fewer than 10 years were excluded [37, 38]. A total of 2,494 women consented to participate in the study, and 23 were excluded from final analysis due to the presence of preexisting ductal carcinoma in situ (DCIS) or invasive breast carcinoma [38]. The trial was undertaken to evaluate the problems of accrual, acute symptomatic toxicity, compliance, and safety as a basis for subsequent large national, multicenter trials designed to test whether tamoxifen can prevent breast cancer. However, the trial has also been analyzed for breast cancer incidence [38].

Acute symptomatic toxicity was low for participants on tamoxifen or placebo, and compliance remained correspondingly high: 77 % of women on tamoxifen and 82 % of women on placebo remained on medication at 5 years, as predicted. There was a significant increase in hot flashes (34 % vs. 20 %), mostly in premenopausal women (P < 0.005); vaginal discharge (16 % vs. 4 %; P < 0.005); and menstrual irregularities (14 % vs. 9 %; P < 0.005), respectively. At the most recent follow-up, 320 women had discontinued tamoxifen and 176 had discontinued placebo prior to the study's completion (P < 0.005).

Until their report in 1994 [37], the Marsden group observed no thromboembolic episodes; a detailed analysis of other coagulation parameters in a sequential subset of women also found no significant changes in protein S, protein C, or cross-linked fibrinogen degradation products. At 70 months, no significant difference in the incidence of deep vein thrombosis or pulmonary embolism was observed between groups. A significant fall in total plasma cholesterol occurred within 3 months and was sustained over 5 years of treatment [39–41]. The decrease affected low-density lipoprotein, with no change in apolipoproteins A and B or high-density lipoprotein cholesterol.

In contrast, tamoxifen exerted antiestrogenic or estrogenic effects on bone density, depending on menopausal status. In premenopausal women, early findings demonstrated a small but significant (P < 0.05) loss of bone in both the lumbar spine and hip at 3 years [41]. In contrast, postmenopausal women had increased bone mineral density in the spine (P < 0.005) and hip (P < 0.001) compared to nontreated women.

Finally, the Marsden group made an extensive study of gynecological complications associated with tamoxifen treatment in healthy women. Since ovarian and uterine assessment by transvaginal ultrasound became available sometime after the trial's start, many subjects did not have a baseline evaluation. Ovarian screening demonstrated a significantly increased risk (P < 0.005) of detecting benign ovarian cysts in premenopausal women who had received tamoxifen for more than 3 months compared to controls. There were no changes in ovarian appearance in postmenopausal women [37]. A careful examination of the uterus with transvaginal ultrasonography using color Doppler imaging in women taking tamoxifen showed that the organ was usually larger; moreover, women with histological abnormalities had significantly thicker endometria [42]. Of particular interest in this regard was the observation that 20 mg of tamoxifen daily exerted a time-dependent proliferation of the endometrium in premenopausal and early postmenopausal women. This effect appeared to be mediated by the stromal component, since no cases of cancer or even epithelial hyperplasia were observed among the tamoxifen-treated group in the Italian study with 33 women [43].

Although the vanguard study has provided invaluable information about the biological effects of tamoxifen in healthy women, the trial was not designed to answer the question of whether tamoxifen prevents breast cancer. In spite of this, an analysis of breast cancer incidence was reported at a median follow-up of 70 months, when 42 % of the participants had completed therapy or withdrawn [38]. During the study, 336 women on tamoxifen and 305 on placebo received hormone-replacement

Fig. 7.3 The study design for the NSABP/NCI P-1 trial. On the *left* are the risk factors, according to the Gail model of breast cancer risk assessment based on which the participants of the study were selected

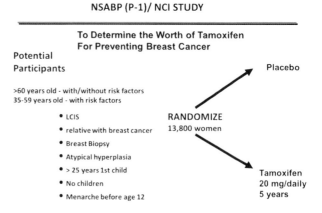

therapy. No difference in the incidence of breast cancer was observed between the groups. There were 34 carcinomas in the tamoxifen group and 36 in the placebo group-a relative risk of 1.06. Of the 70 cancers, only 8 were ductal carcinoma in situ. An analysis of the subset of women on hormone-replacement therapy did not demonstrate an interaction with tamoxifen treatment.

NSABP/NCI P-1 Study

This study opened in the United States and Canada in May of 1992 with an accrual goal of 16,000 women to be recruited at 100 North American sites. It closed after accruing 13,338 in 1997 due to the high-risk status of the participants. The study design is illustrated in Fig. 7.3. Those eligible for entry included any woman over the age of 60 or women between the ages of 35 and 59 whose 5-year risk of developing breast cancer, as predicted by the Gail model [14], was equal to that of a 60-year-old woman. Additionally, any woman over age 35 with a diagnosis of lobular carcinoma in situ (LCIS) treated by biopsy alone was eligible for entry to the study. In the absence of LCIS, the risk factors necessary to enter the study varied with age, such that a 35-year-old woman must have had a relative risk (RR) of 5.07, whereas the required RR for a 45-year-old woman was 1.79. Routine endometrial biopsies to evaluate the incidence of endometrial carcinoma in both arms of the study were also performed.

The breast cancer risk of women enrolled in the study was extremely high, with no age group having an RR of less than 4—including the over-60s group. Recruitment was also balanced, with about one-third younger than 50 years, one-third between 50 and 60 years, and one-third older than 60 years. Secondary end points of the study included the effect of tamoxifen on the incidence of fractures and cardiovascular deaths. Most importantly, the study planned to provide the first information about the role of genetic markers in the etiology of breast cancer. It was hoped to establish whether tamoxifen has a role to play in the treatment of women who are found to carry somatic mutations in the BRCA-1 gene. This did not occur as the number of patients with BRCA-1/2 mutations was not significant in the population [44].

The first results of the NSABP study were reported in September 1998, after a mean follow-up of 47.7 months [45]. There were a total of 368 invasive and noninvasive breast cancers in the participants: 124 in the tamoxifen group and 224 in the placebo group. A 49 % reduction in the risk of invasive breast cancer was seen in the tamoxifen group, and a 50 % reduction in the risk of noninvasive breast cancer was observed. A subset analysis of women at risk due to a diagnosis of LCIS demonstrated a 56 % reduction in this group. The most dramatic reduction was seen in women at risk due to atypical hyperplasia, where risk was reduced by 86 %.

The benefits of tamoxifen were observed in all age groups, with a relative risk of breast cancer ranging from 0.45 in women aged 60 and older to 0.49 for those in the 50- through 59-year-old age group, and 0.56 for women aged 49 and younger. A benefit for tamoxifen was also observed for women with all levels of breast cancer risk within the study, indicating that the benefits of tamoxifen are not confined to a particular lower risk or higher risk subset. Benefits were observed in women at risk on the basis of family history and those whose risk was due to other factors.

As expected, the effect of tamoxifen occurred on the incidence of ER-positive tumors, which were reduced by 69 % per year. The rate of ER-negative tumors in the tamoxifen group (1.46 per 1,000 women) did not significantly differ from the placebo group (1.20 per 1,000 women). Tamoxifen reduced the rate of invasive cancers of all sizes, but the greatest difference between the groups was the incidence of tumors 2.0 cm or less. Tamoxifen also reduced the incidence of both node-positive and node-negative breast cancer. The beneficial effects of tamoxifen were observed for each year of follow-up in the study. After year 1, the risk was reduced by 33 % and, in year 5, by 69 %.

Tamoxifen also reduced the incidence of osteoporotic fractures of the hip, spine, and radius by 19 %. However, the difference approached, but did not reach, statistical significance. This reduction was greatest in women aged 50 and older at study entry. No difference in the risk of myocardial infarction, angina, coronary artery bypass grafting, or angioplasty was noted between groups.

The study confirmed the association between tamoxifen and endometrial carcinoma (Figs. 7.4 and 7.5). The relative risk of endometrial cancer in the tamoxifen group was 2.5. The increased risk was seen in women aged 50 and older, whose relative risk was 4.01 (Fig. 7.5). There was no significance in the incidence of endometrial carcinoma in tamoxifen- or placebo-treated premenopausal women. All endometrial cancers in the tamoxifen group were grade 1 and none of the women on tamoxifen died of endometrial cancer. There was 1 endometrial cancer death in the placebo group. Although there is no doubt that tamoxifen increases the risk of endometrial cancer, it is important to recognize that this increase translates to an incidence of 2.3 women per 1,000 per year who develop endometrial carcinoma. More women in the tamoxifen group developed deep vein thrombosis (DVT) than in the placebo group (Fig. 7.6). Again, this excess risk was confined to women

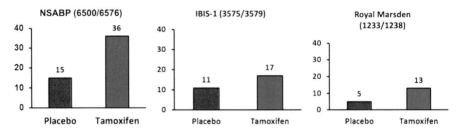

Fig. 7.4 The correlation between the increase in endometrial carcinoma incidence and tamoxifen treatment. In all three clinical trials show an increase in the incidence of endometrial carcinomas in tamoxifen-treated cohorts

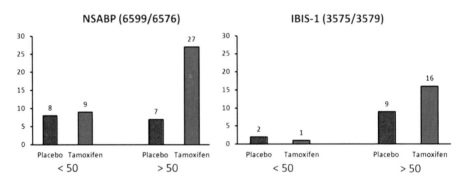

Fig. 7.5 The correlation between increase of endometrial carcinoma incidence and the age of the patient. The results of all three clinical trials showed that the increase in endometrial carcinoma significant incidence occurred in postmenopausal patients (>50 years of age) treated with tamoxifen in comparison to premenopausal patients (<50 years of age)

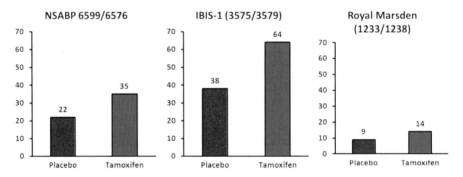

Fig. 7.6 Incidence of deep vein thrombosis (*DVT*) is significantly increased in tamoxifen-treated patients

aged 50 and older. The relative risk of DVT in the older age group was 1.71. (95 % CI 0.85–3.58). An increase in pulmonary emboli was also seen in the older women taking tamoxifen, with a relative risk of approximately 3 (Fig. 7.7). Three deaths

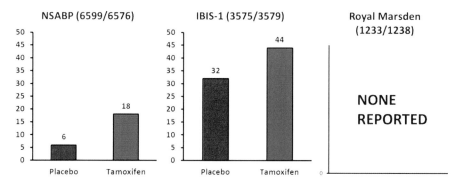

Fig. 7.7 Incidence of pulmonary embolism is increased in tamoxifen-treated patients. Observed in NSABP/P-1 and IBIS trials, but none were reported in the Royal Marsden trials

from pulmonary emboli occurred in the tamoxifen arm, but all were in women with significant comorbidities. An increased incidence of stroke (RR 1.75) was also seen in the tamoxifen group, but this did not reach statistical significance.

An assessment of the incidence of cataract formation was made using patient self-report. A small increase in cataracts was noted in the tamoxifen group—a rate of 24.8 women per 1,000 compared to 21.7 in the placebo group. There was also an increased risk of cataract surgery in the women on tamoxifen. These differences were marginally, statistically significant, and observed in the older patients in the study. This finding emphasizes the ocular safety of tamoxifen first predicted by Harper and Walpole in the 1960s [25], but as will be seen in Chap. 8, raloxifene does not have this effect. These findings emphasize the need to assess the patient's overall health status before making a decision to use tamoxifen for breast cancer risk reduction.

An assessment of quality of life showed no difference in depression scores between groups [46]. Hot flashes were noted in 81 % of the women on tamoxifen compared to 69 % of the placebo group, and the tamoxifen-associated hot flashes appeared to be of greater severity than those in the placebo group. Moderately bothersome or severe vaginal discharge was reported by 29 % of the women in tamoxifen group and 13 % in the placebo group [47]. No differences in the occurrence of irregular menses, nausea, fluid retention, skin changes, or weight gain or loss were reported.

Italian Study

The third tamoxifen prevention study, performed in Italy, began in October 1992 and randomized 5,408 women aged 35–70 to 20 mg of tamoxifen daily for 5 years [48]. Women were required to have had a hysterectomy for a nonneoplastic condition to obviate concerns about an increased risk of endometrial carcinoma.

There was no requirement that participants be at risk for breast cancer development, and in fact, those who underwent premenopausal oophorectomy with hysterectomy actually had a slightly reduced risk of breast cancer development. Women with endometriosis, cardiac disease, and deep venous thrombosis were excluded from the study. Although 5,408 women were randomized into this study, 1,422 withdrew and only 149 completed 5 years of treatment.

The incidence of breast cancer did not differ between groups, with 19 cases in the tamoxifen group and 22 in the placebo group. Tumor characteristics, including size, grade, lymph node status, and receptor status, also did not differ between groups.

The incidence of thrombophlebitis was increased in the tamoxifen group. A total of 64 events were reported, 38 in the tamoxifen group and 18 in the placebo group (P = 0.0053). However, 42 of these were superficial phlebitis.

No differences in the incidence of cerebrovascular ischemic events were observed [48].

In 2003, a brief communication was published on the Italian Study that also compared the effectiveness of tamoxifen in cohorts of women who were using hormone-replacement therapy (HRT) or not. The results showed no significant difference between women taking tamoxifen or placebo in women who never used HRT and were in low-risk group (P = 0.44), and among women in the same cohort but in the high-risk group, there was a nonsignificant difference in favor of tamoxifen (P = 0.099). In the cohort of women that have used HRT during the trial and were in the low-risk group, there was also no statistically significant difference in women taking tamoxifen or placebo (P = 0.31); however, in the high-risk group there was a significant difference in favor of tamoxifen (P = 0.009).

The International Breast Cancer Intervention Study (IBIS-I)

The IBIS-I trial was a double-blind placebo-controlled randomized trial of tamoxifen [49]. Women at high risk (7,152) of breast cancer, between ages of 35 and 7 years were randomized into two groups. Women were randomized either into the placebo group (3,574) or women treated with 20 mg daily tamoxifen (3,578). A total of 13 patients were excluded from the study, and the remaining were followed up for 5 years. The primary outcome measure was the incidence of breast cancer. After a median 50-month follow-up, 69 breast cancer cases were reported in the 5,378 women group treated with tamoxifen, and 101 cases in the 3,566 women placebo group, thus indicating a 32 % reduction (P = 0.013). Endometrial cancer was increased not significantly (11 vs. 2, P = 0.2) (Fig. 7.4), and thromboembolic events were significantly increased in the tamoxifen-treated group (43 vs. 17, P = 0.001) (Fig. 7.7). Based on these results, the authors concluded that preventive administration of tamoxifen is contradicted in women at high risk of thromboembolic disease. Tamoxifen should be stopped as an antithrombotic measure after surgeries or immobilization. However, tamoxifen does reduce the incidence of breast cancer by about a third, and non-breast-cancer causes of death are not increased by tamoxifen [49].

Follow-Up of Chemoprevention Studies with Tamoxifen

The main result from all the studies is that once tamoxifen is stopped, the antitumor effects sustained, systemic symptomology disappears, but the major side effect of an increase in endometrial cancer continues to accumulate in postmenopausal women [50–52]. Again it is tempting to speculate that the nascent breast cancer have been altered to survive in an environment of continuous tamoxifen, acquired resistance evolves, and then a woman's own estrogen causes apoptosis and tumoricidal actions in the "prepared" breast cancer cells after tamoxifen is stopped. This concept is discussed in detail in Chap. 9.

Tamoxifen again became a pioneering medicine but this time as the first drug to be FDA approved to reduce the risk of developing cancer, specifically ER-positive breast cancer. However, the translational research on endometrial cancer risk with tamoxifen [12, 53] demanded a safer solution to chemoprevention with SERMs. A strategy was already in place (Chap. 5) to move forward the first SERM to prevent osteoporosis and prevent breast cancer at the same time without the risk of endometrial cancer being increased. Keoxifene, the failed breast cancer drug, became raloxifene.

Two Approaches to the Chemoprevention of Breast Cancer

The successful clinical completion of the chemoprevention studies in women at high risk of developing breast cancer during the late 1990s resulted in FDA approval of tamoxifen for risk reduction in pre- and postmenopausal women in 1998. Despite reservations about tamoxifen and its toxicology (Chap. 6) for chemoprevention, the drug remains a cheap and lifesaving drug for the treatment of breast cancer worldwide. The data of endometrial cancer, deep vein thrombosis, and pulmonary embolism appear mainly in postmenopausal women [50]. However, the drug has both efficacy and an excellent safety profile in premenopausal women.

A recent review of the literature [54] concluded that "the risk of endometrial cancer, deep vein thrombosis and pulmonary embolism is low in women <50 years who take tamoxifen for breast cancer prevention. The risk decreases from the active to follow-up phase of treatment. Education and counseling are the cornerstones of breast cancer chemoprevention."

Nevertheless, despite the safety issues being low in premenopausal women, no other country has approved tamoxifen for chemoprevention in women with a high risk of developing breast cancer. However, the National Institute of Clinical

Excellence in the UK recommended tamoxifen be offered to reduce the incidence
of breast cancer in high risk women through the National Health Service in the UK
in early 2013.

Chemoprevention of breast cancer did, however, expanded dramatically
throughout the 1990s based upon the laboratory work conducted with the discovery
of selective estrogenic and antiestrogenic actions of estrogen target sites around the
body. This work at the Wisconsin Clinical Cancer Center (Chap. 5) would subsequently be known in the literature as selective ER modulation. The strategic view
described earlier (Chap. 5) was further refined to create a roadmap for drug
development by the pharmaceutical industry. Simply stated, the proposal was to
develop multifunctional medicines to aim at reducing the morbidity and mortality
of a major disease affecting millions of women after menopause but, at the same
time, reducing the risk of breast cancer. In 1990, this proposal was published in
Cancer Research, the flagship journal of the American Association for Cancer
Research [7]. This was the B.F. Cain Memorial Lecture for laboratory advances
in cancer research that were having therapeutic impact in clinical applications and
refined the original SERM concept (Chap. 5).

> We have obtained valuable clinical information about this group of drugs that can be
> applied in other disease states. Research does not travel in straight lines, and observations in
> one field of science often become major discoveries in another. Important clues have been
> garnered about the effects of tamoxifen on bone and lipids; it is possible that derivatives
> could find targeted applications to retard osteoporosis or atherosclerosis. The ubiquitous
> application of novel compounds to prevent diseases associated with the progressive
> changes after menopause may, as a side effect, significantly retard the development of
> breast cancer. The target population would be postmenopausal women in general, thereby
> avoiding the requirement to select a high-risk group to prevent breast cancer.

Raloxifene: Abandoned and Resurrected

Raloxifene, originally called keoxifene, was first reported by scientists at Eli Lilly,
Indianapolis, to be an antiestrogen with a high affinity for the estrogen receptor
(ER) [55]. Much like its earlier analog, LY117018, raloxifene has only mild
estrogen-like properties in the uterus [56].In fact, at very high doses, LY117018
can even block the antiuterotropic effects of a variety of steroidal and nonsteroidal
compounds in the rat [57]. The drug has antitumor effects in the rat, but is less
potent than tamoxifen [23, 58]. Although the original direction for raloxifene's
clinical development was breast cancer therapy, Eli Lilly chose to abandon this
approach toward the end of the 1980s. However, the discovery that raloxifene might
prevent osteoporosis, [59] prevent breast cancer, [23] and, at the same time, have
minor estrogen-like effects in the uterus laid the foundation for the subsequent
confirmation of bone data in animals [56]. These discoveries also led to the
completion of clinical trials that demonstrated maintenance of bone density in
postmenopausal women at risk for osteoporosis [60].

Table 7.2 The Raloxifene Oncology Advisory Committee formed by Eli Lilly

The Raloxifene Oncology Advisory Committee[a]
Alberto Costa, M.D.—European Institute for Oncology, Milan (Breast Surgeon, Co-PI Italian Tamoxifen Prevention Trial)
V. Craig Jordan, Ph.D., D.Sc.—Northwestern University Medical School, Chicago (Committee Chairperson)
Marc E. Lippman, M.D.—Georgetown University Medical School, Washington DC (Director, Lombardi Comprehensive Cancer Center)
Monica Morrow, M.D.—Northwestern University Medical School, Chicago (Breast Surgeon, Director, Lynn Sage Breast Cancer Program)
Larry Norton, M.D.—Memorial Sloan-Kettering Cancer Center, New York (Head, Division of Oncology)
Trevor J. Powels, FRCP, Ph.D.—Royal Marsden Hospital, London (Medical Oncologist, PI Royal Marsden, Tamoxifen Prevention Study)

[a]Responsible for the evaluation and adjudication of breast cancer cases in the 10,533 patients participating in randomized, placebo-controlled trials to prevent osteoporosis

As part of a safety profile for any estrogen-like drug for the prevention of osteoporosis, raloxifene had to be evaluated for breast safety. To this end, Eli Lilly organized an independent oncology advisory committee to adjudicate all breast cancers diagnosed in the randomized, placebo-controlled trials for the prevention of osteoporosis. The committee (Table 7.2) was assembled to provide expertise in diagnosis, breast cancer prevention, and breast medical oncology. Committee members met every 6 months to review pathology, mammograms, and patient records to determine whether disease was preexisting at the time of entry to the trial and whether the cancer was invasive or noninvasive. All patients who developed breast cancer in all trials were adjudicated blind, and the results were then collated and analyzed by Biostatistician Steven Eckert of Eli Lilly.

The pivotal registration trial to establish the efficacy and value of raloxifene for the treatment and prevention of osteoporosis was called Multiple Outcomes of Raloxifene Evaluation (MORE) [61]. The MORE trial was a randomized double-blind trial that recruited 7,705 postmenopausal women (mean age 66.5 years) with osteoporosis defined as prior vertebral fractures or femoral neck or a spine T score 2.5SD or more below that of non-osteoporotic women. Participants were randomized to placebo or two raloxifene treatment groups: 60 or 120 mg daily.

Based on the positive results from the MORE trial, raloxifene is currently FDA approved for the prevention of osteoporosis. Raloxifene, 60 mg daily, produces a 1–2 % increase in postmenopausal bone density—an increase equivalent to that noted with tamoxifen. Raloxifene also reduces fractures by about 30–40 %. In addition, raloxifene is also approved to prevent osteoporosis in Europe and in more than a dozen other countries.

As part of the evaluation of osteoporosis in the MORE trial, there were several preplanned additional outcomes measures: histologically confirmed breast cancer, transvaginal ultrasonography to evaluate uterine effects of raloxifene in 1,781 randomly chosen participants, and an assessment of DVT and pulmonary embolism by chart review.

The MORE trial, analyzed at 3 years of follow-up, documented 27 cases of breast cancer in the control (2,576 women) but only a total of 13 cases in these treated with raloxifene (5,129 women). In other words, 126 women would need to be treated to prevent osteoporosis to prevent one case of breast cancer: the original hypothesis and roadmap [7, 62] was valid [63]!

Most importantly, the decrease in the risk of breast cancer was confined to ER-positive disease; there was a 90 % decrease in ER-positive breast cancer but no change in ER-negative breast cancer. Unlike previous experience with tamoxifen in postmenopausal women, there was no increase in the risk of endometrial cancer during raloxifene treatment. However, there was a threefold increase in venous thrombotic disease equivalent to that reported for both tamoxifen and estrogen in postmenopausal women. It is recommended that raloxifene, tamoxifen, or estrogen replacement is not taken by women with a history of thromboembolic disorders. The analysis of the MORE trail for breast cancer incidences at 3 years was confirmed with a 4 years reanalysis [64], demonstrating a 72 % decrease in the incidence of invasive breast cancer compared to placebo. The decision was made to revise and extend the MORE trial with Continuing Outcomes Relevant to Evista (CORE) trial.

During the 8 years of the MORE/CORE trials, the incidence of invasive breast cancer and ER-positive breast cancer was reduced by 66 % and 76 % respectively with no increase in the risk of endometrial cancer ($P < 0$), no endometrial hyperplasia ($P > 0.99$), and no vaginal bleeding ($P = 0.087$).

However, the fact that raloxifene was proven to reduce the risk of breast cancer but not increase the risk of endometrial cancer mandated that tamoxifen (the FDA-approved standard of care) and raloxifene must be tested head to head in postmenopausal women at high risk for the prevention of breast cancer.

The scene was now set for the NCI/NSAP P-2 study to go forward in high-risk postmenopausal women that would put tamoxifen versus raloxifene with a primary end point: the prevention of breast cancer. No placebo arm was recruited as it was considered unethical not to use tamoxifen, the approved drug of choice known to reduce the risk of breast cancer by 50 %.

However, wisely, the MORE trial was simultaneously extended out to 8 years of raloxifene treatment for women at risk for osteoporosis. All women who volunteered to continue on raloxifene (60 mg daily) had previously taken either 60 or 120 mg raloxifene. A total of 3,510 women were in the raloxifene are compared to 1,703 women in placebo arm [65]. During the CORE trial invasive breast cancer was decreased by 59 % and ER-positive breast cancer by 66 % compared to placebo. Overall, for the continued MORE/CORE trial, invasive breast cancer was reduced by 66 % and ER-positive breast cancer by 76 %.

Although the study of long-term raloxifene in the MORE/CORE trail was necessary because the treatment and prevention of osteoporosis requires continuous treatment (no drug - no benefit), the data was to be important once the results of the STAR trail were evaluated (Chap. 8).

Conclusion

In the 20 years between the 1990s and 2010, not one but two agents were shown to reduce the incidence of invasive breast cancer in postmenopausal women at high risk to develop the disease. Raloxifene was approved for the prevention of osteoporosis in high-risk women with a dramatic reduction in the incidence of breast cancer as a beneficial side effect. The side effect of endometrial cancer with tamoxifen was solved. Overall, a triumph for translational research, the creation of a roadmap to follow and a new drug group called the SERMs.

Postscript. The first study that I ever completed and presented at the International Steroid Hormone Congress in Mexico City in 1974 was on the prevention of rat mammary carcinogenesis with tamoxifen. Arthur Walpole and I had previously discussed the results and we both appreciated the significance of the data for women's health. But the idea and these data were 20 years too soon! Tamoxifen was not even FDA approved for the treatment of breast cancer until December 1977, and this was for metastatic breast cancer. There was a long way to go before the NCI would fund Dr. Fisher's NSABP trial and it would start in 1992. Over the years our Tamoxifen Teams provided most of the translational information about safety (endometrial cancer), strategies with long-term therapy and bone safety. The story of "who did what" in the laboratory at Wisconsin to "set the scene" for the exploitation of SERMs has been told in the Postscript to Chap. 5.

References

1. Lacassagne A (1936) Hormonal pathogenesis of adenocarcinoma of the breast. Am J Cancer 27:217–225
2. Jordan VC (2003) Tamoxifen: a most unlikely pioneering medicine. Nat Rev Drug Discov 2:205–213
3. Jordan VC (2006) Tamoxifen (ICI46,474) as a targeted therapy to treat and prevent breast cancer. Br J Pharmacol 147(Suppl 1):S269–S276
4. Scottish Cancer Trials Office (MRC), Edinburgh (1987) Adjuvant tamoxifen in the management of operable breast cancer: the Scottish Trial. Report from the Breast Cancer Trials Committee. Lancet 2:171–175
5. Fisher B, Costantino J, Redmond C et al (1989) A randomized clinical trial evaluating tamoxifen in the treatment of patients with node-negative breast cancer who have estrogen-receptor-positive tumors. N Engl J Med 320:479–484
6. Jordan VC (1984) Biochemical pharmacology of antiestrogen action. Pharmacol Rev 36:245–276
7. Lerner LJ, Jordan VC (1990) Development of antiestrogens and their use in breast cancer: eighth Cain memorial award lecture. Cancer Res 50:4177–4189
8. Jordan VC (2006) The science of selective estrogen receptor modulators: concept to clinical practice. Clin Cancer Res 12:5010–5013
9. Jordan VC (2007) Chemoprevention of breast cancer with selective oestrogen-receptor modulators. Nat Rev Cancer 7:46–53

10. Jordan VC (2009) A century of deciphering the control mechanisms of sex steroid action in breast and prostate cancer: the origins of targeted therapy and chemoprevention. Cancer Res 69:1243–1254
11. EBCTG (2011) Relevance of breast cancer hormone receptors and other factors to the efficacy of adjuvant tamoxifen: patient-level meta-analysis of randomised trials. Lancet 378:771–784
12. Gottardis MM, Robinson SP, Satyaswaroop PG, Jordan VC (1988) Contrasting actions of tamoxifen on endometrial and breast tumor growth in the athymic mouse. Cancer Res 48:812–815
13. Fornander T, Rutqvist LE, Cedermark B et al (1989) Adjuvant tamoxifen in early breast cancer: occurrence of new primary cancers. Lancet 1:117–120
14. Gail MH, Brinton LA, Byar DP et al (1989) Projecting individualized probabilities of developing breast cancer for white females who are being examined annually. J Natl Cancer Inst 81:1879–1886
15. Huggins C, Grand LC, Brillantes FP (1961) Mammary cancer induced by a single feeding of polymucular hydrocarbons, and its suppression. Nature 189:204–207
16. Gullino PM, Pettigrew HM, Grantham FH (1975) N-nitrosomethylurea as mammary gland carcinogen in rats. J Natl Cancer Inst 54:401–414
17. Dao TL (1962) The role of ovarian hormones in initiating the induction of mammary cancer in rats by polynuclear hydrocarbons. Cancer Res 22:973–981
18. Jordan VC (1976) Effect of tamoxifen (ICI 46,474) on initiation and growth of DMBA-induced rat mammary carcinomata. Eur J Cancer 12:419–424
19. Turcot-Lemay L, Kelly PA (1980) Characterization of estradiol, progesterone, and prolactin receptors in nitrosomethylurea-induced mammary tumors and effect of antiestrogen treatment on the development and growth of these tumors. Cancer Res 40:3232–3240
20. Jordan VC, Allen KE, Dix CJ (1980) Pharmacology of tamoxifen in laboratory animals. Cancer Treat Rep 64:745–759
21. Wilson AJ, Tehrani F, Baum M (1982) Adjuvant tamoxifen therapy for early breast cancer: an experimental study with reference to oestrogen and progesterone receptors. Br J Surg 69:121–125
22. Jordan VC (1983) Laboratory studies to develop general principles for the adjuvant treatment of breast cancer with antiestrogens: problems and potential for future clinical applications. Breast Cancer Res Treat 3(Suppl):S73–S86
23. Gottardis MM, Jordan VC (1987) Antitumor actions of keoxifene and tamoxifen in the N-nitrosomethylurea-induced rat mammary carcinoma model. Cancer Res 47:4020–4024
24. Lacassagne A (1955) Endocrine factors concerned in the genesis of experimental mammary carcinoma. J Endocrinol 13:ix–xviii
25. Harper MJ, Walpole AL (1967) A new derivative of triphenylethylene: effect on implantation and mode of action in rats. J Reprod Fertil 13:101–119
26. Terenius L (1971) Structure-activity relationships of anti-oestrogens with regard to interaction with 17-beta-oestradiol in the mouse uterus and vagina. Acta Endocrinol (Copenh) 66:431–447
27. Jordan VC (1975) Prolonged antioestrogenic activity of ICI 46, 474 in the ovariectomized mouse. J Reprod Fertil 42:251–258
28. Bittner JJ (1939) Relation of nursing to the extra-chromosomal theory of breast cancer in mice. Am J Cancer 35:90–97
29. Lathrop AE, Loeb L (1916) Further investigations on the origin of tumors in mice. III. On the part played by internal secretion in the spontaneous development of tumors. J Cancer Res 1:1–19
30. Hynes NE, Groner B, Michalides R (1984) Mouse mammary tumor virus: transcriptional control and involvement in tumorigenesis. Adv Cancer Res 41:155–184
31. Peters G, Brookes S, Placzek M et al (1989) A putative int domain for mouse mammary tumor virus on mouse chromosome 7 is a 5' extension of int-2. J Virol 63:1448–1450

32. Jordan VC, Lababidi MK, Mirecki DM (1990) Anti-oestrogenic and anti-tumour properties of prolonged tamoxifen therapy in C3H/OUJ mice. Eur J Cancer 26:718–721

33. Jordan VC, Lababidi MK, Langan-Fahey S (1991) Suppression of mouse mammary tumorigenesis by long-term tamoxifen therapy. J Natl Cancer Inst 83:492–496

34. Welsch CW, Goodrich-Smith M, Brown CK, Miglorie N, Clifton KH (1981) Effect of an estrogen antagonist (tamoxifen) on the initiation and progression of gamma-irradiation-induced mammary tumors in female Sprague–Dawley rats. Eur J Cancer Clin Oncol 17:1255–1258

35. Cuzick J, Baum M (1985) Tamoxifen and contralateral breast cancer. Lancet 2:282

36. Powles TJ, Hardy JR, Ashley SE et al (1989) A pilot trial to evaluate the acute toxicity and feasibility of tamoxifen for prevention of breast cancer. Br J Cancer 60:126–131

37. Powles TJ, Jones AL, Ashley SE et al (1994) The Royal Marsden Hospital pilot tamoxifen chemoprevention trial. Breast Cancer Res Treat 31:73–82

38. Powles T, Eeles R, Ashley S et al (1998) Interim analysis of the incidence of breast cancer in the Royal Marsden Hospital tamoxifen randomised chemoprevention trial. Lancet 352:98–101

39. Jones AL, Powles TJ, Treleaven JG et al (1992) Haemostatic changes and thromboembolic risk during tamoxifen therapy in normal women. Br J Cancer 66:744–747

40. Powles TJ, Tillyer CR, Jones AL et al (1990) Prevention of breast cancer with tamoxifen—an update on the Royal Marsden Hospital pilot programme. Eur J Cancer 26:680–684

41. Powles TJ, Hickish T, Kanis JA, Tidy A, Ashley S (1996) Effect of tamoxifen on bone mineral density measured by dual-energy x-ray absorptiometry in healthy premenopausal and post-menopausal women. J Clin Oncol 14:78–84

42. Kedar RP, Bourne TH, Powles TJ et al (1994) Effects of tamoxifen on uterus and ovaries of postmenopausal women in a randomised breast cancer prevention trial. Lancet 343:1318–1321

43. Decensi A, Fontana V, Bruno S et al (1996) Effect of tamoxifen on endometrial proliferation. J Clin Oncol 14:434–440

44. King MC, Wieand S, Hale K et al (2001) Tamoxifen and breast cancer incidence among women with inherited mutations in BRCA1 and BRCA2: National Surgical Adjuvant Breast and Bowel Project (NSABP-P1) Breast Cancer Prevention Trial. JAMA 286:2251–2256

45. Fisher B, Costantino JP, Wickerham DL et al (1998) Tamoxifen for prevention of breast cancer: report of the National Surgical Adjuvant Breast and Bowel Project P-1 Study. J Natl Cancer Inst 90:1371–1388

46. Ganz PA (2001) Impact of tamoxifen adjuvant therapy on symptoms, functioning, and quality of life. J Natl Cancer Inst Monogr 30:130–134

47. Day R, Ganz PA, Costantino JP et al (1999) Health-related quality of life and tamoxifen in breast cancer prevention: a report from the National Surgical Adjuvant Breast and Bowel Project P-1 Study. J Clin Oncol 17:2659–2669

48. Veronesi U, Maisonneuve P, Costa A et al (1998) Prevention of breast cancer with tamoxifen: preliminary findings from the Italian randomised trial among hysterectomised women. Italian Tamoxifen Prevention Study. Lancet 352:93–97

49. Cuzick J, Forbes J, Edwards R et al (2002) First results from the International Breast Cancer Intervention Study (IBIS-I): a randomised prevention trial. Lancet 360:817–824

50. Fisher B, Costantino JP, Wickerham DL et al (2005) Tamoxifen for the prevention of breast cancer: current status of the National Surgical Adjuvant Breast and Bowel Project P-1 study. J Natl Cancer Inst 97:1652–1662

51. Cuzick J, Forbes JF, Howell A (2006) Re: Tamoxifen for the prevention of breast cancer: current status of the National Surgical Adjuvant Breast and Bowel Project P-1 study. J Natl Cancer Inst 98:643, author reply 643–644

52. Powles TJ (1999) Re: Tamoxifen for prevention of breast cancer: report of the National Surgical Adjuvant Breast and Bowel Project P-1 Study. J Natl Cancer Inst 91:730

53. Jordan VC, Morrow M (1994) Should clinicians be concerned about the carcinogenic potential of tamoxifen? Eur J Cancer 30A:1714–1721

54. Iqbal J, Ginsburg OM, Wijeratne TD et al (2012) Endometrial cancer and venous thromboembolism in women under age 50 who take tamoxifen for prevention of breast cancer: a systematic review. Cancer Treat Rev 38:318–328
55. Black LJ, Jones CD, Falcone JF (1983) Antagonism of estrogen action with a new benzothiophene derived antiestrogen. Life Sci 32:1031–1036
56. Black LJ, Sato M, Rowley ER et al (1994) Raloxifene (LY139481 HCI) prevents bone loss and reduces serum cholesterol without causing uterine hypertrophy in ovariectomized rats. J Clin Invest 93:63–69
57. Jordan VC, Gosden B (1983) Inhibition of the uterotropic activity of estrogens and antiestrogens by the short acting antiestrogen LY117018. Endocrinology 113:463–468
58. Clemens JA, Bennett DR, Black LJ, Jones CD (1983) Effects of a new antiestrogen, keoxifene (LY156758), on growth of carcinogen-induced mammary tumors and on LH and prolactin levels. Life Sci 32:2869–2875
59. Jordan VC, Phelps E, Lindgren JU (1987) Effects of anti-estrogens on bone in castrated and intact female rats. Breast Cancer Res Treat 10:31–35
60. Delmas PD, Bjarnason NH, Mitlak BH et al (1997) Effects of raloxifene on bone mineral density, serum cholesterol concentrations, and uterine endometrium in postmenopausal women. N Engl J Med 337:1641–1647
61. Ettinger B, Black DM, Mitlak BH et al (1999) Reduction of vertebral fracture risk in postmenopausal women with osteoporosis treated with raloxifene: results from a 3-year randomized clinical trial. Multiple Outcomes of Raloxifene Evaluation (MORE) Investigators. JAMA 282:637–645
62. Jordan VC (1988) Chemosuppression of breast cancer with tamoxifen: laboratory evidence and future clinical investigations. Cancer Invest 6:589–595
63. Cummings SR, Eckert S, Krueger KA et al (1999) The effect of raloxifene on risk of breast cancer in postmenopausal women: results from the MORE randomized trial. Multiple Outcomes of Raloxifene Evaluation. JAMA 281:2189–2197
64. Cauley JA, Norton L, Lippman ME et al (2001) Continued breast cancer risk reduction in postmenopausal women treated with raloxifene: 4-year results from the MORE trial. Multiple outcomes of raloxifene evaluation. Breast Cancer Res Treat 65:125–134
65. Martino S, Cauley JA, Barrett-Connor E et al (2004) Continuing outcomes relevant to Evista: breast cancer incidence in postmenopausal osteoporotic women in a randomized trial of raloxifene. J Natl Cancer Inst 96:1751–1761

Chapter 8
Tamoxifen and Raloxifene Head to Head: The STAR Trial

Abstract The toxicological concern with the potential of tamoxifen to increase the incidence of endometrial cancer or hepatocellular carcinoma mandated a new approach to chemoprevention. The SERM raloxifene does not have the toxicological concern of tamoxifen and is approved for the treatment and prevention of osteoporosis but at the same time reduces breast cancer incidence. The Study of Tamoxifen and Raloxifene (STAR) demonstrated that the two SERMs were equivalent in reducing breast cancer incidence but raloxifene had a better safety profile. However, tamoxifen can reduce breast cancer incidence during therapy for 5 years, and this is maintained for at least a decade after treatment. In contrast, raloxifene must be given continuously.

The STAR trial recruitment and evaluation was unprecedented in the history of clinical cancer trials (Fig. 8.1). The STAR trial was a phase III, double-blind trial that screened 184,480 postmenopausal women (mean age 58.5 years) for a full year with breast cancer risk over 1.65 %, and 19,747 were subsequently randomized to receive either tamoxifen (20 mg daily) or raloxifene (60 mg daily) for 5 years (Fig. 8.2). The primary aim of the trial was to assess the occurrence of invasive breast cancer in postmenopausal high-risk women with raloxifene and compare the preventive efficacy with, by then an established drug, tamoxifen. The secondary aim was to establish the efficacy of raloxifene treatment, such as cardiovascular, bone density, and general toxicities. Three groups of women were eligible: postmenopausal women over 60, irrespective of their risk of breast cancer; postmenopausal women who were diagnosed previously with lobular carcinoma in situ (LCIS); and postmenopausal women between the ages of 35 and 59, who have a high risk of developing breast cancer based on the presence of a combination of risk factors. The risk factors were assessed by using a modified Gail model that was used in the NSABP/P-1 trial. The main risk factors included age; number of first-degree relatives who have been diagnosed with breast cancer; whether the woman has had any children and the age of the first delivery; history of biopsies, especially if the results have shown atypical hyperplasia; and the age of the woman's first menstrual period.

P.Y. Maximov et al., *Tamoxifen*, Milestones in Drug Therapy, 135
DOI 10.1007/978-3-0348-0664-0_8, © Springer Basel 2013

Fig. 8.1 STAR trial recruitment scheme. A total of 19,747 postmenopausal women were selected based on their eligibility to participate in the study

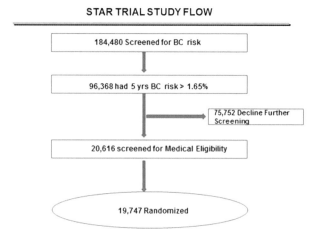

STAR TRIAL STUDY FLOW

184,480 Screened for BC risk

96,368 had 5 yrs BC risk > 1.65%

75,752 Decline Further Screening

20,616 screened for Medical Eligibility

19,747 Randomized

Fig. 8.2 STAR trial randomization scheme. A total of 19,747 selected women were randomized to be treated with either 20 mg of tamoxifen daily or 60 mg of raloxifene daily

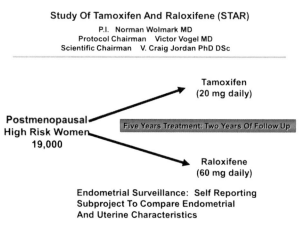

Study Of Tamoxifen And Raloxifene (STAR)
P.I. Norman Wolmark MD
Protocol Chairman   Victor Vogel MD
Scientific Chairman   V. Craig Jordan PhD DSc

Tamoxifen
(20 mg daily)

Postmenopausal
High Risk Women
19,000

Five Years Treatment: Two Years Of Follow Up

Raloxifene
(60 mg daily)

Endometrial Surveillance: Self Reporting
Subproject To Compare Endometrial
And Uterine Characteristics

A preplanned analysis was triggered when a total of 327 incidents of invasive breast cancers occurred. The trial was conducted beginning 1 July 1999 and was assessed at a cutoff date of 31 December 2005. The data reported initially were 6 years and 5 months after the STAR trial initiated recruitment [1].

There were a total of 168 invasive breast cancers in the raloxifene-treated group and 163 invasive breast cancers in the tamoxifen-treated group (Fig. 8.3). A control arm was not considered to be appropriate as tamoxifen was the FDA-approved medicine and the standard of care, but an estimate of invasive breast cancer in a hypothetical control arm based on the level of risk in an equivalent number of women not treated with a SERM was estimated at 312 (Fig. 8.3). Thus, both tamoxifen and raloxifene are producing about a 50 % decrease in breast cancer incidence. There were however fewer noninvasive breast cancer (57 cases) in the tamoxifen-treated group compared with the raloxifene-treated group (80 cases), but this was barely statistically significant (P = 0.052) (Fig. 8.4). However, a later

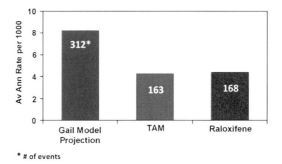

Fig. 8.3 The results of invasive breast cancer reduction in STAR trial. Raloxifene virtually was equivalent to tamoxifen in reducing the incidence of invasive breast cancer by 50 %, as compared to the projected untreated control. It was considered unethical to use untreated control as an approved breast cancer treatment with tamoxifen already was available at the time

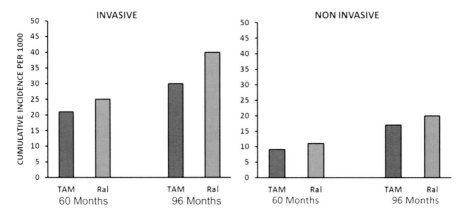

Fig. 8.4 Cumulative incidence of invasive breast cancer and noninvasive breast cancer in women treated with tamoxifen and raloxifene and followed up at 60 and 96 months post randomization

statistical study was initiated to assess the actual benefit/risk for breast cancer prevention for postmenopausal women [2]. The data were pooled from the Women's Health Initiative, STAR trial, and End Results Program and were used to develop a benefit/risk assessment index, which could be used for assessing the chemoprevention benefits with either raloxifene or tamoxifen. The results of the statistical analysis demonstrated that benefit/risk index was dependent on age, race, and history of hysterectomy. Postmenopausal women with no hysterectomy treated with raloxifene generally have better index than those treated with tamoxifen and so do premenopausal women with prior hysterectomy.

In contrast, there were fewer endometrial cancer (23 cases) in patients treated with raloxifene then those treated with tamoxifen (36 cases), though this does not reach statistical significance ($P < 0.07$) (Fig. 8.5). However, this is deceptive as tamoxifen has a fundamentally different effect on the uterus than raloxifene.

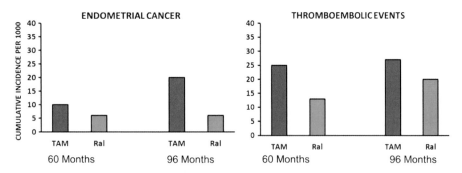

Fig. 8.5 Cumulative incidence of uterine cancers and thromboembolic events in women treated with either tamoxifen or raloxifene and followed up at 60 and 96 months post randomization

Table 8.1 The rates of developed cataracts and cataract surgeries during STAR trial. A total of 8,341 women were treated with tamoxifen and 8,336 were treated with raloxifene

Cataracts and cataract surgery	Events		Rate per 1,000	
	Tamoxifen	Raloxifene	Tamoxifen	Raloxifene
Developed cataracts	739	603	14.58	11.69
Cataracts followed by surgery	575	462	11.18	8.85

Women elected to have 244 hysterectomies on tamoxifen can be compared to 111 hysterectomies in patients taking raloxifene. Similarly, there were fewer thrombotic events (P = 0.01) (Fig. 8.5), cataracts (P = 0.002), and cataract surgeries (P = 0.03) in women being treated with raloxifene (Table 8.1).

Therefore, overall, tamoxifen and raloxifene are equivalent during the treatment phase, for reducing the risk of breast cancer in high-risk postmenopausal women, but raloxifene appears to have a better safety profile than tamoxifen during treatment. However, this is where the pharmacology becomes interesting.

A subsequent analysis of the STAR trial at 90 months after initiating recruitment was reported [3]. Interestingly, the efficacy of raloxifene and tamoxifen did not remain equivalent in the post treatment phase of the study. The 5-year "pulse" of tamoxifen treatment seemed to have changed the breast cancer tissue or changed the tumor environment so that even 5 years after the therapy cessation, the occurrence of breast cancer was still prevented [4]. Similar results were shown in animals, where the number of breast tumors in tamoxifen-treated rats never reached the same levels as in control animals [5]. The efficacy of raloxifene to reduce the incidence of invasive breast cancer decreases so that within 2–3 years after treatment, raloxifene only retain 76 % of the ability of tamoxifen to prevent the occurrence of invasive breast cancer in post treatment period. However, based on the Martino study [6], raloxifene should be considered as a continuous therapy and should not be stopped at 5 years.

Concerning safety with raloxifene, there was now a significant decrease in the incidence of endometrial cancers (P = 0.003), thrombotic events (P = 0.007),

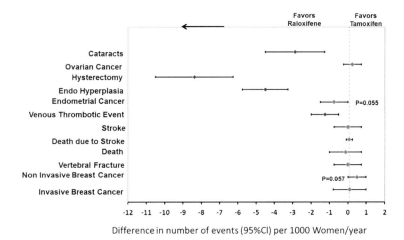

Fig. 8.6 Efficacy and important outcomes in favor of raloxifene and tamoxifen in the STAR trial

(Fig. 8.6) cataracts, and cataract operations (RR = 0.80; 95 % CI, 0.72–0.89 and RR = 0.79; 95 % CI, 0.70–0.90, respectively) (Fig. 8.6). As a summary of the efficacy and important outcomes of the STAR trial, Fig. 8.6 addresses outcomes in favor of either raloxifene or tamoxifen.

Raloxifene was approved by the FDA for the reductions of incidence of breast cancer in high-risk postmenopausal women and breast cancer in postmenopausal women with osteoporosis on 24 July 2007 (the day before my birthday - nice present!).

Postscript. During the past 40 years, the idea of preventing breast cancer in women at high risk for developing the disease has advanced from just that, an idea [7] to become a practical reality with not one but two FDA-approved medicines. Forty years ago, there was no tamoxifen, only ICI 46,474, a failed "morning-after pill" that was reinvented as an antiestrogen throughout the 1970s, and a strategy was established to enable progress to move forward in the clinic for both chemoprevention and long-term adjuvant therapy with an antihormonal agent [8]. Indeed, at that time, the word "chemoprevention" was not even in the English language. It was still for Michael Sporn to invent the idea of using chemicals to prevent cancer [9, 10] and establish the word chemoprevention. Raloxifene the failed "breast cancer drug" was conceptually reinvented as the first SERM to treat osteoporosis and prevent breast cancer at the University of Wisconsin Comprehensive Cancer Center.

At the start of the STAR trial, Dr. Norman Wolmark, principal investigator of the NCI grant and Chairperson of the NSABP, appointed me as the scientific chair for the clinical trial. His goal was to recruit a qualified scientist to address unanticipated issues of importance to our patients, should they arise. My expertise was translational research on both SERMs. Fortunately, and remarkably, no cases arose during the tenure of the STAR trial (in contrast to the NCI/NSABP P-1 trial).

The question was asked to me more than once: "How will you feel if raloxifene proves to be superior to tamoxifen in the STAR trial?" "Delighted" would be my reply as the scientific foundations for the applications of both SERMs (and the concept of the new SERM drug group—Chap. 5) had both emerged from my laboratory. Tamoxifen, a failed contraceptive, was reinvented to become a potential chemopreventive at the Worcester Foundation and as a long-term adjuvant therapy at the University of Leeds in the early 1970's [11, 12]. Raloxifene was a failed breast cancer drug originally called keoxifene that was abandoned in the late 1980s by the pharmaceutical industry but reinvented in my laboratory at the Wisconsin Clinical Cancer Center as a potential candidate medicine with the goal: "prevent diseases associated with the progressive changes after menopause may, as a side effect, significantly retard the development of breast cancer" [13]. Our laboratory data was subsequently confirmed [14], and clinical testing for raloxifene to treat and prevent osteoporosis advanced from about 1992 through clinical testing by the pharmaceutical industry.

The evaluation of the use of two SERMs with different characteristics in the STAR trial taught important lessons in translational research. In the laboratory during the 1980s, it was clear that the structurally related polyhydroxylated compounds LY117,018 and LY156,758 were short acting and rapidly excreted drugs compared to tamoxifen [15–17]. Much higher daily doses of rapidly excreted antiestrogens were necessary for effective antitumor action [5, 17], and the antiestrogenic effects of the polyhydroxylated compounds disappeared rapidly once the drug is stopped. In contrast, tamoxifen accumulates. Thus, large daily doses of raloxifene are necessary to achieve the same efficacy as tamoxifen, and this is true with raloxifene (tamoxifen is used at a standard dose of 20 mg daily; the MORE trial used 60 vs. 120 mg daily of raloxifene). Additionally, the relative clearance rate of raloxifene and tamoxifen would have implications for a correlation between compliance and the actions of the SERMs to be chemopreventive agents in breast cancer. Tamoxifen accumulates but the drug can still be detected in the circulations 6 weeks after the last dose. Raloxifene is cleared rapidly within a few days of the last dose. Thus, missing a few tamoxifen tablets is of little consequence to the efficacy of the drug, but regularly missing raloxifene doses exposes the patient to estrogen-induced proliferation of nascent breast tumors. There is also another important aspect of tamoxifen's pharmacology that is only recently being understood. Long-term adjuvant tamoxifen therapy [18, 19] and chemoprevention [20–22] retain antitumor actions long after tamoxifen is stopped. This was noted in the NSABP P-1 trail [21] and in the NSABP/STAR P-2 trial [3]. In contrast, raloxifene was unable to maintain long-term antitumor effects in the STAR trial [3], confirming the earlier laboratory data [5, 17]. It was this finding that prompted the conclusion of recommendations from the NSABP: "It is unlikely that the optimal durations of raloxifene for chemoprevention will be evaluated in a breast cancer prevention setting; however, the use of raloxifene in treating and preventing osteoporosis is approved for an indefinite period time. Therefore, continuing raloxifene therapy beyond 5 years might be an approach that would preserve its full chemopreventive activity" [3].

References

1. Vogel VG, Costantino JP, Wickerham DL et al (2006) Effects of tamoxifen vs raloxifene on the risk of developing invasive breast cancer and other disease outcomes: the NSABP Study of Tamoxifen and Raloxifene (STAR) P-2 trial. JAMA 295:2727–2741

2. Freedman AN, Yu B, Gail MH et al (2011) Benefit/risk assessment for breast cancer chemoprevention with raloxifene or tamoxifen for women age 50 years or older. J Clin Oncol 29:2327–2333

3. Vogel VG, Costantino JP, Wickerham DL et al (2010) Update of the National Surgical Adjuvant Breast and Bowel Project Study of Tamoxifen and Raloxifene (STAR) P-2 Trial: preventing breast cancer. Cancer Prev Res (Phila) 3:696–706

4. Early Breast Cancer Trialists' Collaborative Group (1998) Tamoxifen for early breast cancer: an overview of the randomised trials. Lancet 351:1451–1467

5. Jordan VC, Allen KE (1980) Evaluation of the antitumour activity of the non-steroidal antioestrogen monohydroxytamoxifen in the DMBA-induced rat mammary carcinoma model. Eur J Cancer 16:239–251

6. Martino S, Cauley JA, Barrett-Connor E et al (2004) Continuing outcomes relevant to Evista: breast cancer incidence in postmenopausal osteoporotic women in a randomized trial of raloxifene. J Natl Cancer Inst 96:1751–1761

7. Lacassagne A (1936) Hormonal pathogenesis of adenocarcinoma of the breast. Am J Cancer 27:217–225

8. Jordan VC (2008) Tamoxifen: catalyst for the change to targeted therapy. Eur J Cancer 44:30–38

9. Sporn MB, Dunlop NM, Newton DL, Smith JM (1976) Prevention of chemical carcinogenesis by vitamin A and its synthetic analogs (retinoids). Fed Proc 35:1332–1338

10. Sporn MB (1976) Approaches to prevention of epithelial cancer during the preneoplastic period. Cancer Res 36:2699–2702

11. Jordan VC (1976) Effect of tamoxifen (ICI 46,474) on initiation and growth of DMBA-induced rat mammary carcinomata. Eur J Cancer 12:419–424

12. Jordan VC (1974) Antitumour activity of the antiestrogen ICI 46,474 (Tamoxifen) in the dimethylbenzanthracene (DMBA)-induced rat mammary carcinoma model. J Steroid Biochem 5:354

13. Lerner LJ, Jordan VC (1990) Development of antiestrogens and their use in breast cancer: eighth Cain memorial award lecture. Cancer Res 50:4177–4189

14. Black LJ, Sato M, Rowley ER et al (1994) Raloxifene (LY139481 HCI) prevents bone loss and reduces serum cholesterol without causing uterine hypertrophy in ovariectomized rats. J Clin Invest 93:63–69

15. Jordan VC, Gosden B (1983) Inhibition of the uterotropic activity of estrogens and antiestrogens by the short acting antiestrogen LY117018. Endocrinology 113:463–468

16. Jordan VC, Gosden B (1983) Differential antiestrogen action in the immature rat uterus: a comparison of hydroxylated antiestrogens with high affinity for the estrogen receptor. J Steroid Biochem 19:1249–1258

17. Gottardis MM, Jordan VC (1987) Antitumor actions of keoxifene and tamoxifen in the N-nitrosomethylurea-induced rat mammary carcinoma model. Cancer Res 47:4020–4024

18. EBCTCG (2005) Effects of chemotherapy and hormonal therapy for early breast cancer on recurrence and 15-year survival: an overview of the randomised trials. Lancet 365:1687–1717

19. Davies C, Godwin J, Gray R et al (2011) Relevance of breast cancer hormone receptors and other factors to the efficacy of adjuvant tamoxifen: patient-level meta-analysis of randomised trials. Lancet 378:771–784

20. Cuzick J, Forbes JF, Sestak I et al (2007) Long-term results of tamoxifen prophylaxis for breast cancer – 96-month follow-up of the randomized IBIS-I trial. J Natl Cancer Inst 99:272–282

21. Fisher B, Costantino JP, Wickerham DL et al (2005) Tamoxifen for the prevention of breast cancer: current status of the National Surgical Adjuvant Breast and Bowel Project P-1 study. J Natl Cancer Inst 97:1652–1662

22. Powles TJ, Ashley S, Tidy A et al (2007) Twenty-year follow-up of the Royal Marsden randomized, double-blinded tamoxifen breast cancer prevention trial. J Natl Cancer Inst 99:283–290

Chapter 9
Acquired Resistance to Tamoxifen: Back to the Beginning

Abstract The clinical acceptance and validation of the therapeutic strategy of long-term adjuvant tamoxifen treatment mandated an examination of acquired drug resistance under laboratory conditions. The first model in vivo of acquired resistance of ER-positive breast cancer cells transplanted into immune deficient mice demonstrated tamoxifen-stimulated tumor growth after about 2 years of continuous treatment. When tamoxifen was stopped, tumors also grew with physiologic estradiol. The model showed that no estrogen (similar to the use of aromatase inhibitors) or a pure antiestrogen to destroy ER (fulvestrant) presaged this therapeutic approach in clinical trials a decade later. However, the long-term retransplantation of breast tumors with acquired tamoxifen resistance for at least 5 years demonstrated a vulnerability of these tumors. Tamoxifen-stimulated tumor growth but physiologic estrogen now caused tumor regression and apoptosis. The new biology of estrogen-induced apoptosis now is used to explain the decrease in mortality after adjuvant tamoxifen is stopped in patients and also the value of conjugated equine estrogens to reduce breast cancer incidence in women treated in their 60s.

Introduction

The idea that the determination of the estrogen receptor (ER) content in the breast tumor of a patient with metastatic breast cancer would predict response to ablative endocrine surgery (oophorectomy, adrenalectomy, hypophysectomy) became a clinical reality and requirement for each breast cancer patient in the mid-1970s [1]. This was established on a National Cancer Institute sponsored meeting in Bethesda, Maryland, at the Holiday Inn in 1974. The rationale was that if the ER was not present in the tumor, then the patient should not have ablative surgery. This would be 30 % of all patients and there would be no response. There would be a response of about 60 % in patients with an ER-positive tumor. Tamoxifen, however, was not considered in these deliberations as it was not yet in clinical trial in America.

P.Y. Maximov et al., *Tamoxifen*, Milestones in Drug Therapy,
DOI 10.1007/978-3-0348-0664-0_9, © Springer Basel 2013

Tamoxifen was Food and Drug Administration (FDA) approved and available to treat metastatic breast cancer in December 1977. By then, the ER had evolved into the target for tamoxifen action [2] and has subsequently become a drug to be used as a potential long-term adjuvant therapy. There was laboratory data to indicate there was potential for tamoxifen as the first chemopreventive for breast cancer.

The fact that all metastatic breast tumors with ER did not respond to tamoxifen treatment, and those tumors that do respond, do so for about 1–2 years [3], created a classification of intrinsic resistance where treatment fails to control tumor growth at the 2-month evaluation point and acquired resistance where the tumor eventually escapes from estrogen blockade of the ER by tamoxifen and grows autonomously.

The prevalent theory in the 1970s for acquired resistance to endocrine therapy was that tumors were heterogeneous and those cells containing ER were controlled and died out, and the ER-negative tumor cells overgrew and become dominant. Thus, a tumor would evolve from ER positive to become ER negative. However, this was inconsistent with clinical experience by the medical oncology community. Select breast cancer could respond to, the then standard of care, high-dose diethylstilbestrol (DES). However, when therapy fails evidenced by tumor regrowth, a withdrawal response can occur by stopping (DES) treatment. Once the tumor regrows again the clinician would try high-dose androgen or progestin therapy. Responses occurred again. This whole process of alternating endocrine therapies is called the endocrine treatment cascade and is used successfully to this day in selected patients before using cytotoxic combination chemotherapy. The practice of medicine therefore was not consistent with the theory that resistance occurred with a trend to ER-negative cell populations: the theory must therefore be incorrect. The solution to the problem was to come from studies utilizing athymic mice to grow human breast cancer cell lines and from the study acquired resistance to tamoxifen.

The MCF-7 Breast Cancer Cell Line

The important cell line MCF-7 created by Soule and coworkers [4]at the Michigan Cancer Foundation (MCF) was from a pleural effusion from a nun, Sister Catherine Frances, initially treated with high-dose DES (tamoxifen was not available at that time). The cell line is ER positive [5] and became the "work horse" in the laboratory for the study of hormone-dependent breast cancer. Tamoxifen blocked spontaneous growth of MCF-7 cells in culture [6] and estradiol reversed the tamoxifen blockade. Estrogen did not however enhance growth in culture but it did in athymic mice [7] leading to the idea that a second factor in vivo was required. Within the decade of the 1980s, the Katzenellenbogen laboratory would discover that the ubiquitous phenol red indicator used in culture media contained a potent estrogenic contaminant [8, 9] (Fig. 1.7, Chap. 1).

Nevertheless, it was probably fortunate that the ER-positive MCF-7 cells were always grown in an estrogen-containing environment to maintain their hormone-responsive characteristics. Without estrogen in the media, the estrogen-responsive cells die [10].

The value of the MCF-7 cell line to breast cancer research has been reviewed previously [11]. Throughout the 1980s and 1990s, numerous reports of tamoxifen resistance or resistance to raloxifene-like molecules or pure antiestrogens were published using MCF-7 cells in vitro or with other ER-positive cells [12–23]. We will, however, focus here on the importance of the transplantation of MCF-7 cells into athymic mice to create a breakthrough in deciphering acquired drug resistance. Shafie and Granthan [24] first showed that MCF-7 tumors grow in athymic mice with estradiol treatment, but not with tamoxifen treatment. Osborne [25] demonstrated that tamoxifen would control estrogen-stimulated MCF-7 growth in athymic mice but eventually the MCF-7 derived tumors would grow despite tamoxifen treatment [26]. Osborne concluded that part of the action of tamoxifen was tumoristatic; therefore, long-term treatment was necessary[26] . This was consistent with original data generated in carcinogen-induced rat mammary cancer models [27]. However, the finding that MCF-7 tumors with acquired resistance to tamoxifen grew *because* of estrogen or tamoxifen treatment not despite the tamoxifen was a discovery [28]. The tumors were transplantable and had adapted a mechanism for the tamoxifen-ER complex to cause growth somewhat similar to estrogen. Additionally, the resistance (tamoxifen-stimulated growth) is not athymic mouse specific, i.e., some strange metabolic difference or difference in NK cells. Tamoxifen-stimulated MCF-7 tumor growth occurs in either athymic rats or beige (NK deficient) mice [29]. Unfortunately (or as it turned out fortunately!), cell lines of tamoxifen-resistant tumors could not be transferred and retain the tamoxifen-resistant growth phenotype in vitro. However, to explain the estrogen-like action of tamoxifen, an interesting hypothesis emerged in the early 1990s to explain tamoxifen-stimulated growth via the generation of estrogenic isomers of tamoxifen metabolites. This will be described briefly, as an interesting chemical approach was used to address the proposed molecular mechanism of acquired tamoxifen resistance. It is an excellent example of how basic structure-function relationship can resolve important clinical questions in the laboratory.

Tamoxifen Metabolism Hypothesis

Tamoxifen is metabolized to numerous hydroxylated compounds, some with estrogen-like actions and others with antiestrogenic actions (Chap. 3). The metabolism hypothesis with subsequent geometric isomerization to putative estrogens was based on the known estrogenic and antiestrogenic properties of the cis (ICI 47,699) and trans (ICI 46,474) isomers of tamoxifen [30–33]. It was noted that there is less tamoxifen in tumors with acquired resistance [31] and an increase in E 4-hydroxytamoxifen as a putative estrogen. Similar findings were made in patients failing tamoxifen therapy, i.e., lower levels of tamoxifen in the tumor and the ratio of E to Z isomers of 4-hydroxytamoxifen were higher [32]. Additionally [33], metabolite E, a weak estrogen, was identified in patients with tamoxifen refractory tumors. To evaluate the hypothesis a series of non-isomerizable fixed ring derivatives and isomers of 4-hydroxytamoxifen and metabolite E were synthesized. The E isomer of 4-hydroxytamoxifen is actually a very weak antiestrogen (not a full estrogen) [34, 35]. The Z isomer of metabolite E is only a very weak estrogen (Fig. 3.2, Chap. 3).

To address the tamoxifen metabolism hypothesis, further in vivo, a fixed ring version of tamoxifen was synthesized so that any metabolite that were produced could not isomerize to potent estrogens. Fixed ring tamoxifen is equally able to stimulate the acquired tamoxifen treatment tumors as the parent drug [36]. Thus, other resistance mechanisms, based on growth factor driven tumor growth have now become most useful for developing future therapeutic strategies either as second line treatments or if given with tamoxifen initially may prevent resistance occurring in the first place.

Growth Factor-Driven Acquired and Intrinsic Resistance

There is compelling evidence that HER 2/neu can subvert hormone-responsive growth completely in ER-positive cells. Stable transfection of MCF-7 cells with the HER 2/neu gene results in tumor growth in athymic mice not regulated by tamoxifen [37].

Over the past 20 years the Osborne Group in Texas have refined the growth factor driven MCF-7 model in vivo and defined precisely the ways of blocking either the receptors or their tyrosine kinases singly or together to create long-term responses or "cures" in vivo while applying either tamoxifen or estrogen deprivations equivalent to aromatase inhibitors treatment strategies.

In recent years antibodies targeting HER2, or tyrosine kinase inhibitors that target the HER family (1–4) have become available for clinical evaluation. Among anti-HER2 monoclonal antibodies tested, trastuzumab is now a well-known and approved drug that is established though clinical trials as an important component of the first-line treatment of patients with HER2 amplified metastatic breast cancer [38–40]. When trastuzumab is administered in a preoperative setting, this strategy increases the pathological complete response rate [38]. In a large phase III trial investigating adjuvant therapy in HER2 positive early breast cancer, the addition of trastuzumab to chemotherapy increases both the disease-free and overall survival [41]. Aside from trastuzumab there is also pertuzumab, which is a monoclonal antibody against HER2 that blocks dimerization with HER1 and HER3 [42]. Although pertuzumab has therapeutic activity in HER2 positive breast cancer patients, combination therapy with trastuzumab has proven to be more effective [43]. Ertumaxomab is another monoclonal antibody against HER2 that has demonstrated strong immunological responses in HER2 positive breast cancer patients in phase I clinical trial [44].

Aside from monoclonal anti-HER2 antibodies, the use of tyrosine kinase inhibitors to target HER2 is proving to be effective. In particular, lapatinib, a dual tyrosine kinase inhibitor of both HER1 and HER2 and of Akt and mitogen-activated protein kinase (MAPK), has been demonstrated to inhibit cell growth and induce apoptosis in several breast cancer cell lines [45]. Results from phase I and II clinical trials have shown that lapatinib has therapeutic value in a number of tumors, in particular in breast cancer patients [46–48]. In a xenograft mouse model, lapatinib is able to prevent tamoxifen resistance [49], showing the role of increased growth factor signaling pathways in resistance [50] and the potential benefit of targeting the increased growth factor signaling to reverse tamoxifen resistance in the clinic. A systemic review of the databases from clinical trials (including phase III) demonstrates that combination therapy of HER2-positive HR-positive metastatic breast cancers in postmenopausal women with lapatinib and anastrozole is superior to lapatinib monotherapy and superior to tamoxifen treatment [51].

Thus, it is now clear that exogenous inhibitors of the HER-signaling network and other mitogenic pathways can abrogate or improve the response rate of breast cancer with acquired resistance [52].

An Evolving Model of Acquired Resistance to SERMs and Aromatase Inhibitors

The transplantable model of acquired tamoxifen resistance in ER-positive breast cancer cell lines develops within about a year [28, 53]. This is the same time that resistance to tamoxifen treatment occurs in ER-positive metastatic breast cancer. Thus, the model recapitulates acquired resistance to tamoxifen in metastatic breast cancer, and therapeutic studies in the mice mimic the second-line responses of tumors in aromatase inhibitors or fulvestrant after tamoxifen failure in clinical trial [54, 55]. The laboratory-derived tumor of acquired resistance to tamoxifen does not grow without physiologic estrogen action. This is supported by the fact that no estrogen treatment maybe like aromatase inhibitor treatment or a pure antiestrogen ICI 164,384 (the lead compound that resulted in fulvestrant [56, 57]) stops tumor growth [58].

At this time, in the mid-1980s, it was clear that long-term adjuvant tamoxifen therapy for years or indefinitely [59–61] was showing promise for enhanced survival, and there was no early recurrence of micrometastatic disease as a result of the development of early acquired resistance. Something was conceptually wrong with the link between the endocrine treatment of metastatic breast cancer with its greater bulk and the responsiveness of micrometastatic disease that is undetectable during adjuvant therapy.

One plausible explanation was proposed in the early 1990s based on the transplantable model of acquired resistance to tamoxifen maintained through serial transplantation into further generations of tamoxifen-treated year after year in athymic mice. After about 5 years of retransplantation, the tamoxifen-stimulated MCF-7 tumors changed their survival characteristics and responsiveness to estrogen. Physiologic estrogen was no longer a survival signal causing tumor growth in

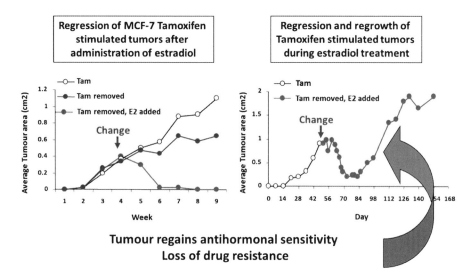

Fig. 9.1 Cyclic changes in sensitivity and resistance of breast tumors grown in vivo after treatments with tamoxifen and estradiol

the animals [28] but rather an inhibitor of tumor growth causing small tamoxifen-stimulated tumors to just melt away [62] (Fig. 9.1). It was suggested that following long-term adjuvant tamoxifen therapy, it was actually the act of stopping tamoxifen that reinforced and enhanced patient survival [63]. A woman's own estrogen was now killing the prepared and sensitized micrometastasis. Further study expanded the hypothesis to become a cyclical event with physiologic estrogen causing the destruction of a novel form of acquired antiestrogen resistance, but then the tumor was again responsive to antihormonal therapies such as aromatase inhibitors or indeed tamoxifen treatment (Fig. 9.1). It was suggested that physiologic estrogen could be used as a salvage therapy [64]. However, this was extremely controversial. The suggestion that administering estradiol to breast cancer patients after failing repeated antihormone therapies for breast cancer was unacceptable to IRBs in the 1990s and especially so to women's advocate groups. Nevertheless, with the therapeutic drift from tamoxifen to the aromatase inhibitors during the first decade of the twenty-first century, acquired resistance to estrogen deprivation became an important scientific issue.

In the 1970s and 1980s, Richard Santen [65, 66] had systematically and rigorously examined the clinical endocrine pharmacology of aminoglutethimide as an inhibitor of estrogen production, but the drug was not specific from the aromatase enzyme and glucocorticoids had to be coadministered. Angela Brodie had pioneered the practical applications of developing specific drugs to destroy the aromatase enzyme first in the 1970s at the Worcester Foundation and subsequently at the University of Maryland. Her discovery of the properties of 4-hydroxyandrostenedione went from the laboratory to clinical trial with approval in Europe [67–70]. The new aromatase inhibitors started to become the antihormonal standard of care with long-term adjuvant therapy so naturally attention turned to the laboratory studies of acquired drug resistance. Santen's group reported that long-term estrogen-deprived (LTED) cells from the MCF-7 line would respond to estrogen in vitro initially claimed to have "acquired hypersensitivity" to minute amounts of estrogen in the environment to accomplish an apparent "estrogen-independent growth response" [71, 72]. Santen would subsequently show that LTED cells would respond to estrogen with apoptosis [73]. This was an explanation of Haddow's original chemical therapy for breast cancer, i.e., high-dose estrogen to treat postmenopausal patients with metastatic breast cancer [74, 75]. However, the new twist was that the antihormone therapies has now sensitized breast cancer cells to low doses of estrogen therapy, perhaps in the physiologic range. This concept could be used in the clinic as a salvage therapy and to explain the paradoxal new data with the estrogen replacement (CEE) in the Women's Health Initiative (WHI) of hysterectomized women [76]. There were fewer breast cancers!

Back to the Beginning

Paul Ehrlich created the first chemical therapy (chemotherapy) when he discovered Salvarsan for the treatment of syphilis in the later part of the nineteenth century. In the early years of the twentieth century, he turned his attentions to treating cancer and chose to develop animal models to facilitate drug testing. He had created this successful translational research process with his work on syphilis, so why not build on success? The year before his death in 1915, Ehrlich conceded defeat stating, "I have wasted 15 years of my life on experimental cancer research."

Sir Alexander Haddow accepted the challenge in the 1940s when he found that carcinogenic polycyclic hydrocarbons cause tumor regression in animal models. Clearly, it was not going to be possible to use these same hydrocarbons in patients, but he reasoned that the new synthetic estrogens diethylstilbestrol and the triphenylethylenes had multiple phenyl rings, so he tested them. Tumor regressions occurred in the animals, so high-dose estrogen therapy was tested in patients and produced therapeutic effect in about 30 % of metastatic breast cancer in postmenopausal women over 60 [74]. High-dose estrogen therapy remained the palliative treatment of choice until tamoxifen become the standard of care, and because it was safer and therefore more versatile, its applications extended to long-term adjuvant therapy and chemoprevention during the 1980s [3, 77].

Returning to high-dose estrogen therapy pre-tamoxifen, Haddow was the inaugural Karnofsky Memorial Lecturer at ASCO [78, 79]. In his lecture, Haddow expressed his concern about progress in cancer therapeutics. He did not believe there would ever be a cancer-specific target as Erlich had proposed; cancer was self. Haddow also reasoned that unlike the story of antibiotics which could be tested in the laboratory to determine the correct antibiotic for the appropriate treatment of the actual disease, this did not happen in cancer therapy. The crude cancer therapies were nonspecific and tried on the patient as the only way to determine whether the tumor was sensitive or not. He stated:

Table 9.1 Objective response rates in postmenopausal women with metastatic breast cancer undergoing high dose estrogen therapy. The patients were divided based on years after menopause (Basil Stoll. Breast Cancer Management Early and Late. William Herman Medical Books Ltd., London pp. 133–146)

Age since menopause	Patient #'s	% Regression
Postmenopausal 0–5 years	63	9 %
Postmenopausal > 5 years	344	35 %

> the need exists for some method of prior screening to indicate the optimal choice (of chemotherapy) in particular cases ... efforts thus far have been disappointing.

He also stated:

> ... the extraordinary extent of tumour regression observed in perhaps 1 % of post-menopausal cases (with oestrogen) has always been regarded as of major theoretical importance, and it is a matter for some disappointment that so much of the underlying mechanisms continues to elude us ... [79]

The one bright glimmer of hope reason was the fact that high-dose DES was extremely effective in some breast cancers. Haddow, it should be noted, also used his preliminary data [74] to conduct a multicentric clinical trial through the Royal Society of Medicine. He had a discovery:

> When the various reports were assembled at the end of that time, it was fascinating to discover that rather general impression, not sufficiently strong from the relatively small numbers in any single group, became reinforced to the point of certainty; namely, the beneficial responses were three times more frequent in women over the age of 60 years than in those under that age; that oestrogens may, on the contrary, accelerate the course of mammary cancer in younger women, and that their therapeutic use should be restricted to cases 5 years beyond the menopause. Here was an early and satisfying example of the advantages which may accrue from cooperative clinical trial.

This observation in clinical practice was supported by Dr. Basil Stoll whose personal experience with high-dose DES for the treatment of metastatic breast cancer in postmenopausal women replicated Haddow's observations (Table 9.1). Thus, estrogen deprivation is the key to success for estrogen therapy, both for the clinical use of high-dose therapy and for the interpretation of the CEE trial alone in the WHI [76]. The women in the WHI trial were an average 68 years of age! But can we now seek a mechanism for the chain of events that causes the estrogen-ER complex to trigger apoptosis?

Mechanisms of Estrogen-Induced Apoptosis

Studies of the molecular mechanisms of estradiol-induced apoptosis have occurred only during the last decade. The study by Santen's group showed that estrogen increases Fas ligand in LTED MCF-7 [73] cells but, by contrast, estradiol increases Fas receptor in apoptotic long-term tamoxifen-resistant (phase II) MCF-7 tumors [80], both pointing to an extrinsic mechanism through "death receptors." However, these early studies were not time dependent but only snapshots of the apoptosis process at random times.

During the early 1990s, a couple of important estrogen-deprived cell lines were cloned from a cell population of MCF-7:WS8s following long-term (>1 year) estrogen deprivation in phenol-red-free media containing triple charcoal stripped serum. The two cell lines MCF-7:5C [81] and MCF-7:2A [82] were created in the anticipation of eventually being able to elucidate resistance to aromatase inhibitors, but they were placed in liquid nitrogen and stored for that day.

Lewis and coworkers [83] focused efforts in vitro on the MCF-7:5C cell line to describe the development of early apoptotic responses to estradiol. Rapid apoptotic events occurred at the intrinsic mitochondrial level with release of cytochrome C and a rise in proapoptotic gene products (BAX, BIM, and NOXA). Apoptosis was completely blocked by both fulvestrant (that destroys the cellular ER) and 4-hydroxytamoxifen, though the latter SERM did not affect the cell cycle in MCF-7:5C cells (i.e., these cells are resistant to SERMs). Flow cytometry was used to confirm the development of estrogen-induced apoptosis with increased annexin V and DAPI staining was used to confirm apoptosis by microscopy.

The MCF-7:2A cells only slowly go through apoptosis during the second week of estradiol treatment but this can be accelerated by using buthionine sulfoximine (BSO) to prevent glutathione synthesis [84]. The reduction of mechanisms to protect cells from reactive oxygen species is clearly an important protective measure to ensure survival of aromatase resistant cells.

The unique cell lines that are so sensitive either to estradiol-induced growth MCF-7:WS8 or rapidly apoptotic MCF-7:5C cells and slowly apoptotic MCF-7:2A cells have formed the foundations for an extensive study of the mechanistic studies of basal gene levels of activations between estrogen-responsive and estrogen-independent cell growth and the timed gene responses of all those cell lines over a 96-h period and the rate of gene activation of the MCF-7:2A cells over the second week of estrogen exposure [85].

Eric Ariazi at the Fox Chase Cancer Center working with Heather Cunliffe at Translational Genomics in Arizona created a superb Agilent gene array database for a "movie" of pathway analysis in the life and death of breast cancer cells. Essentially the study [85] creates a sequenced cooperative enrichment analysis of inflammatory responses, ER signaling, inflammation, and unfolded protein responsiveness in the endoplasmic reticulum during the timed move to full apoptosis. Ping Fan has described AP-1 synthesis and activation to initiate apoptosis through the accumulation of reactive oxygen species (ROS), all of which can be blocked by 4-hydroxytamoxifen or paradoxically a cSrc inhibitor [86]. But with the cascade of caspases created by estrogen action in MCF-7:5C cells and its modulations by arachidonic acid [85], the question must be asked: "What is it about the ER that triggers apoptosis in the correctly conditioned estrogen-deprived cells?" To address the question and find an answer, one must first examine the relationship between the ligand, the ER and the actual shape of the ER complex. It is this interrogation that exposed the mechanism of the "Haddow paradox" [79].

A New Classification of Estrogens

The crystallization of the human ER ligand-binding domain with estradiol, raloxifene [87] diethylstilbestrol and 4-hydroxytamoxifen [88] precisely revealed the nature of the structural changes in the ER complex to create a mechanism of estrogen action that neatly dovetailed with the structure-activity relationships first described for modulation with the prolactin gene by the ER complex [35, 89–92] and the studies of the modulation of the transforming growth factor-alpha (TGF-α) gene by mutant ER-α in the 1990s [93, 94] and the 2000s [95–98]. Simply summarized, these studies defined the interaction of antiestrogenic side chains, correctly positioned to interact, neutralize, or shield the exposed amino acid 351 once the activation function-2 (AF-2) binding site for coactivators on helix 12 has been pushed open like the jaws of a crocodile. Pharmacologically, the angular triphenylethylenes that form the backbone of the SERMs only become antiestrogenic at appropriate target sites like the breast or uterus with a correctly positioned side chain.

But it was Geoffrey Greene [88] who used the phrase "the bulky antiestrogenic side chain" that created our next conceptual advance, as the antiestrogenic side chain was a finger like alkylaminoethoxy side chain, a trivial amount of molecular "bulk." However, Greene was including the nonplanar phenyl ring! We hypothesized that the planar and angular nonsteroidal estrogens would fit the ER ligand-binding domain differently. All estrogens were not equal. A precise biological assay of two different cell lines derived using the ER-negative MDA-MB-231 cell line either stably transfected with wild-type ER or the asp 351gly mutant. Planar (class I) estrogens such as DES and estradiol and nonplanar (class II) triphenylethylene estrogens were compared and contrasted to switch on or off the TGF-α gene. The results were a simple yes/no answer. A planar estrogen (class I) would easily fit in the binding pocket of the LBD to activate AF 2 coactivator binding formed from a closed helix 12 sealing the ligand inside. Both cell lines would activate TGF-α. In contrast, the estrogen-like activity of 4-hydroxytamoxifen with a short antiestrogenic side chain results from the negatively charged aspartate 351 communicating with AF-1 to cause estrogen action (weak as it is) and activation of the TGF-α gene. In the cells with the asp351gly mutation, there would be no activation of TGF-α [99]. A triphenylethylene estrogen had some estrogen action with wild-type ER and an exposed asp 351, but with the asp 351 gly mutant with no charge, there was none [99]. It was proof that the shape of the ER complex with a triphenylethylene had a pushed back helix 12. Simply stated, crocodile jaws closed for a class I estrogen, jaws open for a class II estrogen. In the paper, it was stated that the authors had no idea what this would mean in biology [99] but there was a claim that it could be important. We showed the effect was reproducible by classifying the estrogen-like contaminant of the nonsteroidal didesmethyl methoxychlor (DDM) as a class 2 estrogen [100].

However, the fact that 4-hydroxytamoxifen completely blocked the action of estradiol to cause apoptosis in MCF-7:5C cells opened the door to prove that shape mattered for the estrogen-ER complex to trigger apoptosis. Did the "jaws of the crocodile" need to be closed to trigger apoptosis?

The first clue that the hypothesis was going to prove to be correct and control apoptosis was that the triphenylethylene estrogen-ER complexes were shown not to be destroyed in MCF-7 cells like estradiol, but to accumulate like 4-hydroxytamoxifen. The ER complex for these nonplanar estrogens was like an antiestrogen! The shape of the ER with different types of estrogen did, in fact, control an important biological process—estrogen-induced apoptosis! Further studies exhaustively demonstrated that the triphenylethylenes stimulated the growth of MCF-7 cells just like estradiol, but with less potency, and confirmed and massively expanded earlier studies that triphenylethylene estrogens did block apoptosis. Triphenylethylene complex with ER did not bind the coactivator SRC-3 as avidly at the promoter regions of estrogen-responsive genes [101], and these data beautifully confirmed the observation in complimentary studies that SRC-3 was important for estrogen-induced apoptosis [102]. By studying SRC3-interacting proteins, one could decipher the early events in estrogen-induced apoptosis in vitro [102].

However, during this conversation with nature to decipher the mechanism of estrogen-induced apoptosis, one very important fact was inconsistent. If estrogenic triphenylethylenes block estrogen-induced apoptosis in a cell like MCF-7:5C in the laboratory, then why did Haddow observe his best responses with estrogen-induced tumor regress with estrogenic triphenylethylenes used for the treatment of metastatic breast cancer in late postmenopausal women [74]? A clinical reality with tumor regression with estrogen trumps a laboratory study every time! This inconsistency was solved with that the triphenylethylenes kill the cells in culture in 2 weeks. The time course is extended with class II angular estrogens so the triggering process is only occurring slowly. In the patient the long-term retention and storage of triphenylethylenes in a woman's body fat provides a continuous high estrogen environment to produce optimal antitumor actions. This was discovered by one of my current PhD stidents Dr. IfeyinwaObiorah. A conversation with nature does work!

Final Thoughts on Four Decades of Discovery to Advance the Value of the ER Target in Breast Cancer

We begin and end our story with the actions of synthetic estrogens to kill breast cancer cells that have been prepared for sacrifice through estrogen deprivations. The best current example of the value of this knowledge in women's health are the results of the Women's Health Initiative with conjugated equine estrogens alone in hysterectomized women to reduce breast cancer incidence and mortality for women in their mid-60s [76]. The 40 years starting with the development of tamoxifen from a failed contraceptive to being the gold standard that saved the lives of millions of women through the prudent application of the laboratory principle of long-term adjuvant therapy [2] resulted in the mandatory laboratory study of acquired drug resistance to long-term tamoxifen therapy. Acquired resistance would surely occur, but no one could have predicted the development of tamoxifen-stimulated breast cancer growth or the evolution of acquired resistance to expose a fatal vulnerability in breast cancer so that physiologic estrogen triggered apoptosis. Each discovery was in the hands of young scientists as generations of Tamoxifen Teams that turned ideas into lives saved. Progress occurred through their outstanding skill in the laboratory and the philosophy that if Nature gives us the "wrong answer" to our question, Nature does not lie. The answer is the true answer to the question that must be considered as the solution to the problem to be solved.

Postscript. During his Ph.D. training, Doug Wolf discovered multiple valuable clues to understand SERMs, drug resistance, and estrogen-induced apoptosis, but at the time all of this was speculative with no real basis in scientific fact. The two discoveries that Doug contributed were both serendipity. In fact, all advances are serendipity in basic science, but it is the recognition of the new knowledge that becomes the key to discovery. One spots the clue and expands on the observation because it is a "conversation with Nature." The unimaginative scientist throws the clue away as it does not fit the model of what is correct or incorrect in their mind at the time.

In a search for mechanisms to explain acquired tamoxifen resistance, Doug was focused in two directions in his Ph.D. thesis. The two main questions were as follows: "Is acquired drug resistance to tamoxifen because a mutation of the estrogen receptor occurs to change the pharmacology of tamoxifen from an antiestrogen to an estrogen?" and secondly "What growth factor receptors and receptor signal transduction pathways are responsible for estradiol-stimulated growth of tumors with acquired tamoxifen resistance and does tamoxifen use the same pathways as estradiol?"

To address the issue of a mutation of the ER enhancing the estrogen-like effects of tamoxifen, Doug created a number of tamoxifen-stimulated tumor lines and screened them for ER mutations [62]. All tumor lines had wild-type ER except one with a large proportion of an ER with an asp 351 tyr mutation [62, 103]. We had no idea at the time what this was going to mean for understanding the mechanics of SERM action but it was destined to be profound. Bill Catherino, an M.D., Ph.D. student in my laboratory at Wisconsin, subsequently created the BC-2 stably transfected cell line in MDA-MB-231 cells using a cDNA for the mutant receptor [104]. Anna Levenson, a postdoctoral fellow and then a research assistant professor at Northwestern used a transforming growth factor (TGF)-α target (discovered by Mei Huey Jeng) [105] to compare and contrast the estrogenic and antiestrogenic action of tamoxifen and raloxifene. The asp351tyr ER turned out to be the first and, to date, the only natural mutation of the human ER to change the pharmacology of a nonsteroidal antiestrogen from a complete antiestrogen to an estrogen [93, 106]. We were mystified why a mutation buried in the ligand-binding domain (LBD) of the ER could influence the pharmacology of raloxifene, but the reason became clear with the subsequent publications of the crystal structure of the raloxifene-ER LBD [87]. However, if one examines the X-ray crystallography in the papers it is almost impossible to interpret in "the real world" of protein-protein interactions. That is for the outside! The fact that we realized that Asp 351 was a surface amino acid on the ER complex was the key to finding the "antiestrogen region" was had predicted in paper published 15 years earlier [90, 107]. But the discovery was by chance and this chance created opportunities for a productive scientific collaboration. I had been invited to Signal Pharmaceuticals in California to discuss a new SERM, but as I was waiting for my taxi to take me to my hotel, I started to wander the corridors and struck up a conversation with a young man Jim Zapf who was "playing" on his computer. "What do you do?" says I. Jim replied, "I do docking of ligands with the ER ligand binding domain." "OK," I said. "How good is your program? Can you show me the outside of the ER complex dimer— this is what other proteins see?" "No problem," Jim replies. "Let me ask you this. Color in where helix 12 is with the estradiol or raloxifene ER complex?" In a second or two I exclaim, "It really is the crocodile model of estrogen and antiestrogen action." We had proposed this 15 years earlier [90]. "OK so where is aspartate 351 in the estradiol ER complex?" I inquired. Jim replies, "It's here under helix 12 on the surface of the complex but it does not play a role." As we switch to the raloxifene-ER complex, the significance of aspartate 351 was clear through its interaction with the "antiestrogenic side chain" of raloxifene. The pyrolidine ring shields and neutralized the aspartate producing a complete antiestrogen, but tamoxifen has a side chain that is a few Å shorter and cannot do the job completely and is promiscuous with estrogen-like actions. This chance meeting resulted in collaboration and a half a dozen publications of ER modulation. We subsequently interrogated the ligand asp 351 interactions (Chap. 5, Postscript) and this was reviewed by Levenson [108]. Anait Levenson proved herself to be an exceptional scientist.

One of the Doug's other tasks was to utilize the Marco Gottardis athymic mouse model of acquired resistance to tamoxifen [28] to discover the growth factor pathways, responsible for estradiol or tamoxifen-stimulated tumor growth. At this time, in the early 1990s, growth factor signaling was the fashion [109] and primarily spearheaded by Dr. Marc E. Lippman who had just become the director of the Lombardi Cancer Center in Washington, DC. He had moved, with all his staff, from the National Cancer Institute in Bethesda where he was the head of the Breast program. Doug's project was simple. Grow up some of the tamoxifen-stimulated tumors with tamoxifen in athymic mice and then switch to either tamoxifen or physiologic estrogen released from subcutaneous capsules. Then, harvest growing tumors and measure all known growth factors and their receptors to answer the question: "Is estrogen or tamoxifen induced-growth stimulated by the same or different growth factors?" The tumors did not grow with physiologic estradiol; they disappeared—they just melted away in a few weeks! I suggested that the long-term tamoxifen exposure had somehow accelerated a natural sensitivity to estrogen-induced tumor cell death. It was the explanations of Haddow's landmark observation in patients 50 years before [74, 78]! These data at Wisconsin [63] were presented at the St. Gallen Breast Cancer Conference in 1992 and were replicated at Northwestern by a superb team of resident surgeons Kathy Yao, Eun-Sook Lee, Dave Bentram, Gale England, a medical oncology fellow Ruth O'Regan, and my

Ph.D. student Jennifer MacGregor Shafer [64]. Their data showed that Doug's work was reproducible and the phenomenon occurred over a 5-year period (i.e., in the last 2 years of transplantation in tamoxifen-treated mice). Gale England showed this beautifully in her notebook and Dave Bentram stepped in to perform biotransplant tumor experiments requested by the referees for Kathy Yao's paper [64]. They thought the animals had changed, not the tumor. Dave showed that it was the tumor, not the animals. These data opened a new door of discovery for the next decade with the exploitation of the principle of successfully treating patients with acquired antihormone therapy with low doses of estradiol [110], the study of mechanisms [73, 80, 83, 85, 111] that answered Haddow's statement of dismay in his 1971 Karnofsky lecture:

> ... the extraordinary extent of tumour regression observed in perhaps 1 % of post-menopausal cases (with oestrogen) has always been regarded as of major theoretical importance, and it is a matter for some disappointment that so much of the underlying mechanisms continues to elude us ...

I was thrilled to be selected as the 38th winner of the Karnofsky Memorial Lecture and selected as my title, "The paradoxical actions of estrogen in breast cancer: survival or death?" As Haddow and I were (are) British and my Tamoxifen Team have, through serendipity, now discovered the molecular mechanism of estrogen-induced apoptosis, this seemed to me to be the appropriate tribute to his pioneering advance in chemical therapy.

Our subsequent work also provided the basis for the explanation of the antitumor effects of physiologic estrogen when used as estrogen replacement therapy [76]. A valuable conversation with nature that could have been so easily abandoned in 1993 with the "wrong answer" from Doug's experiment that could not reproduce estrogen response in Marco's Model. But two other twists were necessary to advance our Tamoxifen Team tale.

It is worth emphasizing the significant role that Dr. Joan Lewis-Wambi played in this story, our knowledge of estrogen-induced apoptosis and the cell model she breathed life into—by chance. Dr. Shun-Yuan Jiang created both the MCF-7:5C [81] cells and MCF-7:2A cells [82]. Both cell lines were cloned out of populations that were estrogen deprived for almost a year. The majority of cells died but some survived and grew under estrogen-free conditions. The MCF-7:5C [81] are ER positive and PgR negative, and we reported they did not respond to estrogen or antiestrogens. Joan Lewis almost 10 years later was given the task of studying these cells at a time that it was clear that the aromatase inhibitors would be an essential treatment option for breast cancer patients in the medical oncologists' armamentarium. What did she do? She changed the serum conditions to grow our MCF-7:5C cells and did not follow the essential tradition of repeating exactly what Shun-Yuan had done in her paper [81]. Amazingly, the MCF-7:5C cells grew spontaneously, but apoptosis occurred rapidly with physiologic estrogen in vitro and in vivo. We had never had a cell line that responded to estrogen as a cidal stimulus—and now we did [112]. She created a pivotal paper on the intrinsic mechanism of apoptosis [83] and followed this up with a super description of the delayed apoptosis (estrogen took a week longer to cause cell death in the MCF-7:2A cells) observed in the 2A cells that could be advanced to immediate cell death with estrogen if glutathione synthesis was blocked [84]. I should document that her husband Dr. Chris Wambi was conducting research on the redox role of glutathione using buthionine sulfoximine (BSO) to stop glutathione synthesis, and it was this husband and wife team that found our mechanism of cell survival that could be neutralized so that estrogen now caused rapid cell death. This is a good husband/wife synergy in science.

Without these cell models, our expanding experience and publications with acquired tamoxifen and raloxifene resistance in vivo, we could not have successfully competed for our Department of Defense Center of Excellence Grant. These studies and models passed on one to another over decades by my trainees significantly advanced women health and helped families stay together longer through the increased survival of women either with breast cancer or at risk of breast cancer.

Debra Tonetti came to work in my laboratory with a background in PKC alpha. After settling for a year she requested to continue to work on PKC alpha to determine its effect following transfection into T47D:A18 cells. Her studies on tumor growth in athymic animals showed that estrogen rapidly killed cells. Her excellent series of studies [113–116] laid the foundation for a new line of investigation to find non-estrogenic synthetic compounds that can safely kill breast cancer specifically.

References

1. McGuire WL, Carbone PP, Vollmer EP, United States. National Cancer Institute. Breast Cancer Treatment Committee (1975) Estrogen receptors in human breast cancer. Raven Press, New York
2. Jordan VC (2008) Tamoxifen: catalyst for the change to targeted therapy. Eur J Cancer 44:30–38
3. Ingle JN, Ahmann DL, Green SJ et al (1981) Randomized clinical trial of diethylstilbestrol versus tamoxifen in postmenopausal women with advanced breast cancer. N Engl J Med 304:16–21
4. Soule HD, Vazguez J, Long A et al (1973) A human cell line from a pleural effusion derived from a breast carcinoma. J Natl Cancer Inst 51:1409–1416
5. Brooks SC, Locke ER, Soule HD (1973) Estrogen receptor in a human cell line (MCF-7) from breast carcinoma. J Biol Chem 248:6251–6253
6. Lippman ME, Bolan G (1975) Oestrogen-responsive human breast cancer in long term tissue culture. Nature 256:592–593
7. Shafie SM (1980) Estrogen and the growth of breast cancer: new evidence suggests indirect action. Science 209:701–702
8. Berthois Y, Katzenellenbogen JA, Katzenellenbogen BS (1986) Phenol red in tissue culture media is a weak estrogen: implications concerning the study of estrogen-responsive cells in culture. Proc Natl Acad Sci U S A 83:2496–2500
9. Bindal RD, Katzenellenbogen JA (1988) Bis(4-hydroxyphenyl)[2-(phenoxysulfonyl)phenyl] methane: isolation and structure elucidation of a novel estrogen from commercial preparations of phenol red (phenolsulfonphthalein). J Med Chem 31:1978–1983
10. Welshons WV, Jordan VC (1987) Adaptation of estrogen-dependent MCF-7 cells to low estrogen (phenol red-free) culture. Eur J Cancer Clin Oncol 23:1935–1939

11. Levenson AS, Jordan VC (1997) MCF-7: the first hormone-responsive breast cancer cell line. Cancer Res 57:3071–3078

12. Nawata H, Bronzert D, Lippman ME (1981) Isolation and characterization of a tamoxifen-resistant cell line derived from MCF-7 human breast cancer cells. J Biol Chem 256:5016–5021

13. Miller MA, Lippman ME, Katzenellenbogen BS (1984) Antiestrogen binding in antiestrogen growth-resistant estrogen-responsive clonal variants of MCF-7 human breast cancer cells. Cancer Res 44:5038–5045

14. Bronzert DA, Greene GL, Lippman ME (1985) Selection and characterization of a breast cancer cell line resistant to the antiestrogen LY 117018. Endocrinology 117:1409–1417

15. van den Berg HW, Lynch M, Martin J et al (1989) Characterisation of a tamoxifen-resistant variant of the ZR-75-1 human breast cancer cell line (ZR-75-9a1) and ability of the resistant phenotype. Br J Cancer 59:522–526

16. Wiseman LR, Johnson MD, Wakeling AE et al (1993) Type I IGF receptor and acquired tamoxifen resistance in oestrogen-responsive human breast cancer cells. Eur J Cancer 29A:2256–2264

17. Brunner N, Frandsen TL, Holst-Hansen C et al (1993) MCF7/LCC2: a 4-hydroxytamoxifen resistant human breast cancer variant that retains sensitivity to the steroidal antiestrogen ICI 182,780. Cancer Res 53:3229–3232

18. Lykkesfeldt AE, Madsen MW, Briand P (1994) Altered expression of estrogen-regulated genes in a tamoxifen-resistant and ICI 164,384 and ICI 182,780 sensitive human breast cancer cell line, MCF-7/TAMR-1. Cancer Res 54:1587–1595

19. Borras M, Jin L, Bouhoute A et al (1994) Evaluation of estrogen receptor, antiestrogen binding sites and calmodulin for antiestrogen resistance of two clones derived from the MCF-7 breast cancer cell line. Biochem Pharmacol 48:2015–2024

20. Brunner N, Boysen B, Jirus S et al (1997) MCF7/LCC9: an antiestrogen-resistant MCF-7 variant in which acquired resistance to the steroidal antiestrogen ICI 182,780 confers an early cross-resistance to the nonsteroidal antiestrogen tamoxifen. Cancer Res 57:3486–3493

21. Larsen SS, Madsen MW, Jensen BL, Lykkesfeldt AE (1997) Resistance of human breast-cancer cells to the pure steroidal anti-estrogen ICI 182,780 is not associated with a general loss of estrogen-receptor expression or lack of estrogen responsiveness. Int J Cancer 72:1129–1136

22. Parisot JP, Leeding KS, Hu XF et al (1999) Induction of insulin-like growth factor binding protein expression by ICI 182,780 in a tamoxifen-resistant human breast cancer cell line. Breast Cancer Res Treat 55:231–242

23. Chan CM, Lykkesfeldt AE, Parker MG, Dowsett M (1999) Expression of nuclear receptor interacting proteins TIF-1, SUG-1, receptor interacting protein 140, and corepressor SMRT in tamoxifen-resistant breast cancer. Clin Cancer Res 5:3460–3467

24. Shafie SM, Grantham FH (1981) Role of hormones in the growth and regression of human breast cancer cells (MCF-7) transplanted into athymic nude mice. J Natl Cancer Inst 67:51–56

25. Osborne CK, Hobbs K, Clark GM (1985) Effect of estrogens and antiestrogens on growth of human breast cancer cells in athymic nude mice. Cancer Res 45:584–590

26. Osborne CK, Coronado EB, Robinson JP (1987) Human breast cancer in the athymic nude mouse: cytostatic effects of long-term antiestrogen therapy. Eur J Cancer Clin Oncol 23:1189–1196

27. Jordan VC, Allen KE (1980) Evaluation of the antitumour activity of the non-steroidal antioestrogen monohydroxytamoxifen in the DMBA-induced rat mammary carcinoma model. Eur J Cancer 16:239–251

28. Gottardis MM, Jordan VC (1988) Development of tamoxifen-stimulated growth of MCF-7 tumors in athymic mice after long-term antiestrogen administration. Cancer Res 48:5183–5187

29. Gottardis MM, Wagner RJ, Borden EC, Jordan VC (1989) Differential ability of antiestrogens to stimulate breast cancer cell (MCF-7) growth in vivo and in vitro. Cancer Res 49:4765–4769

30. Harper MJ, Walpole AL (1966) Contrasting endocrine activities of cis and trans isomers in a series of substituted triphenylethylenes. Nature 212:87

31. Osborne CK, Coronado E, Allred DC et al (1991) Acquired tamoxifen resistance: correlation with reduced breast tumor levels of tamoxifen and isomerization of trans-4-hydroxytamoxifen. J Natl Cancer Inst 83:1477–1482

32. Osborne CK, Wiebe VJ, McGuire WL et al (1992) Tamoxifen and the isomers of 4-hydroxytamoxifen in tamoxifen-resistant tumors from breast cancer patients. J Clin Oncol 10:304–310

33. Wiebe VJ, Osborne CK, McGuire WL, DeGregorio MW (1992) Identification of estrogenic tamoxifen metabolite(s) in tamoxifen-resistant human breast tumors. J Clin Oncol 10:990–994

34. Murphy CS, Langan-Fahey SM, McCague R, Jordan VC (1990) Structure-function relationships of hydroxylated metabolites of tamoxifen that control the proliferation of estrogen-responsive T47D breast cancer cells in vitro. Mol Pharmacol 38:737–743

35. Jordan VC, Koch R, Langan S, McCague R (1988) Ligand interaction at the estrogen receptor to program antiestrogen action: a study with nonsteroidal compounds in vitro. Endocrinology 122:1449–1454

36. Wolf DM, Langan-Fahey SM, Parker CJ et al (1993) Investigation of the mechanism of tamoxifen-stimulated breast tumor growth with nonisomerizable analogues of tamoxifen and metabolites. J Natl Cancer Inst 85:806–812

37. Benz CC, Scott GK, Sarup JC et al (1992) Estrogen-dependent, tamoxifen-resistant tumorigenic growth of MCF-7 cells transfected with HER2/neu. Breast Cancer Res Treat 24:85–95

38. Slamon DJ, Leyland-Jones B, Shak S et al (2001) Use of chemotherapy plus a monoclonal antibody against HER2 for metastatic breast cancer that overexpresses HER2. N Engl J Med 344:783–792

39. Marty M, Cognetti F, Maraninchi D et al (2005) Randomized phase II trial of the efficacy and safety of trastuzumab combined with docetaxel in patients with human epidermal growth factor receptor 2-positive metastatic breast cancer administered as first-line treatment: the M77001 study group. J Clin Oncol 23:4265–4274

40. Gasparini G, Gion M, Mariani L et al (2007) Randomized Phase II Trial of weekly paclitaxel alone versus trastuzumab plus weekly paclitaxel as first-line therapy of patients with Her-2 positive advanced breast cancer. Breast Cancer Res Treat 101:355–365

41. Robert N, Leyland-Jones B, Asmar L et al (2006) Randomized phase III study of trastuzumab, paclitaxel, and carboplatin compared with trastuzumab and paclitaxel in women with HER-2-overexpressing metastatic breast cancer. J Clin Oncol 24:2786–2792

42. Bernard-Marty C, Lebrun F, Awada A, Piccart MJ (2006) Monoclonal antibody-based targeted therapy in breast cancer: current status and future directions. Drugs 66:1577–1591

43. Cortes J, Fumoleau P, Bianchi GV et al (2012) Pertuzumab monotherapy after trastuzumab-based treatment and subsequent reintroduction of trastuzumab: activity and tolerability in patients with advanced human epidermal growth factor receptor 2-positive breast cancer. J Clin Oncol 30:1594–1600

44. Kiewe P, Hasmuller S, Kahlert S et al (2006) Phase I trial of the trifunctional anti-HER2 x anti-CD3 antibody ertumaxomab in metastatic breast cancer. Clin Cancer Res 12:3085–3091

45. Konecny GE, Pegram MD, Venkatesan N et al (2006) Activity of the dual kinase inhibitor lapatinib (GW572016) against HER-2-overexpressing and trastuzumab-treated breast cancer cells. Cancer Res 66:1630–1639

46. Gomez HL, Doval DC, Chavez MA et al (2008) Efficacy and safety of lapatinib as first-line therapy for ErbB2-amplified locally advanced or metastatic breast cancer. J Clin Oncol 26:2999–3005

47. Nelson MH, Dolder CR (2006) Lapatinib: a novel dual tyrosine kinase inhibitor with activity in solid tumors. Ann Pharmacother 40:261–269

48. Cameron D, Casey M, Press M et al (2008) A phase III randomized comparison of lapatinib plus capecitabine versus capecitabine alone in women with advanced breast cancer that has progressed on trastuzumab: updated efficacy and biomarker analyses. Breast Cancer Res Treat 112:533–543

49. Xia W, Bacus S, Hegde P et al (2006) A model of acquired autoresistance to a potent ErbB2 tyrosine kinase inhibitor and a therapeutic strategy to prevent its onset in breast cancer. Proc Natl Acad Sci U S A 103:7795–7800

50. Shou J, Massarweh S, Osborne CK et al (2004) Mechanisms of tamoxifen resistance: increased estrogen receptor-HER2/neu cross-talk in ER/HER2-positive breast cancer. J Natl Cancer Inst 96:926–935

51. Riemsma R, Forbes CA, Amonkar MM et al (2012) Systematic review of lapatinib in combination with letrozole compared with other first-line treatments for hormone receptor positive(HR+) and HER2+ advanced or metastatic breast cancer (MBC). Curr Med Res Opin 28(8):1263–1279

52. Maximov PY, Lewis-Wambi JS, Jordan VC (2009) The paradox of oestradiol-induced breast cancer cell growth and apoptosis. Curr Signal Transduct Ther 4:88–102

53. Schafer JM, Lee ES, O'Regan RM et al (2000) Rapid development of tamoxifen-stimulated mutant p53 breast tumors (T47D) in athymic mice. Clin Cancer Res 6:4373–4380

54. Osborne CK, Pippen J, Jones SE et al (2002) Double-blind, randomized trial comparing the efficacy and tolerability of fulvestrant versus anastrozole in postmenopausal women with advanced breast cancer progressing on prior endocrine therapy: results of a North American trial. J Clin Oncol 20:3386–3395

55. Howell A, Robertson JF, Quaresma Albano J et al (2002) Fulvestrant, formerly ICI 182,780, is as effective as anastrozole in postmenopausal women with advanced breast cancer progressing after prior endocrine treatment. J Clin Oncol 20:3396–3403

56. Wakeling AE, Bowler J (1987) Steroidal pure antioestrogens. J Endocrinol 112:R7–R10

57. Wakeling AE, Dukes M, Bowler J (1991) A potent specific pure antiestrogen with clinical potential. Cancer Res 51:3867–3873

58. Gottardis MM, Jiang SY, Jeng MH, Jordan VC (1989) Inhibition of tamoxifen-stimulated growth of an MCF-7 tumor variant in athymic mice by novel steroidal antiestrogens. Cancer Res 49:4090–4093

59. Tormey DC, Jordan VC (1984) Long-term tamoxifen adjuvant therapy in node-positive breast cancer: a metabolic and pilot clinical study. Breast Cancer Res Treat 4:297–302

60. Scottish Cancer Trials Office (MRC), Edinburgh (1987) Adjuvant tamoxifen in the management of operable breast cancer: the Scottish Trial. Report from the Breast Cancer Trials Committee. Lancet 2:171–175

61. Fisher B, Brown A, Wolmark N et al (1987) Prolonging tamoxifen therapy for primary breast cancer. Findings from the National Surgical Adjuvant Breast and Bowel Project clinical trial. Ann Intern Med 106:649–654

62. Wolf DM, Jordan VC (1994) Characterization of tamoxifen stimulated MCF-7 tumor variants grown in athymic mice. Breast Cancer Res Treat 31:117–127

63. Wolf DM, Jordan VC (1993) A laboratory model to explain the survival advantage observed in patients taking adjuvant tamoxifen therapy. Recent Results Cancer Res 127:23–33

64. Yao K, Lee ES, Bentrem DJ et al (2000) Antitumor action of physiological estradiol on tamoxifen-stimulated breast tumors grown in athymic mice. Clin Cancer Res 6:2028–2036

65. Santen RJ, Samojlik E, Wells SA (1980) Resistance of the ovary to blockade of aromatization with aminoglutethimide. J Clin Endocrinol Metab 51:473–477

66. Santen RJ, Worgul TJ, Samojlik E et al (1981) A randomized trial comparing surgical adrenalectomy with aminoglutethimide plus hydrocortisone in women with advanced breast cancer. N Engl J Med 305:545–551

67. Brodie AM, Schwarzel WC, Brodie HJ (1976) Studies on the mechanism of estrogen biosynthesis in the rat ovary–I. J Steroid Biochem 7:787–793

68. Brodie AM, Schwarzel WC, Shaikh AA, Brodie HJ (1977) The effect of an aromatase inhibitor, 4-hydroxy-4-androstene-3,17-dione, on estrogen-dependent processes in reproduction and breast cancer. Endocrinology 100:1684–1695

69. Brodie AM, Garrett WM, Hendrickson JR et al (1981) Inactivation of aromatase in vitro by 4-hydroxy-4-androstene-3,17-dione and 4-acetoxy-4-androstene-3,17-dione and sustained effects in vivo. Steroids 38:693–702

70. Coombes RC, Goss P, Dowsett M et al (1984) 4-hydroxyandrostenedione in treatment of postmenopausal patients with advanced breast cancer. Lancet 2:1237–1239

71. Masamura S, Santner SJ, Heitjan DF, Santen RJ (1995) Estrogen deprivation causes estradiol hypersensitivity in human breast cancer cells. J Clin Endocrinol Metab 80:2918–2925

72. Shim WS, Conaway M, Masamura S et al (2000) Estradiol hypersensitivity and mitogen-activated protein kinase expression in long-term estrogen deprived human breast cancer cells in vivo. Endocrinology 141:396–405

73. Song RX, Mor G, Naftolin F et al (2001) Effect of long-term estrogen deprivation on apoptotic responses of breast cancer cells to 17beta-estradiol. J Natl Cancer Inst 93:1714–1723

74. Haddow A, Watkinson JM, Paterson E, Koller PC (1944) Influence of synthetic oestrogens on advanced malignant disease. Br Med J 2:393–398

75. Kennedy BJ, Nathanson IT (1953) Effects of intensive sex steroid hormone therapy in advanced breast cancer. J Am Med Assoc 152:1135–1141

76. Anderson GL, Chlebowski RT, Aragaki AK et al (2012) Conjugated equine oestrogen and breast cancer incidence and mortality in postmenopausal women with hysterectomy: extended follow-up of the Women's Health Initiative randomised placebo-controlled trial. Lancet Oncol 13:476–486

77. Jordan VC (2003) Tamoxifen: a most unlikely pioneering medicine. Nat Rev Drug Discov 2:205–213

78. Haddow A (1971) Cancer research: the great debate. N Engl J Med 285:24–28

79. Haddow A, David A (1970) Karnofsky memorial lecture. Thoughts on chemical therapy. Cancer 26:737–754

80. Osipo C, Gajdos C, Liu H et al (2003) Paradoxical action of fulvestrant in estradiol-induced regression of tamoxifen-stimulated breast cancer. J Natl Cancer Inst 95:1597–1608

81. Jiang SY, Wolf DM, Yingling JM et al (1992) An estrogen receptor positive MCF-7 clone that is resistant to antiestrogens and estradiol. Mol Cell Endocrinol 90:77–86

82. Pink JJ, Jiang SY, Fritsch M, Jordan VC (1995) An estrogen-independent MCF-7 breast cancer cell line which contains a novel 80-kilodalton estrogen receptor-related protein. Cancer Res 55:2583–2590

83. Lewis JS, Meeke K, Osipo C et al (2005) Intrinsic mechanism of estradiol-induced apoptosis in breast cancer cells resistant to estrogen deprivation. J Natl Cancer Inst 97:1746–1759

84. Lewis-Wambi JS, Kim HR, Wambi C et al (2008) Buthionine sulfoximine sensitizes antihormone-resistant human breast cancer cells to estrogen-induced apoptosis. Breast Cancer Res 10:R104

85. Ariazi EA, Cunliffe HE, Lewis-Wambi JS et al (2011) Estrogen induces apoptosis in estrogen deprivation-resistant breast cancer through stress responses as identified by global gene expression across time. Proc Natl Acad Sci U S A 108:18879–18886

86. Fan P, McDaniel RE, Kim HR et al (2012) Modulating therapeutic effects of the c-Src inhibitor via oestrogen receptor and human epidermal growth factor receptor 2 in breast cancer cell lines. Eur J Cancer 48(18):3488–3498

87. Brzozowski AM, Pike AC, Dauter Z et al (1997) Molecular basis of agonism and antagonism in the oestrogen receptor. Nature 389:753–758

88. Shiau AK, Barstad D, Loria PM et al (1998) The structural basis of estrogen receptor/coactivator recognition and the antagonism of this interaction by tamoxifen. Cell 95:927–937

89. Jordan VC, Koch R, Mittal S, Schneider MR (1986) Oestrogenic and antioestrogenic actions in a series of triphenylbut-1-enes: modulation of prolactin synthesis in vitro. Br J Pharmacol 87:217–223

90. Lieberman ME, Gorski J, Jordan VC (1983) An estrogen receptor model to describe the regulation of prolactin synthesis by antiestrogens in vitro. J Biol Chem 258:4741–4745

91. Lieberman ME, Jordan VC, Fritsch M et al (1983) Direct and reversible inhibition of estradiol-stimulated prolactin synthesis by antiestrogens in vitro. J Biol Chem 258:4734–4740

92. Jordan VC, Lieberman ME (1984) Estrogen-stimulated prolactin synthesis in vitro. Classification of agonist, partial agonist, and antagonist actions based on structure. Mol Pharmacol 26:279–285

93. Levenson AS, Catherino WH, Jordan VC (1997) Estrogenic activity is increased for an antiestrogen by a natural mutation of the estrogen receptor. J Steroid Biochem Mol Biol 60:261–268

94. Levenson AS, Tonetti DA, Jordan VC (1998) The oestrogen-like effect of 4-hydroxytamoxifen on induction of transforming growth factor alpha mRNA in MDA-MB-231 breast cancer cells stably expressing the oestrogen receptor. Br J Cancer 77:1812–1819

95. Bentrem D, Dardes R, Liu H et al (2001) Molecular mechanism of action at estrogen receptor alpha of a new clinically relevant antiestrogen (GW7604) related to tamoxifen. Endocrinology 142:838–846

96. MacGregor Schafer J, Liu H, Bentrem DJ et al (2000) Allosteric silencing of activating function 1 in the 4-hydroxytamoxifen estrogen receptor complex is induced by substituting glycine for aspartate at amino acid 351. Cancer Res 60:5097–5105

97. Liu H, Park WC, Bentrem DJ et al (2002) Structure-function relationships of the raloxifene-estrogen receptor-alpha complex for regulating transforming growth factor-alpha expression in breast cancer cells. J Biol Chem 277:9189–9198

98. Liu H, Lee ES, Deb Los Reyes A et al (2001) Silencing and reactivation of the selective estrogen receptor modulator-estrogen receptor alpha complex. Cancer Res 61:3632–3639

99. Jordan VC, Schafer JM, Levenson AS et al (2001) Molecular classification of estrogens. Cancer Res 61:6619–6623

100. Bentrem D, Fox JE, Pearce ST et al (2003) Distinct molecular conformations of the estrogen receptor alpha complex exploited by environmental estrogens. Cancer Res 63:7490–7496

101. Maximov P, Sengupta S, Lewis-Wambi JS et al (2011) The conformation of the estrogen receptor directs estrogen-induced apoptosis in breast cancer: A hypothesis. Horm Mol Biol Clin Investig 5:27–34

102. Hu ZZ, Kagan BL, Ariazi EA et al (2011) Proteomic analysis of pathways involved in estrogen-induced growth and apoptosis of breast cancer cells. PLoS One 6:e20410

103. Wolf DM, Jordan VC (1994) The estrogen receptor from a tamoxifen stimulated MCF-7 tumor variant contains a point mutation in the ligand binding domain. Breast Cancer Res Treat 31:129–138

104. Catherino WH, Wolf DM, Jordan VC (1995) A naturally occurring estrogen receptor mutation results in increased estrogenicity of a tamoxifen analog. Mol Endocrinol 9:1053–1063

105. Jeng MH, Jiang SY, Jordan VC (1994) Paradoxical regulation of estrogen-dependent growth factor gene expression in estrogen receptor (ER)-negative human breast cancer cells stably expressing ER. Cancer Lett 82:123–128

106. Levenson AS, Jordan VC (1998) The key to the antiestrogenic mechanism of raloxifene is amino acid 351 (aspartate) in the estrogen receptor. Cancer Res 58:1872–1875

107. Jordan VC (1984) Biochemical pharmacology of antiestrogen action. Pharmacol Rev 36:245–276

108. Levenson AS, MacGregor Schafer JI, Bentrem DJ et al (2001) Control of the estrogen-like actions of the tamoxifen-estrogen receptor complex by the surface amino acid at position 351. J Steroid Biochem Mol Biol 76:61–70

109. Dickson RB, Lippman ME (1995) Growth factors in breast cancer. Endocr Rev 16:559–589

110. Ellis MJ, Gao F, Dehdashti F et al (2009) Lower-dose vs high-dose oral estradiol therapy of hormone receptor-positive, aromatase inhibitor-resistant advanced breast cancer: a phase 2 randomized study. JAMA 302:774–780

111. Liu H, Lee ES, Gajdos C et al (2003) Apoptotic action of 17beta-estradiol in raloxifene-resistant MCF-7 cells in vitro and in vivo. J Natl Cancer Inst 95:1586–1597

112. Lewis JS, Osipo C, Meeke K, Jordan VC (2005) Estrogen-induced apoptosis in a breast cancer model resistant to long-term estrogen withdrawal. J Steroid Biochem Mol Biol 94:131–141

113. Tonetti DA, Chisamore MJ, Grdina W et al (2000) Stable transfection of protein kinase C alpha cDNA in hormone-dependent breast cancer cell lines. Br J Cancer 83:782–791

114. Chisamore MJ, Ahmed Y, Bentrem DJ et al (2001) Novel antitumor effect of estradiol in athymic mice injected with a T47D breast cancer cell line overexpressing protein kinase Calpha. Clin Cancer Res 7:3156–3165

115. Lin X, Yu Y, Zhao Y et al (2006) Overexpression of PKCα is required to impact estradiol inhibition and tamoxifen-resistance in a T47D human breast cancer tumor model. Carcinogenesis 27:1538–1546

116. Zhang Y, Zhao H, Asztalos S et al (2009) Estradiol-induced regression in T47D:A18/PKCalpha tumors requires the estrogen receptor and interaction with the extracellular matrix. Mol Cancer Res 7:498–510

Chapter 10
The Legacy of Tamoxifen

Abstract Tamoxifen, the first targeted therapy to treat breast cancer, has dramatically changed medicine. Study of the pharmacology of tamoxifen created a successful adjuvant treatment strategy to save lives, created the first chemopreventive to prevent any cancer in humans, and was the pioneering selective estrogen receptor modulator (SERM) that resulted in the new drug group, the SERMs. New agents such as lasofoxifene and bazedoxifene show promise in the range of beneficial effects they demonstrate in clinical trial to treat multiple diseases in women. Additionally, new agents and approaches with conjugated equine estrogen are being explored to prevent hot flashes, thereby enhancing the likelihood that compliance with SERMs improves.

Introduction

During the 1970s and 1980s, the pharmaceutical industry worked diligently to study the structure-activity relationships of nonsteroidal antiestrogens to find a competitor for tamoxifen. The list includes droloxifene (3-hydroxytamoxifen), trioxifene, LY117,018, toremifene, and idoxifene [1]. Clinical trials were, in the main, unable to show any significant advantages over tamoxifen. The bench mark to predict success was less uterotrophic activity and LY117,018, which as a result evolved to become raloxifene via LY156,758. Toremifene was registered for the treatment of metastatic breast cancer but is not approved for adjuvant therapy in the United States. There has been interest in the use of toremifene for the treatment of prostate cancer [2, 3]. Tamoxifen, uniquely, remained the sole agent of choice as an adjuvant therapy for about 20 years.

ICI Pharmaceutical Division chose another direction to solve the "estrogenic tickle" of tamoxifen with a plan for the development of fulvestrant as an injectable pure antiestrogen.

P.Y. Maximov et al., *Tamoxifen*, Milestones in Drug Therapy,
DOI 10.1007/978-3-0348-0664-0_10, © Springer Basel 2013

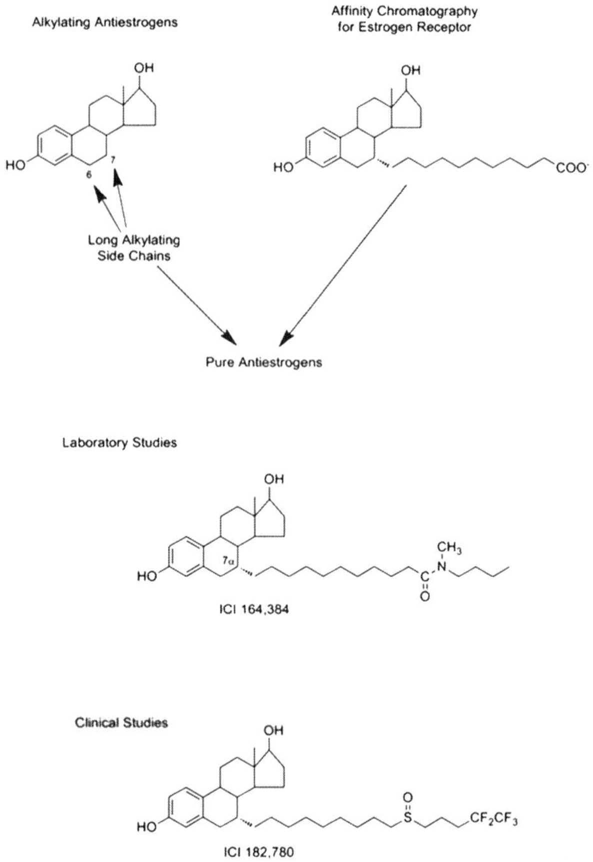

Fig. 10.1 The progress of two unrelated ideas coming together to create a new drug group: the pure antiestrogens. Estradiol derivatives substituted at 6 and 7 positions were created to deliver an alkylating agent via the ER to DNA. In contrast, estradiol was attached to long hydrocarbon chains on the Sephadex column to purify the ER. Both aspects of estradiol chemistry came together to create the pure antiestrogens at ICI Pharmaceuticals Division in the early 1980s

Pure Antiestrogens

The possibility that a pure antiestrogen could be developed with high binding affinity for the ER combines the observation that MER 25, the first antiestrogen, has virtually no estrogenic properties in any animal species [4], with the knowledge that binding affinity and biological activity are separate functions of the same molecule [5]. The antiestrogens ICI164,384 and ICI182,780 are derivatives of estradiol with an optimal binding affinity for the ER, but these structural analogs are unique because they do not have any estrogenic properties and they have a novel subcellular mechanism of action [6] (Fig. 10.1). The serendipitous discovery of pure antiestrogens occurred through two essentially unsuccessful research endeavors that converged thus providing the optimal intellectual environment for new drug discovery. Derivatives of estradiol or estrone substituted in the 6 and 7 positions were being evaluated as potential alkylating antiestrogens in the late 1970s through an ICI-Leeds University joint research scheme [7]. Independently, scientists in France were attempting to purify the ER using estradiol linked at the 7 position through a ten-membered carbon side chain to

Sephadex columns [8]. Dr. Alan Wakeling brought both of these independent ideas together to discover the structure-function relationships of a new class of compounds that have no estrogenic properties in any test system [9–11]. The pure antiestrogen ICI 164,384 has been used extensively in laboratory studies [6], but the more potent ICI182,780 [11] is currently approved for the treatment of breast cancer in postmenopausal women metastatic breast cancer.

The compound is used as a 250-mg injectable 1-month sustained release preparation with therapeutic equivalence to anastrozole following failure of tamoxifen therapy [12, 13]. However, the endocrine option of fulvestrant has never achieved "first-line" status and as such never been evaluated as an adjuvant therapy. Nevertheless, 2-week injection strategies deserve mention.

The idea of combining an aromatase inhibitor with fulvestrant versus an aromatase inhibitor alone has merit from laboratory studies but has produced one result which was an improvement for the combination versus the aromatase inhibitor alone. By contrast, a second trial using the same treatment [14] protocol showed no difference for the combination versus the aromatase inhibitor alone [15]. It seems that the trial that showed no improvement for the combination [15] had a higher population of patients who had been exposed to tamoxifen treatment previously. Another issue is dosage. The pharmacokinetics of fulvestrant from the 250-mg depot injection is poor with low circulating levels [16]. To address this critically important issue, the CONFIRM trial has compared 250 versus 500 mg monthly injections [17]. The higher dose provides a superior response so this should now be considered to be the dosage of choice.

Angela Brodie's dedicated and pioneering work [18–20] was essential as proof of principle that a selective aromatase inhibitor could be discovered with clinical efficacy. The problem with her discovery, 4-hydroxyandrostenedione, was that it was an injectable rather than a more convenient oral preparation. However, the fact that the failed "morning-after pill" ICI46,474 was transformed successfully into the "gold standard" tamoxifen for the adjuvant treatment of breast cancer provided a new target (the aromatase enzyme) to improve antihormonal therapy in breast cancer. With profits expanding from sales of tamoxifen in the United States after 1990, the key issue for the successful drug development of an aromatase inhibitor would be satisfied: profits. The patent from tamoxifen would be running out in America by 2000, and aromatase inhibitors would be substituted, but only for the postmenopausal patients. Three orally active third-generation aromatase inhibitors were subsequently successfully developed for adjuvant therapy: anastrozole, letrozole, and exemestane. Each was demonstrated to have a small but consistent improvement over 5 years of tamoxifen alone whether given instead of tamoxifen in postmenopausal patients, after 5 years of tamoxifen, or switching after a couple of years of tamoxifen [22–29]. There has even been a successful trial of exemestane as a prevention in postmenopausal high-risk women [30]. However, it is hard to see how this approach would be superior to a sophisticated third-generation SERM functioning as a multifunctional medicine in women's health.

The advantages of aromatase inhibitors for postmenopausal patients are clear in large population trials and for healthcare systems. Patents for aromatase inhibitors are now running out or have run out and cheap generics are becoming available.

The aromatase inhibitors were initially priced extremely high compared to tamoxifen to compensate for each only securing about 1/3 of the original tamoxifen market. A disease-free survival advantage is noted for adding an aromatase inhibitor to the treatment plan compared to tamoxifen alone [31] and concerns about endometrial cancer and blood clots are diminished. Current clinical studies to improve endocrine response rates seek to exploit emerging knowledge about the molecular mechanisms of antihormone resistance to aromatase inhibitors [32]. Combinations of letrozole and lapatinib, an inhibitor of the HER2 pathway, show some advantages over letrozole alone in ER-positive and HER-positive metastatic breast cancer [33]. A similar improvement in responsiveness to aromatase inhibitors is noted with a combination with the mTor inhibitor everolimus [34–36]. None of this would have come about but for the 20 years of experience using tamoxifen as the pioneer.

SERM Successes

A failed "morning-after pill," ICI46,474, becomes tamoxifen and a failed "breast cancer drug," LY156,758, becomes raloxifene to give us the science of selective estrogen receptor modulators (SERMs). There two "wrongs" gave women's health a path that was the "right" research track. As a result the lives of millions of women were improved worldwide. The women who survived through tamoxifen treatment provided strength and support for their families, and the drug continues to fulfill that role in society. Grandmothers now see their grandchildren grow up and mothers see their children married to have families of their own. Women who use raloxifene to prevent osteoporosis have fewer breast cancers, perhaps 20,000 fewer breast cancers if the half a million women taking the drug continue to do so for a decade. Less morbidity occurs with less treatment of cancer and possibly less deaths from breast cancer in the long run.

What is perhaps unique is that without tamoxifen there would be no raloxifene as there had to be a leader to beat. What is unusual is that the pharmacological basis for the development of two orphan drugs from two separate drug companies in separate continents should spring from the same laboratory. The Tamoxifen Team laboratory chose to move, after being talent spotted from Leeds University, to Switzerland and then Wisconsin. These were the opportunities presented and seized upon to be in the right place at exactly the right time, trained and ready to exploit the stream of scientific discoveries that charged medicine twice by the 1990s.

SERMs did not end with raloxifene and the principle created successes and failures over the years. We will close with the pharmacological success of SERMs despite the unsuccessful struggle in this harsh economic climate to create a viable economic model for new compounds. But that initially was the start of both tamoxifen and raloxifene; the key to success was first to market with tamoxifen earning billions over the past 40 years after being abandoned as being financially unviable and raloxifene earning billions too after being totally abandoned for clinical development for half a decade!

The market for the prevention of osteoporosis is much bigger than breast cancer so considerable effort has gone into the development of SERMs for this indication. We will not consider arzoxifene as it has been tested unsuccessfully as a breast cancer therapy and its effectiveness in osteoporosis is proven, but there are consistent decreases in breast cancer incidence. Development is terminated because of toxicity with increased risk of endometrial cancer. We will consider ospemifene and lasofoxifene as agents modeled on earlier antiestrogens and bazedoxifene as a SERM with an interesting twist—combination with conjugated equine estrogen.

Lasofoxifene (CP-336156, Fablyn)

Lasofoxifene is interesting as its structure has its origins to the early days of the 1960s when Lednicer and coworkers [37–39] were seeking the optimal postcoital contraceptive (Fig. 10.2). Nafoxidine was the result that then evolved into a potential breast cancer drug that failed [40]. The search for SERMs defined and refined the possible structural components necessary for the new target—osteoporosis. The discovery and preliminary preclinical pharmacology of CP-33156 were first reported in 1998 and since then there has been a steady stream of important publications about this interesting compound. David Thompson's group has contributed most of the new knowledge describing the actions of CP-33156 in the rat with a particular focus on bone, circulating cholesterol, and the uterus [41–44]. The crystallography of lasofoxifene with the ligand-binding domain (LBD) of the ER is resolved [45]. The conformations of the complex is consistent with prior structure of 4-hydroxytamoxifen [46] and raloxifene [47] which adopt the antagonist conformation with helix 12 pushed back and unable to seal the lasofoxifene into the LBD.

An extremely interesting aspect of the pharmacology of lasofoxifene is the enhanced bioavailability of the levorotatory (l-) enantiomer being more potent in terms of ER binding affinity. The potency in vivo is enhanced because the (l) isomer lasofoxifene is a poor substrate for glucuronidation.

A whole range of clinical trials with lasofoxifene have been completed for the prevention of osteoporosis [48, 49] with beneficial effects of significantly reducing strokes, coronary heart disease, and breast cancer [50] without increasing endometrial cancer. These are all the properties originally proposed for the potential of SERMs [51].

Finally one interesting aspect of lasofoxifene is the enhanced improvement in vaginal atrophy observed with treatment and increased vaginal lubrication [52]. However, despite the fact that lasofoxifene is approved for the treatment and prevention of osteoporosis in the European Union at doses 1/100 of those used for raloxifene, the SERM still is unable to control hot flashes. This is a serious barrier to compliance and quality of life. However, the road to development of the SERM bazedoxifene has produced an interesting solution.

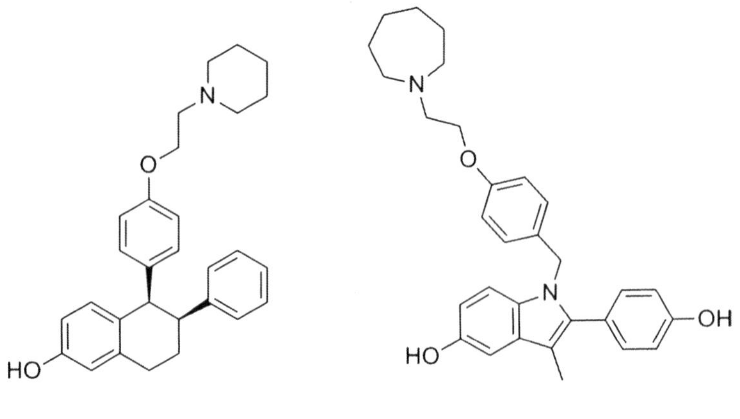

Fig. 10.2 Chemical structures of new SERMs lasofoxifene and bazedoxifene

Bazedoxifene (TSE-424, WAY-140424)

Bazedoxifene is an indole derivative, almost obviously developed from the earlier compound zindoxifene (Fig. 10.2) by attaching an alkylaminoethoxy phenyl side chain in the appropriate "antiestrogen" position of the molecule. The original metabolites of zindoxifene were actually estrogenic in laboratory tests [53] and zindoxifene was without activity for the treatment of breast cancer [54]. Initial laboratory studies with bazedoxifene showed activity as an antiestrogen in MCF-7 breast cancer cells but also was effective in causing cell death [55] in aromatase-resistant breast cancer cells derived from the MCF-7 cell line [56]. Bazedoxifene is a typical SERM which maintains bone density in the ovariectomized rat [57] and the cynomolgus monkey over an 18-month treatment period [58]. Clinical studies demonstrate the value of bazedoxifene from the treatment and potential of osteoporosis. But it is the pairing of bazedoxifene with conjugated equine estrogen (CEE) that enhances effects of lowering lipids and improving bone density while reducing vasomotor effects [59]. In fact, a comparison with lasofoxifene and raloxifene suggests a unique gene profiling for bazedoxifene and CEE on breast cancer cells [60].

Ospemifene (FC-1271a)

This triphenylethylene is a metabolite of toremifene with a unique glycol side chain. This transformation by deamination of the side chain of a nonsteroidal antiestrogen was first noted with tamoxifen when metabolite Y was first discovered [61, 62]. The same transformation occurs with toremifene. Ospemifene is a typical SERM in the rat [63]. Lowering cholesterol, building bone, and blocking estrogen stimulated uterine weight. A range of studies have demonstrated a lack of genotoxicity [64] significant antitumor actions in mice [65] and ability to block the growth of premalignant lesions in a mouse model of DCIS [66]. Indeed the pharmacological effects of ospemifene have been documented in rhesus macaque monkeys [67] as well as humans.

Refining the SERM Concept Further

The fact that there are two ERs, ERα and ERβ [68], naturally has caused a search for ER-specific subtype drugs. Most of our knowledge of the role of each ER subtype has come from a study of knockout mice for one or the other ER [69]. Pharmacologically the main difference between the ER seems to be the AF-1 region [70]. The ligand-binding pockets of ERα and ERβ are very similar with two amino acids Leu and Met in ERα replaced by Met and Leu in ERβ [71].

Despite the difficulties that need to be advanced for subtype-specific agents in very similar proteins, the quest for new medicines has been a priority; changing the antiestrogenic dimethylaminoethoxy side chain to an acrylic side chain creates ERα-specific activity in stimulating endometrial cancer cells [72]. The ERβ-specific agonist SERBA-1 caused involution of the mouse prostate with no effects on ventral prostrate or testicular weight [73]. The Wyeth ERβ-specific agonist ERβ-041 has a dramatic effect in preclinical models of adjuvant-induced arthritis [74]. Most importantly numerous pharmaceutical companies are addressing the issue of controlling hot flashes for a more acceptable SERM. Both Eli Lilly and Johnson & Johnson [75, 76] have compounds shown to control changes in skin temperature in the morphine-dependent rat models.

However, the SERM principle has now been applied to all members of the nuclear receptor superfamily to create selective nuclear receptor modulation to treat diseases with greater specificity not previously believed to be possible. There are now selective androgen receptor modulators (SARMs) [77], selective progesterone receptor modulators (SPRMs) [78], selective glucocorticoid receptor modulators (SGRMs) [79], selective mineralocorticoid receptor modulators (SMRMs) [80], selective thyroid receptor modulators (STRMs) [81], and selective peroxisome proliferator-activated receptor modulators (SPPARMs) [82]. The idea of switching on and off target sites around the body to improve human health and survival is very appealing as we increase longevity.

However, as we bring our story to a close, it is perhaps ironic to reflect that all this progress in a new pharmacology of receptor action was made possible by a potent postcoital contraceptive in the rat, originally designed to prevent life. Much good came from that failed contraceptive tamoxifen that has dramatically enhanced life expectancy, prevented breast cancers, created the SERMs, and dramatically enhanced the prospects of a longer healthier life.

Postscript. Breast cancer is the most prevalent cancer of women and death rates are only secondary to lung cancer. However, lung cancer has a known cause, smoking; the targeting of women by the advertising industry in the 1980s to encourage smoking as a positive lifestyle advance has had consequences with a rising mortality. Breast cancer has no such cause and effect solution to prevent the disease. Yet despite the huge problem of "where to start" in treatment and prevention of breast cancer, the last four decades of research has heralded a new era in personalized medicine for cancer in general, in large part because of the breakthroughs in breast cancer treatment.

The understanding of the links between hormones and breast cancer was to mature for over a century [83] but was, as with all breakthroughs, dependent on the fashions in research. Change occurred in 1971 with passing of the National Cancer Act. This important political step was to articulate a plan to sponsor research and translate the profound breakthroughs that would result into improved patient care. This would be achieved through a nationwide system of clinical cancer centers where laboratory scientists and clinical scientists would interact daily to decrease the mortality from cancer. I have had the privilege of either directing breast cancer programs (University of Wisconsin Comprehensive Cancer Center at Madison, Wisconsin. Then with Monica Morrow, M.D., perhaps the most accomplished breast cancer surgeon in the world; at the Robert H. Lurie Comprehensive Cancer Center, Northwestern University, Chicago), as the vice president of Medical Science (Fox Chase Cancer Center, Philadelphia) or as the scientific director (Georgetown University Lombardi Comprehensive Cancer Center, Washington, DC). But it was the experience of the first cancer center I experienced at the University of Wisconsin (Madison) that was critical for my development as a cancer scientist. The opportunity to be recruited was the reason I went to America. This was a wonderful place to learn and develop my ideas. I had the pleasure of working with Director Paul Carbone, Lasker Prize winner (for the development of MOPP and the treatment of Hodgkin's disease) and also the head of the Eastern Cooperative Group. I was talent spotted because of what I could achieve if given the chance to develop tamoxifen to its full potential. This clearly was a success and the wonderful environment of talented scientific colleagues and first-rate graduate students gave medicine SERMs. But it is my interaction with Harold Rusch the inaugural and then former director of the clinical cancer center that I cherish the most. Harold had his office next to mine and we talked every day. He taught me valuable lessons in scientific leadership and the requirement to advance the career development of one's staff. To this day I answer my phone with "How can I help you?" His book "Something Attempted, Something Done" must be read. He was also the first director of the McArdle Laboratory and built it to be a world-class center of excellence in cancer research. Through the tragedy of his daughter's death from breast cancer, he became one of this nation's strongest advocates for clinical cancer centers to take ideas to the clinic to save lives. There had to be a path to clinical trials and patient care, and he was strategically situated on the President's Cancer Panel to advocate change. He became the first director of the Wisconsin Clinical Cancer Center and then recruited Paul Carbone to continue the task. I was honored when Harold told me that on his death he would like me to speak at his memorial service. He had been diagnosed with prostate cancer and had but a short time to live. To me it was important to obtain a letter of gratitude for all Dr. Rusch had achieved for cancer research in the United States. I went to the President of the United States. This letter was received just in time at a ceremony at Dr. Rusch's home with the letter read and presented by Donna Shala, then chancellor of the University of Wisconsin-Madison. At Harold's memorial service, I read that same letter as my mark of respect for a great yet humble man, who thought of his staff and colleagues always before himself.

With regard to hormones and cancer, the "epicenter" for positive change I believe was the Worcester Foundation for Experimental Biology in Shrewsbury, Massachusetts. This was the home of the oral contraceptive and the founding Director Gregory Pincus [84] created a world-renowned research institution with a principal theme of reproduction research. It was at the Foundation that Pincus turned the dream of oral contraception into a practical reality. His drive and commitment accelerated clinical testing with a progestin which was the culmination of a decade of laboratory investigations. But luck takes control, as often as not. I particularly like the story of the first trials with a synthetic progestin that were found to contain an impurity. The progestin was purified and less effective as a contraceptive. The impurity was an estrogen so the combined oral contraceptives "so to speak" was conceived. But by the late 1960s, fashions in research were changing and cancer research was to move center stage. With the passing of the National Cancer Act in 1971 came opportunity for funding. For one of us (VCJ), who was a visiting scientist at the Foundation (1972–1974), from the University of Leeds, England, this was an important time and valuable to learn and exchange ideas. But the opportunities from the environment of the Foundation catalyzed the conversion of ICI46,474 to tamoxifen (with a *big* push from Lois Trench).

The philosophy of the Foundation was to advance new ideas and concepts. The first systematic studies with tamoxifen as a breast cancer drug were started [85] but remarkably, in a laboratory not more than 100 yards away from mine, Angela and Harvey Brodie were taking the first steps to create 4-hydroxyandronestedione [18] as the first specific aromatase inhibitor successfully tested in patients [21]. Angela's tenacity and vision was critical for the future development of new aromatase inhibitors. The subsequent pharmaceutical development of tamoxifen as the first long-term adjuvant endocrine therapy targeted to the ER and chemopreventive made the improvements with aromatase inhibitors certain. Tamoxifen and the aromatase inhibitors all continue to reduce mortality. These are the therapeutic cornerstones of the modern era of targeted treatments for breast cancer. All the successes in hormones and breast cancer started at the Foundation to be a practical approach to the treatment and prevention.

Furthermore, it is remarkable to note that the scientists at the Worcester Foundation had already changed the world with the oral contraceptive and M. C. Chang had conducted seminal studies on in vitro fertilization with the discovery of sperm capacitation within the uterus. This knowledge was used first in animals. I liked the stories I heard that Chang had taken sperm and egg from a mink and a stoat that normally would never mate to create a *stink*! The animal work was necessary to set the stage for the birth of Louise Brown at 11:47 p.m., 25 July 1978 (coincidentally my birthday). By 8 June 1980, health authorities in Virginia announced the first US-built clinic using the Edwards-Steptoe's method. Society has much to be grateful for from the research on hormones initiated in the confines of a couple of acres of land in Massachusetts and the vision of Gregory Pincus. There are four major advances in women's health: the oral contraceptive, in vitro fertilization, a clinical plan for tamoxifen, and the first specific aromatase inhibitor!

References

1. Gradishar WJ, Jordan VC (1997) Clinical potential of new antiestrogens. J Clin Oncol 15:840–852
2. Stein S, Zoltick B, Peacock T et al (2001) Phase II trial of toremifene in androgen-independent prostate cancer: a Penn cancer clinical trials group trial. Am J Clin Oncol 24:283–285
3. Raghow S, Hooshdaran MZ, Katiyar S, Steiner MS (2002) Toremifene prevents prostate cancer in the transgenic adenocarcinoma of mouse prostate model. Cancer Res 62:1370–1376
4. Lerner LJ, Holthaus FJ Jr, Thompson CR (1958) A non-steroidal estrogen antiagonist 1-(p-2-diethylaminoethoxyphenyl)-1-phenyl-2-p-methoxyphenyl ethanol. Endocrinology 63:295–318
5. Jordan VC, Collins MM, Rowsby L, Prestwich G (1977) A monohydroxylated metabolite of tamoxifen with potent antioestrogenic activity. J Endocrinol 75:305–316
6. Wakeling AE (1994) A new approach to breast cancer therapy-total estrogen ablation with pure antiestrogens. In: Jordan VC (ed) Long-term tamoxifen treatment for breast cancer. University of Wisconsin Press, Madison, pp 219–234
7. Jordan VC, Fenuik L, Allen KE et al (1981) Structural derivatives of tamoxifen and oestradiol 3-methyl ether as potential alkylating antioestrogens. Eur J Cancer 17:193–200
8. Bucourt R, Vignau M, Torelli V (1978) New biospecific adsorbents for the purification of estradiol receptor. J Biol Chem 253:8221–8228
9. Wakeling AE, Bowler J (1987) Steroidal pure antioestrogens. J Endocrinol 112:R7–R10
10. Bowler J, Lilley TJ, Pittam JD, Wakeling AE (1989) Novel steroidal pure antiestrogens. Steroids 54:71–99
11. Wakeling AE, Dukes M, Bowler J (1991) A potent specific pure antiestrogen with clinical potential. Cancer Res 51:3867–3873
12. Osborne CK, Pippen J, Jones SE et al (2002) Double-blind, randomized trial comparing the efficacy and tolerability of fulvestrant versus anastrozole in postmenopausal women with advanced breast cancer progressing on prior endocrine therapy: results of a North American trial. J Clin Oncol 20:3386–3395
13. Howell A, Robertson JF, Quaresma Albano J et al (2002) Fulvestrant, formerly ICI 182,780, is as effective as anastrozole in postmenopausal women with advanced breast cancer progressing after prior endocrine treatment. J Clin Oncol 20:3396–3403
14. Mehta RS, Barlow WE, Albain KS et al (2012) Combination anastrozole and fulvestrant in metastatic breast cancer. N Engl J Med 367:435–444
15. Bergh J, Jonsson PE, Lidbrink EK et al (2012) FACT: an open-label randomized phase III study of fulvestrant and anastrozole in combination compared with anastrozole alone as first-line therapy for patients with receptor-positive postmenopausal breast cancer. J Clin Oncol 30:1919–1925
16. Howell A, DeFriend DJ, Robertson JF et al (1996) Pharmacokinetics, pharmacological and anti-tumour effects of the specific anti-oestrogen ICI 182780 in women with advanced breast cancer. Br J Cancer 74:300–308
17. Di Leo A, Jerusalem G, Petruzelka L et al (2010) Results of the CONFIRM phase III trial comparing fulvestrant 250 mg with fulvestrant 500 mg in postmenopausal women with estrogen receptor-positive advanced breast cancer. J Clin Oncol 28:4594–4600
18. Brodie AM, Schwarzel WC, Shaikh AA, Brodie HJ (1977) The effect of an aromatase inhibitor, 4-hydroxy-4-androstene-3,17-dione, on estrogen-dependent processes in reproduction and breast cancer. Endocrinology 100:1684–1695

19. Brodie AM, Longcope C (1980) Inhibition of peripheral aromatization by aromatase inhibitors, 4-hydroxy- and 4-acetoxy-androstene-3,17-dione. Endocrinology 106:19–21
20. Brodie AM, Marsh D, Brodie HJ (1979) Aromatase inhibitors – IV. Regression of hormone-dependent, mammary tumors in the rat with 4-acetoxy-4-androstene-3,17-dione. J Steroid Biochem 10:423–429
21. Coombes RC, Goss P, Dowsett M et al (1984) 4-hydroxyandrostenedione in treatment of postmenopausal patients with advanced breast cancer. Lancet 2:1237–1239
22. Baum M, Budzar AU, Cuzick J et al (2002) Anastrozole alone or in combination with tamoxifen versus tamoxifen alone for adjuvant treatment of postmenopausal women with early breast cancer: first results of the ATAC randomised trial. Lancet 359:2131–2139
23. Howell A, Cuzick J, Baum M et al (2005) Results of the ATAC (Arimidex, Tamoxifen, Alone or in Combination) trial after completion of 5 years' adjuvant treatment for breast cancer. Lancet 365:60–62
24. Thurlimann B, Keshaviah A, Coates AS et al (2005) A comparison of letrozole and tamoxifen in postmenopausal women with early breast cancer. N Engl J Med 353:2747–2757
25. Coates AS, Keshaviah A, Thurlimann B et al (2007) Five years of letrozole compared with tamoxifen as initial adjuvant therapy for postmenopausal women with endocrine-responsive early breast cancer: update of study BIG 1-98. J Clin Oncol 25:486–492
26. Coombes RC, Hall E, Gibson LJ et al (2004) A randomized trial of exemestane after two to three years of tamoxifen therapy in postmenopausal women with primary breast cancer. N Engl J Med 350:1081–1092
27. Boccardo F, Rubagotti A, Puntoni M et al (2005) Switching to anastrozole versus continued tamoxifen treatment of early breast cancer: preliminary results of the Italian Tamoxifen Anastrozole Trial. J Clin Oncol 23:5138–5147
28. Goss PE, Ingle JN, Martino S et al (2003) A randomized trial of letrozole in postmenopausal women after five years of tamoxifen therapy for early-stage breast cancer. N Engl J Med 349:1793–1802
29. Goss PE, Ingle JN, Martino S et al (2005) Randomized trial of letrozole following tamoxifen as extended adjuvant therapy in receptor-positive breast cancer: updated findings from NCIC CTG MA.17. J Natl Cancer Inst 97:1262–1271
30. Goss PE, Ingle JN, Ales-Martinez JE et al (2011) Exemestane for breast-cancer prevention in postmenopausal women. N Engl J Med 364:2381–2391
31. Dowsett M, Cuzick J, Ingle J et al (2010) Meta-analysis of breast cancer outcomes in adjuvant trials of aromatase inhibitors versus tamoxifen. J Clin Oncol 28:509–518
32. Roop RP, Ma CX (2012) Endocrine resistance in breast cancer: molecular pathways and rational development of targeted therapies. Future Oncol 8:273–292
33. Riemsma R, Forbes CA, Amonkar MM et al (2012) Systematic review of lapatinib in combination with letrozole compared with other first-line treatments for hormone receptor positive(HR+) and HER2+ advanced or metastatic breast cancer(MBC). Curr Med Res Opin 28:1263–1279
34. Bachelot T, Bourgier C, Cropet C et al (2012) Randomized phase II trial of everolimus in combination with tamoxifen in patients with hormone receptor-positive, human epidermal growth factor receptor 2-negative metastatic breast sancer with prior exposure to aromatase inhibitors: A GINECO study. J Clin Oncol 30:2718–2724
35. Baselga J, Campone M, Piccart M et al (2012) Everolimus in postmenopausal hormone-receptor-positive advanced breast cancer. N Engl J Med 366:520–529
36. Baselga J, Semiglazov V, van Dam P et al (2009) Phase II randomized study of neoadjuvant everolimus plus letrozole compared with placebo plus letrozole in patients with estrogen receptor-positive breast cancer. J Clin Oncol 27:2630–2637
37. Lednicer D, Babcock JC, Marlatt PE et al (1965) Mammalian antifertility agents. I. Derivatives of 2,3-diphenylindenes. J Med Chem 8:52–57

38. Lednicer D, Lyster SC, Aspergren BD, Duncan GW (1966) Mammalian antifertility agents. 3. 1-aryl-2-phenyl-1,2,3,4-tetrahydro-1-naphthols, 1-aryl-2-phenyl-3,4-dihydronaphthalenes, and their derivatives. J Med Chem 9:172–176

39. Lednicer D, Lyster SC, Duncan GW (1967) Mammalian antifertility agents. IV. Basic 3,4-dihydronaphthalenes and 1,2,3,4-tetrahydro-1-naphthols. J Med Chem 10:78–84

40. Legha SS, Slavik M, Carter SK (1976) Nafoxidine – an antiestrogen for the treatment of breast cancer. Cancer 38:1535–1541

41. Ke HZ, Paralkar VM, Grasser WA et al (1998) Effects of CP-336,156, a new, nonsteroidal estrogen agonist/antagonist, on bone, serum cholesterol, uterus and body composition in rat models. Endocrinology 139:2068–2076

42. Ke HZ, Qi H, Crawford DT et al (2000) Lasofoxifene (CP-336,156), a selective estrogen receptor modulator, prevents bone loss induced by aging and orchidectomy in the adult rat. Endocrinology 141:1338–1344

43. Ke HZ, Qi H, Chidsey-Frink KL et al (2001) Lasofoxifene (CP-336,156) protects against the age-related changes in bone mass, bone strength, and total serum cholesterol in intact aged male rats. J Bone Miner Res 16:765–773

44. Ke HZ, Foley GL, Simmons HA et al (2004) Long-term treatment of lasofoxifene preserves bone mass and bone strength and does not adversely affect the uterus in ovariectomized rats. Endocrinology 145:1996–2005

45. Vajdos FF, Hoth LR, Geoghegan KF et al (2007) The 2.0 A crystal structure of the ERalpha ligand-binding domain complexed with lasofoxifene. Protein Sci 16:897–905

46. Shiau AK, Barstad D, Loria PM et al (1998) The structural basis of estrogen receptor/coactivator recognition and the antagonism of this interaction by tamoxifen. Cell 95:927–937

47. Brzozowski AM, Pike AC, Dauter Z et al (1997) Molecular basis of agonism and antagonism in the oestrogen receptor. Nature 389:753–758

48. Cummings SR, Ensrud K, Delmas PD et al (2010) Lasofoxifene in postmenopausal women with osteoporosis. N Engl J Med 362:686–696

49. Moffett A, Ettinger M, Bolognese M et al (2004) Lasofoxifene, a next generation SERM, is effective in preventing loss of BMD and reducing LDL-C in postmenopausal women. J Bone Miner Res 19:S96

50. LaCroix AZ, Powles T, Osborne CK et al (2010) Breast cancer incidence in the randomized PEARL trial of lasofoxifene in postmenopausal osteoporotic women. J Natl Cancer Inst 102: 1706–1715

51. Lerner LJ, Jordan VC (1990) Development of antiestrogens and their use in breast cancer: eighth Cain memorial award lecture. Cancer Res 50:4177–4189

52. Gennari L (2009) Lasofoxifene, a new selective estrogen receptor modulator for the treatment of osteoporosis and vaginal atrophy. Expert Opin Pharmacother 10:2209–2220

53. Robinson SP, Jordan VC (1987) Reversal of the antitumor effects of tamoxifen by progesterone in the 7,12-dimethylbenzanthracene-induced rat mammary carcinoma model. Cancer Res 47: 5386–5390

54. Jabara AG, Toyne PH, Harcourt AG (1973) Effects of time and duration of progesterone administration on mammary tumours induced by 7,12-dimethylbenz(a)anthracene in Sprague–Dawley rats. Br J Cancer 27:63–71

55. Chan O, Inouye K, Akirav E et al (2005) Insulin alone increases hypothalamo-pituitary-adrenal activity, and diabetes lowers peak stress responses. Endocrinology 146:1382–1390

56. Lewis-Wambi JS, Kim H, Curpan R et al (2011) The selective estrogen receptor modulator bazedoxifene inhibits hormone-independent breast cancer cell growth and down-regulates estrogen receptor alpha and cyclin D1. Mol Pharmacol 80:610–620

57. Kanasaki H, Bedecarrats GY, Kam KY et al (2005) Gonadotropin-releasing hormone pulse frequency-dependent activation of extracellular signal-regulated kinase pathways in perifused LbetaT2 cells. Endocrinology 146:5503–5513

58. Smith S, Minck D, Jolette J et al (2005) Bazedoxifene prevents ovariectomy-induced bone loss in the Cynomolgus monkey. J Bone Miner Res 20:S174

59. Kharode Y, Bodine PV, Miller CP et al (2008) The pairing of a selective estrogen receptor modulator, bazedoxifene, with conjugated estrogens as a new paradigm for the treatment of menopausal symptoms and osteoporosis prevention. Endocrinology 149:6084–6091

60. Chang KC, Wang Y, Bodine PV et al (2010) Gene expression profiling studies of three SERMs and their conjugated estrogen combinations in human breast cancer cells: insights into the unique antagonistic effects of bazedoxifene on conjugated estrogens. J Steroid Biochem Mol Biol 118:117–124

61. Bain RR, Jordan VC (1983) Identification of a new metabolite of tamoxifen in patient serum during breast cancer therapy. Biochem Pharmacol 32:373–375

62. Jordan VC, Bain RR, Brown RR et al (1983) Determination and pharmacology of a new hydroxylated metabolite of tamoxifen observed in patient sera during therapy for advanced breast cancer. Cancer Res 43:1446–1450

63. Qu Q, Zheng H, Dahllund J et al (2000) Selective estrogenic effects of a novel triphenyl-ethylene compound, FC1271a, on bone, cholesterol level, and reproductive tissues in intact and ovariectomized rats. Endocrinology 141:809–820

64. Hellmann-Blumberg U, Taras TL, Wurz GT, DeGregorio MW (2000) Genotoxic effects of the novel mixed antiestrogen FC-1271a in comparison to tamoxifen and toremifene. Breast Cancer Res Treat 60:63–70

65. Wurz GT, Read KC, Marchisano-Karpman C et al (2005) Ospemifene inhibits the growth of dimethylbenzanthracene-induced mammary tumors in Sencar mice. J Steroid Biochem Mol Biol 97:230–240

66. Namba R, Young LJ, Maglione JE et al (2005) Selective estrogen receptor modulators inhibit growth and progression of premalignant lesions in a mouse model of ductal carcinoma in situ. Breast Cancer Res 7:R881–R889

67. Wurz GT, Hellmann-Blumberg U, DeGregorio MW (2008) Pharmacologic effects of ospemifene in rhesus macaques: a pilot study. Basic Clin Pharmacol Toxicol 102:552–558

68. Nilsson S, Gustafsson JA (2011) Estrogen receptors: therapies targeted to receptor subtypes. Clin Pharmacol Ther 89:44–55

69. Nilsson S, Makela S, Treuter E et al (2001) Mechanisms of estrogen action. Physiol Rev 81:1535–1565

70. McInerney EM, Weis KE, Sun J et al (1998) Transcription activation by the human estrogen receptor subtype beta (ER beta) studied with ER beta and ER alpha receptor chimeras. Endocrinology 139:4513–4522

71. Pike AC, Brzozowski AM, Hubbard RE et al (1999) Structure of the ligand-binding domain of oestrogen receptor beta in the presence of a partial agonist and a full antagonist. EMBO J 18:4608–4618

72. Hoekstra WJ, Patel HS, Liang X et al (2005) Discovery of novel quinoline-based estrogen receptor ligands using peptide interaction profiling. J Med Chem 48:2243–2247

73. Norman BH, Dodge JA, Richardson TI et al (2006) Benzopyrans are selective estrogen receptor beta agonists with novel activity in models of benign prostatic hyperplasia. J Med Chem 49:6155–6157

74. Follettie MT, Pinard M, Keith JC Jr et al (2006) Organ messenger ribonucleic acid and plasma proteome changes in the adjuvant-induced arthritis model: responses to disease induction and therapy with the estrogen receptor-beta selective agonist ERB-041. Endocrinology 147:714–723

75. Jain N, Xu J, Kanojia RM et al (2009) Identification and structure-activity relationships of chromene-derived selective estrogen receptor modulators for treatment of postmenopausal symptoms. J Med Chem 52:7544–7569

76. Wallace OB, Lauwers KS, Dodge JA et al (2006) A selective estrogen receptor modulator for the treatment of hot flushes. J Med Chem 49:843–846

77. Mohler ML, Bohl CE, Jones A et al (2009) Nonsteroidal selective androgen receptor modulators (SARMs): dissociating the anabolic and androgenic activities of the androgen receptor for therapeutic benefit. J Med Chem 52:3597–3617

78. Chabbert-Buffet N, Meduri G, Bouchard P, Spitz IM (2005) Selective progesterone receptor modulators and progesterone antagonists: mechanisms of action and clinical applications. Hum Reprod Update 11:293–307
79. Hudson AR, Roach SL, Higuchi RI (2008) Recent developments in the discovery of selective glucocorticoid receptor modulators (SGRMs). Curr Top Med Chem 8:750–765
80. Baxter JD, Funder JW, Apriletti JW, Webb P (2004) Towards selectively modulating mineralocorticoid receptor function: lessons from other systems. Mol Cell Endocrinol 217:151–165
81. Yoshihara HA, Scanlan TS (2003) Selective thyroid hormone receptor modulators. Curr Top Med Chem 3:1601–1616
82. Berger JP, Petro AE, Macnaul KL et al (2003) Distinct properties and advantages of a novel peroxisome proliferator-activated protein [gamma] selective modulator. Mol Endocrinol 17: 662–676
83. Jordan VC (2009) A century of deciphering the control mechanisms of sex steroid action in breast and prostate cancer: the origins of targeted therapy and chemoprevention. Cancer Res 69:1243–1254
84. Speroff L (2009) A good man: Gregory Goodwin Pincus: the man, his story, the birth control pill. Arnica Pub., Portland, xxi, 359 pp
85. Jordan VC (2006) Tamoxifen (ICI46,474) as a targeted therapy to treat and prevent breast cancer. Br J Pharmacol 147(Suppl 1):S269–S276

Appendix A: Four Decades of Discovery in Breast Cancer Research and Treatment: An Interview with V. Craig Jordan

Marc Poirot

The past is never dead. It is not even the past.—William Faulkner

Abstract

V. Craig Jordan is a pioneer in the molecular pharmacology and therapeutics of breast cancer. As a teenager, he wanted to develop drugs to treat cancer, but at the time in the 1960s, this was unfashionable. Nevertheless, he saw an opportunity and, through his mentors, trained himself to reinvent a failed "morning-after pill" to become tamoxifen, the gold standard for the treatment and prevention of breast cancer. It is estimated that at least a million women worldwide are alive today because of the clinical application of Jordan's laboratory research. Throughout his career, he has always looked at "the good, the bad, and the ugly" of tamoxifen. He was the first to raise concerns about the possibility of tamoxifen increasing endometrial cancer. He described selective estrogen receptor modulation (SERM), and he was the first to describe both the bone protective effects and the breast chemopreventive effects of raloxifene. Raloxifene did not increase endometrial cancer and is now used to prevent breast cancer and osteoporosis. The scientific strategy he introduced of using long-term therapy for treatment and prevention caused him to study acquired drug resistance to SERMs. He made the paradoxical discovery that physiological estrogen can be used to treat and to prevent breast

This article is republished in full from Jordan VC (2011) Four decades of discovery in breast cancer research and treatment–an interview with V. Craig Jordan. Interview by Marc Poirot. Int J DevBiol 55(7-9):703-712 with permission.

M. Poirot (✉)
Sterol Metabolism and Therapeutic Innovations in Oncology, INSERM UMR 1037,
University of Toulouse III, Cancer Research Center of Toulouse, Institut Claudius Regaud,
20, rue du pont Saint Pierre, Toulouse Cedex 31052, France
e-mail: marc.poirot@inserm.fr

cancer once exhaustive antihormone resistance develops. His philosophy for his four decades of discovery has been to use the conversation between the laboratory and the clinic to improve women's health.

Abbreviations. AACR, American Association for Cancer Research; ASCO, American Society of Clinical Oncology; CEE, Conjugated equine estrogen, DES, Diethylstilbestrol; DMBA, Dimethylbenzanthracene; EBCTCG, Early Breast Cancer Trialists' Collaborative Group; ECOG, Eastern Cooperative Oncology Group; FDA, Food and Drug Administration; ICI, Imperial Chemical Industries; SERM, Selective estrogen receptor modulator; STAR, Study of Tamoxifen and Raloxifene; TGF-α, Transforming growth factor-alpha; WFEB, Worcester Foundation for Experimental Biology; WHI, Women's Health Initiative.

Tamoxifen, originally classified as a nonsteroidal antiestrogen but now known as the first selective estrogen receptor modulator (SERM), is a pioneering medicine that for more than 20 years was the gold standard for the adjuvant treatment of breast cancer in pre- and postmenopausal patients with ER-positive tumors [1]. Millions of women continue to live longer and healthier lives because of tamoxifen treatment. Tamoxifen is also a pioneering medicine, as it is the first drug to be approved in the United States of America by the Food and Drug Administration (FDA) for the reduction of the incidence of breast cancer in high-risk pre- and postmenopausal women [2].

Craig Jordan grew up with a passion for chemistry, but was specifically intrigued by the prospect of using organic chemistry to design drugs to treat cancer. At the age of 13, his mother allowed him to convert his bedroom into a chemistry laboratory, where he often got into difficulties during his experiments, either setting the curtains on fire as a rather overreactive experiment was being thrown out of the window or destroying the lawn outside. However, he did convince his mother that by using the chemistry of fertilizers, he could regrow the lawn again, but when he did, it came out an interesting shade of blue! Craig had a passion for teaching, and the chemistry and biology teachers at his school, Moseley Hall Grammar School in Cheadle, Cheshire, England, allowed him to have a laboratory to teach biochemistry. It was these same teachers who convinced his parents that he should apply to university. By contrast, Craig was more content with the idea of becoming an organic chemistry technician at the research laboratories of Imperial Chemical Industries (ICI) near where he lived.

Craig was given an opportunity for interview at only one university (Leeds University, West Yorkshire, England), but he succeeded in convincing the two faculty interviewers, Dr. Ronnie Kaye and Dr. Edward Clark, that he should have a chance in the Pharmacology Department. Years later, Craig found out that the reason he was given an interview was that they had been intrigued at the Headmaster's letter, which stated the candidate was "an unusual young man" and then repeated the statement in capitals. On July 18, 2001, Craig received the first honorary Doctor of Medicine degree from the University of Leeds for humanitarian research that has changed healthcare. The citation, presented by the Chancellor Lord Melvyn Bragg, starts: "Craig Jordan is one of the most distinguished medical scientists of the last one hundred years." He was delighted to be able to invite Drs. Clark and Kaye to the luncheon and the ceremony (Fig. A.1). These were the two individuals who talent-spotted Craig; Dr. Kaye was his tutor for his 4 years as an undergraduate, and Dr. Clark persuaded him to become a graduate student armed with the last available Medical Research Council studentship in the United Kingdom for the year 1969 (Fig. A.2). Someone had declined their studentship, thus allowing Craig to do a Ph.D.! Dr. Clark's project, which Craig found so attractive, was the prospect of extracting the ER from the rodent uterus, purifying it and then crystallizing the ER protein with an estrogen and a nonsteroidal antiestrogen. The x-ray crystallography would be completed at the Astbury Department of Biophysics at the University of Leeds, and all the work was estimated to take the 3 years of the scholarship. At that time, the nonsteroidal antiestrogens had failed to fulfill their promise in the pharmaceutical industry as "morning-after pills"; they were perfect in rats, but in women they did exactly the opposite and enhanced fertility by inducing ovulation.

The project in crystallizing the ER did not go as planned, so he rapidly changed his topic with a new title: "A study of the oestrogenic and anti-oestrogenic activities of some substituted triphenylethylenes and triphenylethanes" (Fig. A.3). This was a good strategic research choice, as no one has yet succeeded in crystallizing the whole ER with either an estrogen or antiestrogen. But further difficulties were to arise in Craig's journey to a career in cancer research.

As a Ph.D. student, Craig was talent spotted for an immediate tenure track faculty position because of his skill as a lecturer. He had no publications and his Ph.D. topic was going nowhere. No one was recommending careers in failed contraceptives! During the interview with the University Committee charged with making the appointment, he was told that he would have to go to America to get his BTA (been to America) before he could start the job. First, however, he had to get a Ph. D., and to do that, it had to be examined. However, the university could find no one in the country qualified for the task. Sir Charles Dodds, the discoverer of the synthetic estrogen, diethylstilbestrol (DES), declined with regrets as he had not kept up with the literature for the past 20 years! But here is where luck and chance take control. He was in the right place at the right time and, by meeting the right people, changed medicine.

Dr. Arthur Walpole was head of the Fertility Control Program at ICI's Pharmaceuticals Division and a personal friend of the chairman of Craig's Pharmacology Department. The university reluctantly accepted Dr. Walpole (despite the fact that he was from industry!) to be Craig's examiner, and he was also able to organize a 2-year visit to the Worcester Foundation for Experimental Biology (WFEB) in Shrewsbury, Massachusetts, to study with Dr. Michael Harper on new methods of contraception. Harper and Walpole had completed all the early work on ICI 46,474 as a contraceptive at ICI Pharmaceuticals in the early 1960s. Craig vividly remembers the transatlantic telephone call with Dr. Harper: "Can you come in September?" "Will $12,000 a year be enough?" "Will you work on prostaglandins?" "Yes, yes, yes," he replied and went off to the library to find out what prostaglandins were! But when he got to the WFEB in September 1972, he was told that Dr. Harper had gone to Geneva to be head of Contraception Research

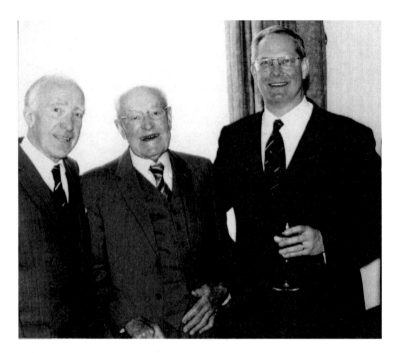

Fig. A.1 Photograph before the ceremony for the degree of Doctor of Medicine *honoris causa* **at Leeds University** on 18 July 2001. Dr. Edward R. Clark, my Ph.D. supervisor (1969–1972) (*left*), and Dr. Ronnie Kaye, head of my degree course (1965–1969) (*center*), formally from the Department of Pharmacology, University of Leeds, England. I am on the *right side* with my signature glass of Burgundy

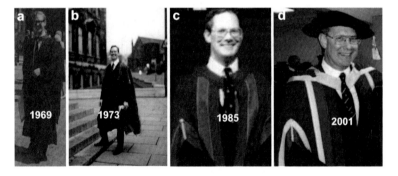

Fig. A.2 I always love dressing up. The University of Leeds is my *alma mater*, and I have attended four ceremonies there: (**a**) Bachelor of Science, First Class Honours, 1969; (**b**) Doctor of Philosophy, 1973; (**c**) Doctor of Science, earned by examination. A select committee evaluated my refereed publications to establish a contribution to science, 1985; (**d**) Honorary Doctor of Medicine for Humanitarian Research, 2001

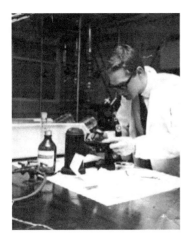
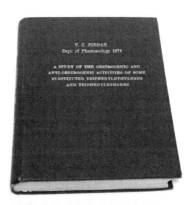

Fig. A.3 My first publicity photograph during the time that I was a Ph.D. student at the Department of Pharmacology, University of Leeds, England, 1969–1972. It was necessary as I had been selected as the Medical Research Council's student representative to the Nobel Prize Winner's meeting in Lindau, Germany, in 1972. I am examining cells from mouse vaginal smears; big science. Also shown is my Ph.D. that nobody wanted to examine

at the World Health Organization. Craig was told to sit down, write up what he would do for the next 2 years, and organize his own laboratory. He was now an independent investigator.

A phone call to Dr. Walpole explained his dilemma at the WFEB, but he felt that there was an opportunity for the failed morning-after pill, ICI 46,474, to be used for the treatment of breast cancer. This call was rewarded by Dr. Walpole arranging for funding and contacts with Ms. Lois Trench at ICI America for Craig to conduct the translational research on the drug that would become tamoxifen. As an independent investigator, the research funding from ICI was an unrestricted research grant, but as Craig was not a cancer research scientist and he was at WFEB, the home of the oral contraceptive, what was the first step to be? Again, it is who you meet. After the National Cancer Act in 1971, the WFEB director had made the decision to bring a cancer research specialist onto the Board of Scientific Advisors to help with future funding opportunities in hormones and cancer research. Dr. Elwood Jensen was the director of the Ben May Laboratory for Cancer Research in Chicago, Illinois, and was credited with the translational research where he described the ER in immature rat estrogen target tissues and then used this knowledge to propose a test for the hormone dependency of metastatic breast cancers. Simply stated, if the ER is absent in the tumor, the patient was unlikely to respond to endocrine ablation (oophorectomy, adrenalectomy, or hypophysectomy), but if the tumor was ER positive, there was a high probability that the tumor would respond to estrogen withdrawal. It was a practical test to avoid morbidity from unnecessary operations that require hospitalization.

Craig spent the day with Dr. Elwood Jensen in November 1972 and told him what he wanted to do with ICI 46,474. Craig subsequently traveled to the Ben May

Laboratory for Cancer Research to be taught techniques of ER analysis and to learn all about the dimethylbenzanthracene (DMBA) rat mammary carcinoma model and then to Dr. Bill McGuire's laboratory in San Antonio, Texas, to learn complementary analytical methods for the ER. Armed with these techniques and resources from ICI throughout the 1970s (his first decade of discovery), he created the laboratory principles of targeting the tumor ER and advocating the use of long-term adjuvant tamoxifen therapy as the appropriate clinical strategy to save lives (Fig. A.4) [3, 4]. This proposition by Craig was not at all popular, as throughout the 1970s and 1980s in the United Kingdom, it was strongly believed there was no correlation between tamoxifen use and the presence of the ER in breast tumors. Additionally, nobody was interested in a new antihormone therapy, as combination cytotoxic chemotherapy was king. It was going to cure cancer. However, Craig persevered and had the courage of his convictions that his laboratory research would save lives. As it turned out, tamoxifen has probably saved more lives than any other cancer therapeutic drug.

Craig also learned an important lesson at the WFEB around the time he was to leave and return to Leeds. A senior scientist at the WFEB, Dr. Eliahu Caspi, invited Craig to his office for an interview to explore the possibility of Craig staying at the WFEB. Craig recalls this was a very frightening experience, for Dr. Caspi had a no-nonsense personality, judged people, and said what he thought. He stated that he had been asked to evaluate my CV, as everybody was of the opinion that I would be a useful asset at the WFEB. He stared at Craig across the desk and said, "You don't have a CV, as you have no publications." After the initial shock, Craig responded, "But I haven't discovered anything yet." The advice Craig received was some of the best advice he had received thus far in his career. He was told "to tell them the story so far and link together several related publications to create a theme." Craig has done this ever since, creating the theme of tamoxifen. In 1998, with the release of the successful chemoprevention trial with tamoxifen, Craig was referred to as the "Father of Tamoxifen" by the *Chicago Tribune*, a title that has stuck to this day.

Although many people published using tamoxifen in their studies as a laboratory tool or used it in the 1960s in reproduction research, Craig's focus from the outset was clear; the goal was to develop a medicine for the treatment and prevention of breast cancer (he conducted the first chemopreventive study in the laboratory in 1974 [7], 3 years before the drug was approved by the FDA for the treatment of metastatic breast cancer in postmenopausal women). Craig stresses that but for the unrestricted support from ICI, meeting the right people and his uncompromising determination (many referred to this at the time as poor career judgment), tamoxifen would probably not have happened. Scientists at ICI did not conduct any studies with the drug as an antitumor agent. Indeed, in late 1972, all of the data with ICI 46,474 was reviewed and the research director terminated clinical trials and stopped the development project. The Marketing Department had decided that a treatment for metastatic breast cancer was not going to generate sufficient revenue.

Arthur Walpole was toward the end of his career and chose to take early retirement, but only agreed to remain an employee if funds could be given to a young man he had met, Craig Jordan, who (as he did) wanted to turn ICI 46,474 into

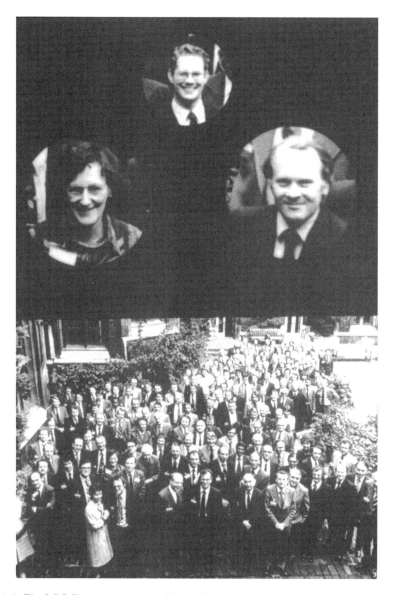

Fig. A.4 The I.C.I. Pharmaceuticals at King's College, Cambridge, Meeting in the summer of 1977. The goal of the meeting was physician education about research being done with tamoxifen. This was the first time I presented in public my ideas about targeting the tumor ER and using long-term treatment with tamoxifen as the best strategy to be applied to adjuvant therapy [5]. *Reviews on Endocrine-related Cancer* (49–55). However, the major presentation that made everything change clinically was in Arizona in 1979 [6]. In the above picture, Michael Baum (*right*), was the Chair of the session at King's College and stated that they had plans to use 2 years of tamoxifen as an adjuvant therapy (*on a hunch*). Helen Stewart (*left*) was considering starting a pilot trial in Scotland using 5 years of adjuvant tamoxifen for the treatment of patients. For the placebo arm, patients would be treated with tamoxifen at first recurrence. If toxicity was acceptable, they would

a drug to treat breast cancer. Walpole and Craig subsequently worked together on an ICI/University joint research scheme when Craig returned as lecturer in the Department of Pharmacology at the University of Leeds in September 1974. Earlier in his career, Dr. Walpole was an accomplished cancer research scientist, but had not been allowed to work in this area by ICI because fertility control was considered to be potentially more lucrative [8]. Dr. Walpole died suddenly on July 2, 1977, before he could witness the success of Craig's laboratory strategy for the treatment and prevention of breast cancer.

The clinical development of tamoxifen was very progressive and validated all your assumptions. Could you tell us how you were involved in the clinical evaluation and how you convinced the company to invest in what may have been very challenging trials?

I think it's fair to say that this was not the real story, but the real story is unbelievable. I have always considered my research as being a conversation between the laboratory and the clinic, and I had the privilege of first introducing tamoxifen to clinical trials' organizations in America. My objective was to provide a scientific rationale for the clinical studies in treatment and prevention. My research and qualifications were required to obtain approval for tamoxifen as a medicine in both Japan and Germany, and I was delighted to be the only person invited from outside of ICI Pharmaceuticals to attend a celebration in 1977, of the Queen's Award for Technological Achievement for tamoxifen. The surprising part about the tamoxifen story is that although patents for the drug were obtained by ICI Pharmaceuticals around the world, in the mid-1960s, these same patents were denied in the United States of America. Thus, all of the work I was completing on the antitumor actions of tamoxifen in the United States was done without patent protection for ICI. Looked at another way, it was clear that all the other pharmaceutical companies had no interest in the clinical development of tamoxifen, because either the drug was not going to work very well or not generate enough revenue. But it was my clinical strategy of long-term adjuvant therapy that saved lives and made revenues [9]. Clinical testing went ahead and when the patents expired in the rest of the world, ICI was awarded the patent for the use of tamoxifen in the treatment of breast cancer in 1985, but backdated to the original patent application in 1965. Now, extended adjuvant therapy was the practical solution for effective treatment. Thus, for the next 20 years, ICI was able to generate

---

Fig. A.4 (continued) move forward to test the idea of early long-term treatment or late treatment at first recurrence. Both trials showed survival advantages for long-term adjuvant tamoxifen. The week after the King's College Meeting, I was at the University of Wisconsin at their Comprehensive Cancer Center to convince clinicians of the Eastern Cooperative Oncology Group (ECOG) that longer was going to be better. At the time, tamoxifen was not on the market in America but I was talent spotted by Paul Carbone, the Head of ECOG and the director of the Comprehensive Cancer Center, to be recruited to the University of Wisconsin, Department of Human Oncology. Eventually, I would be the director of their Breast Cancer Research and Treatment Program

enormous revenues in the United States, as tamoxifen was the standard of care for long-term adjuvant tamoxifen therapy and the only game in town. This money catalyzed the advent of ICI marketing antiandrogens for prostate cancer and the aromatase inhibitors for breast cancer.

Watching your scientific activity since the beginning, you always seem fascinated by the development of small molecules since their conception up to their development. Is that what gives you much fun in your work?

I absolutely love experiments involving the structure-function relationships of the antiestrogens. My basic scientific research has been to create models of gene modulation or replication to determine the structure of the ER antiestrogen complex that subsequently could be interrogated. This passion resulted in a whole series of publications focused on the modulation of the prolactin gene [10–12] which then went through a metamorphosis to study the modulation of the SERM ER complex and the way that the ligand can interact with specific amino acids, thereby switching on or switching off the complex at target genes. We actually found the only natural mutation of the human ER in a laboratory model of tamoxifen-stimulated tumor growth [13]. We engineered the mutant ER into ER-negative breast cancer cells and found it would make the antiestrogen, raloxifene, an estrogen at the transforming growth factor-alpha (TGF-α) target gene. For me, this was important as one amino acid in the ER could change the pharmacology of raloxifene. In other words, this provided a fascinating insight into the relationship of the antiestrogenic side chain and a specific amino acid at the surface of the ER protein [14–17].

Do you think that a drug may have a commercial future in the chemoprevention of cancer?

As you know, we have made enormous progress with advancing the failed breast cancer drug, raloxifene, and millions of women are now benefiting from its use for the treatment of osteoporosis, but with a reduction in breast cancer incidence at the same time. This is the practical reality of our early translational research completed at the University of Wisconsin in the second decade of discovery (1980s). The "Tamoxifen Team" discovered selective estrogen receptor modulation and tamoxifen and raloxifene were both now classified as SERMs [18]. But the realization that tamoxifen could not possibly have widespread use because it increases the risk (though this is very small) of endometrial cancer in postmenopausal women [19], naturally guided us to our new SERM strategy in the late 1980s. We discovered that SERMs maintain bone density [20] and therefore could potentially prevent osteoporosis with the beneficial antiestrogenic side effect of preventing breast cancer [21]. We had solid translational research, as we had found that tamoxifen built bone both in the laboratory [20] and in clinical trial [22]. Raloxifene has a better safety profile and does not increase the risk of endometrial cancer [23], but it does not reduce the risk of coronary heart disease. I think the new SERM, lasofoxifene [24], is very good, as it prevents osteoporosis, breast cancer, coronary heart disease, and strokes, but without an increase of endometrial cancer. The problem is how to

advance in a crowded market with low budgets for marketing. Lasofoxifene is approved but not marketed in the European Union.

No molecule targeting estrogen receptor has, to date, proved to be more efficient than tamoxifen in patients despite the development of a number of promising compounds. How do you explain that? Was it a choice of the pharmaceutical industry because of the cost of the development of such compound?

The issue with tamoxifen is unique. It was clearly lucky that tamoxifen had an acceptable toxicology profile for the treatment of cancer. It came onto the market at a time when the standard of care was combination cytotoxic chemotherapy, so tamoxifen looked good to patients. Tamoxifen was not supposed to succeed but advanced from strength to strength for 20 years. However, things change very rapidly in the arena of patient preference. In the early 1990s, when tamoxifen was being considered for testing as a chemopreventive and the specter of endometrial cancer translated from the laboratory [19] to clinical practice, this was clearly not good news for well women. Worse still, tamoxifen was found to produce DNA adducts in rat liver and initiate rat liver hepatocarcinogenesis [25]. Although liver tumors did not translate to clinical practice, this did not lessen concern, as the drug ended up with a black box label as a human carcinogen. Timing is everything with discovery and competitors could never catch up with clinical testing, despite the fact they may have been safer. We will never know.

To demonstrate that natural or synthetic molecules can prevent the occurrence of cancer is long and expensive. This raises the question of the life of the patents but also the natural molecules, which may not be patentable. Do you think there may be solutions to these problems?

I think it's currently impossible to find a solution to this dilemma. Clearly, the pharmaceutical industry will never advance with 20 year studies because the patents will run out. But here is a controversial point: the success of healthcare has now created the situation of increased longevity, so that drugs that enhance survival through prevention can only make matters worse. What is society to do? How does society find the resources to support an aging population?

You have developed recently a very provocative approach using estrogens for the treatment of breast cancers. This can be considered as a paradoxical use of estrogens? Could you explain us a little bit about that.

The third and fourth decades have been a wonderful surprise in our journey of discovery. We posed the question (based upon the clinical acceptance of long-term antihormonal therapy [9] as the most appropriate adjuvant treatment for breast cancer), what would be the mechanism and the timeframe for acquired antihormone resistance? Our first model clearly showed something unique as far as drug resistance is concerned—SERM-stimulated growth, something that is not seen with any other drug in cancer therapy [26]. This form of resistance occurred within a year or two and was consistent with the development of acquired resistance to tamoxifen in metastatic breast cancer. However, here was the dilemma: this model did not replicate the outstanding success observed with 5 years of adjuvant tamoxifen treatment [27]. In fact, 5 years of treatment continues to enhance decreases in mortality for more than a decade once tamoxifen is stopped. By a series of lucky accidents, one of my students (Doug Wolf) discovered that physiologic estrogen could cause dramatic tumor regression after 5 years of tamoxifen treatment, i.e., serial transplantation of tamoxifen-resistant tumors into generations of tamoxifen-treated mice [28]. This discovery reminded me of the words of Sir Alexander Haddow, FRS in 1970 during the Inaugural Karnofsky Lecture at the American Society of Clinical Oncology (ASCO): "... the extraordinary extent of tumour regression observed in perhaps 1 % of post-menopausal cases (with oestrogen) has always been regarded as of major theoretical importance, and it is a matter for some disappointment that so much of the underlying mechanisms continues to elude us ..." [29]. It is now clear that aggressive estrogen deprivation with aromatase inhibitors or SERMs can rapidly reconfigure breast cancer cells through an evolution of drug resistance, which exposes a vulnerability that could not be anticipated—physiological estrogen-induced apoptosis [30, 31]. When Haddow did his original work using high-dose DES for the treatment of metastatic breast cancer in women during their late 60s and 70s, the best therapeutic results occurred the further away the patient was from the menopause. Antihormone therapy accelerates all of that in breast cancer, so physiologic estrogen can initiate the same triggering mechanism. Indeed, this is possibly the same mechanism that is occurring in the Women's Health Initiative (WHI) by conjugated equine estrogen (CEE) alone actually produces a decrease in the incidence of breast cancer in hysterectomized postmenopausal women [32]. What is particularly interesting about these data is the 6 years of monitoring after CEE is stopped, there is a continued reduction in the incidence of breast cancer, i.e., the estrogen has destroyed the nascent breast cancer cells in the ducts [33]. Our current laboratory work is focused entirely on deciphering the molecular mechanism of estrogen-induced apoptosis [34]. In this way, we may find the vulnerability triggered by the ER estrogen complex for cellular destruction; that vulnerable site in the cancer cell may be the next target for a new class of selective anticancer agents applicable to sites other than breast cancer.

Your contributions to medicine have received a lot of recognition but how does one become the "Diana, Princess of Wales Professor of Cancer Research"?

Life is all about chance meetings. In the mid-1990s, I was invited to organize a Breast Cancer Symposium in Chicago, and Diana was my keynote speaker (Fig. A.5). She came on a 3-day visit to Northwestern University and the Robert H. Lurie Comprehensive Cancer Center. Naturally, it was a very special time and when she left to return to London, we agreed to correspond and I sent her copies of my books on tamoxifen. There was even talk of a return trip for either her or Prince William or Prince Harry to open one of our new research buildings. Regrettably, everything changed with her untimely death in a tragic car accident in Paris on August 31, 1997. An anonymous donation was subsequently made to the Robert

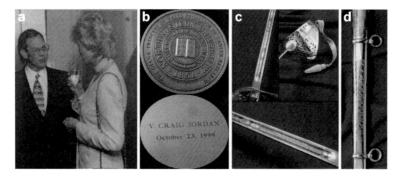

Fig. A.5 The Diana, Princess of Wales Chair of Cancer Research. In June 1996, Diana, the Princess of Wales visited Chicago for 3 days and we first met (**a**) at the evening reception at the home of the President of Northwestern University, Henry Bienen. The Chair was anonymously endowed at the Robert H. Lurie Comprehensive Cancer Center after Diana's untimely death on 31 August 1997. I was inaugurated on 23 October 1999, being presented with a unique Professorial medal (**b**) with copies being sent to her sons Prince William and Harry and also kept by my daughters, Helen and Alexandra. My students presented me with an engraved sword (**c**) to commemorate the event and their names, and the dates of the award of their Ph.D. degrees are engraved on the scabbard (**d**)

H. Lurie Comprehensive Cancer Center, and with letters from Lady Sarah McCorquodale (her sister) and the Earl Spencer (her brother), it was agreed that I would hold a professorship at Northwestern University in her name. Essentially, it was my British citizenship, a British medicine (tamoxifen), and our meeting and correspondence that was important to the family. On October 23, 1999, the Professorship was conferred on me by Henry Bienen, the president of Northwestern University, and over a 2-day period, there was a symposium in my honor by my former Ph.D. students, and during the celebration dinner, attended by representatives from the British Embassy, Barry Furr (the Chief Scientist from ICI), family, friends, and colleagues, my students presented me with an engraved sword (Fig. A.5) with each of the dates of their Ph.D. engraved on the scabbard as battle honors—very moving!

You have contributed more than 600 research and review papers to the literature with more than 23,000 citations and an h-index of 80. If you had to select ten of your research papers and three reviews, which would they be and why?

- Jordan V. C. (1976). *Eur J Cancer* 12: 419–424 [7]. Literally my first cancer research paper with tamoxifen that was rejected in 1974, but with kind and generous comments from one of the reviewers. I persevered and eventually this was one of the papers from my work used to justify the chemoprevention trials.
- Jordan V. C. and Allen K. E. (1980). *Eur J Cancer* 16: 239–251 [4]. The paper makes three points: this is the first refereed article that longer treatment is going to be better than shorter treatment; our discovery of 4-hydroxytamoxifen's

pharmacology as a potent antiestrogen with a binding affinity for ER equivalent to estradiols [35] naturally made us think that this would be a more powerful anticancer agent—not true, cleared too quickly—and finally, we stated that antiestrogen treatment followed by estrogen deprivation would be a good strategy for people—true.

- Gottardis M. M., et al. (1988). *Cancer Res* 48: 812–815 [19]. This was the paper that warned the clinical community that tamoxifen could potentially increase the incidence of endometrial cancer in patients—true.
- Gottardis M. M. and Jordan V. C. (1988). *Cancer Res* 48: 5183–5187 [26]. This was the first report that acquired drug resistance with tamoxifen was unique and stimulated by SERMs—true.
- Love R. R., et al. (1992). *New Engl J Med* 326: 852–856 [22]. This was the randomized clinical trial based on our laboratory evidence and subsequently those of others that tamoxifen would maintain bone density in people. This paper opened the door to raloxifene.
- Levenson A. S. and Jordan V. C. (1998). *Cancer Res* 58: 1872–1875 [14]. A clean demonstration that a mutant ER found in a tamoxifen-stimulated tumor by a previous Ph.D. student (Doug Wolf) could change an antiestrogen to an estrogen. This could be done by a natural process.
- Cummings S. R., et al. (1999). *JAMA* 281: 2189–2197 [23]. Proof of principle that the concept we first articulated back in the late 1980s that you could develop a SERM to prevent osteoporosis and prevent breast cancer at the same time—true.
- Yao K., et al. (2000). *Clin Cancer Res* 6: 2028–2036 [30]. The first refereed publication to demonstrate that drug resistance to tamoxifen evolves and exposes a vulnerability to permit physiologic estrogen to cause tumor regression. Subsequently translated to the clinic—true.
- Vogel V. G., et al. (2006). The Study of Tamoxifen and Raloxifene (STAR): Report of the National Surgical Adjuvant Breast and Bowel Project P-2 Trial. *JAMA*. 295: 2727–2741 [36]. Two discarded drugs from the pharmaceutical industry that were reinvented in the same pharmacology laboratory to become the pioneering chemopreventive agents and FDA-approved—true.
- Vogel V. G., et al. (2010). *Cancer Prev Res* 3: 696–706 [37]. A follow-up of the trial several years after stopping SERM treatment, confirmed the predictions of one of my Ph.D. students (Marco Gottardis) in 1987 that tamoxifen would be the better chemopreventive in the long term.

I've always viewed an invitation to write a review article from a journal as a wonderful opportunity to project your personality, express your views, and, most importantly, reach out to young scientists and graduate students as theirs is the future. Here are my three choices:

- Jordan V. C. (1984). *Pharm Rev* 36: 245–276 [39]. This was my first major review when I first came to America. No one had really treated the topic as an issue in pharmacology, as all of the previous reviews in the 1960s and 1970s were about the control of fertility. I wanted a summary of the mechanisms of action of antiestrogens. It was all of our knowledge up to that point (423 citations).

- Jordan V. C. (2006). *Br J Pharmacol* 147: S269–S276 [40]. I was thrilled to be asked by the British Pharmacological Society to write the story of my research in a Special Issue of our Journal. I got wonderful feedback from students.
- Jordan V. C. (2009). *Cancer Res.* 69: 1243–1254 [41]. I was proud to be asked by the American Association for Cancer Research (AACR) to contribute a review of progress in hormone dependent tumors as a part of a series to celebrate the 100th anniversary of AACR.

I see that you received the David A. Karnofsky Award in 2008 from ASCO, but it is stated in the regulations for the Award that it is given in "recognition of innovative clinical research and developments that have changed the way oncologists think about the general practice of oncology." You are a laboratory scientist and not a clinician; didn't this surprise you?

When I received the telephone call from the chair of the Awards Committee, Gabriel Hortobagyi, I was absolutely dumbfounded, because naturally, I knew I was not a clinician! All previous recipients were clinicians. This is ASCO's highest award, and I was being asked to join the legends of clinical practice. For the first 15 min of my conversation with Gabriel, I examined with him every reason why I should not be their recipient. After 15 min, he became exasperated and said, "Is this a 'Yes, I accept'?" I accepted the honor. Apparently, I learned that the reason the committee selected my work was because as a laboratory scientist and a pharmacologist, I had always been present at clinical breast cancer meetings over the decades, putting forward my point of view in cancer treatment with SERMs. For me, the promise of life was the most important goal. But safety was essential. The involvement I had every day with the clinical evaluation of tamoxifen [22], followed by leadership positions for the evaluation of raloxifene [23], and then as the scientific chair of the Study of Tamoxifen and Raloxifene (STAR) [36, 37] allowed me to deploy the knowledge generated by my "Tamoxifen Team" over decades to save lives and advance women's health [38]. Please remember that when I started this improbable and unlikely journey at the beginning of the 1970s, cancer therapeutics with a targeted agent, chemoprevention, and the drug group, SERMs (or even tamoxifen for that matter!) did not exist. Cancer research was not recommended as a career for the pharmacologist and the pharmacologist would not knowingly venture into women's health. All of the revenues in the pharmaceutical industry were derived from heart drugs and drugs that affected the central nervous system (e.g., tranquilizers).

When I was starting the research for my Ph.D. at Leeds University, Sir Alexander Haddow, FRS in the Inaugural Karnofsky Lecture [29], was dismayed at the prospect for cancer therapeutics. Unlike the success noted with antibiotics for the treatment of different infectious diseases, there were no laboratory tests to establish whether chemotherapy would be effective or not. The physician just had to give it to the patient and see if it worked! Haddow was also not convinced that a cancer-specific drug could be developed because cancer was self. In Haddow's Karnofsky Lecture publication, there was one glimmer of hope: Haddow had used the first chemical therapy to treat any cancer, i.e., high-dose estrogen to treat metastatic breast cancer in women in their late 60s and 70s. He observed that some of the responses just melted the tumors away. But he was dismayed that the mechanisms had remained elusive. I am pleased to say that we have now solved the question surrounding the mechanism of estrogen-induced apoptosis [34].

It is fair to say that the work that has evolved and developed on the treatment and prevention of breast cancer over the past four decades has changed our outlook and replaced pessimism with hope. The first decade of discovery was essential to move forward in the field [9]. It has not only been possible to create change in medical practice, but the laboratory principles all translated to patient care to save or at least extend lives. That is what pharmacology is.

In closing, I must end where we began. I have thanked Drs. Kaye and Clark (Fig. A.1) many times for the opportunity they gave me with a place at Leeds University. The reply I received was usually "we were only doing our job." Good words to remember and live by.

References

1. Jordan VC (2003) Tamoxifen: a most unlikely pioneering medicine. Nat Rev Drug Discov 2:205–213
2. Jordan VC (2007) Chemoprevention of breast cancer with selective oestrogen receptor modulators. Nat Rev Cancer 7:46–53
3. Jordan VC, Koerner S (1975) Tamoxifen (ICI46,474) and the human carcinoma 8S oestrogen receptor. Eur J Cancer 11:205–206
4. Jordan VC, Allen KE (1980) Evaluation of the antitumour activity of the nonsteroidal antioestrogen monohydroxytamoxifen in the DMBA-induced rat mammary carcinoma model. Eur J Cancer 16:239–251
5. Jordan VC (1978) Use of the DMBA-induced rat mammary carcinoma system for the evaluation of tamoxifen as a potential adjuvant therapy. Rev Endocr Relat Cancer Suppl:49–55
6. Jordan VC, Dix CJ, Allen KE (1979) The effectiveness of long term tamoxifen treatment in a laboratory model for adjuvant hormone therapy of breast cancer. In: Salmon SE, Jones SE (eds) Adjuvant therapy of cancer II. Grune & Stratton, Philadelphia, pp 19–26
7. Jordan VC (1976) Effect of tamoxifen (ICI46,474) on initiation and growth of DMBA-induced rat mammary carcinomata. Eur J Cancer 12:419–424
8. Jordan VC (1988) The development of tamoxifen for breast cancer therapy: a tribute to the late Arthur L. Walpole. Breast Cancer Res Treat 11:197–209
9. Jordan VC (2008) Tamoxifen: catalyst for the change to targeted therapy. Eur J Cancer 44:30–38
10. Lieberman ME, Jordan VC, Fritsch M, Santos MA, Gorski J (1983) Direct and reversible inhibition of estradiol-stimulated prolactin synthesis by antiestrogens in vitro. J Biol Chem 258:4734–4740
11. Lieberman ME, Gorski J, Jordan VC (1983) An estrogen receptor model to describe the regulation of prolactin synthesis by antiestrogens in vitro. J Biol Chem 258:4741–4745

12. Jordan VC, Lieberman ME (1984) Estrogen-stimulated prolactin synthesis in vitro classification of agonists, partial agonist and antagonist actions based on structure. Mol Pharm 26:279–285

13. Wolf DM, Jordan VC (1994) The estrogen receptor from a tamoxifen stimulated MCF-7 tumor variant contains a point mutation in the ligand binding domain. Breast Cancer Res Treat 31:129–138

14. Levenson AS, Jordan VC (1998) The key to the antiestrogenic mechanism of raloxifene is Amino Acid 351 (Asp) in the estrogen receptor. Cancer Res 58:1872–1875

15. Macgregor-Schafer JI, Liu H, Bentrem D, Zapf J, Jordan VC (2000) Allosteric silencing of activating function 1 in the 4-hydroxytamoxifen estrogen receptor complex by substituting glycine for aspartate at amino acid 351. Cancer Res 60:5097–5105

16. Liu H, Lee ES, De Los Reyes A, Zapf JW, Jordan VC (2001) Silencing and reactivation of the selective estrogen receptor modulator (SERM)-ER alpha complex. Cancer Res 61:3632–3639

17. Liu H, Park W, Bentrem DJ, McKian KP, De Los Reyes A, Macgregor-Schafer J, Zapf JW, Jordan VC (2002) Structure-function relationships of the raloxifene-estrogen receptor alpha complex for regulating transforming growth factor-alpha expression in breast cancer cells. J Biol Chem 277:9189–9198

18. Jordan VC (2001) Selective estrogen receptor modulation: a personal perspective. (Perspectives in Cancer Research). Cancer Res 61:5683–5687

19. Gottardis MM, Robinson SP, Satyaswaroop PG, Jordan VC (1988) Contrasting actions of tamoxifen on endometrial and breast tumor growth in the athymic mouse. Cancer Res 48:812–815

20. Jordan VC, Phelps E, Lindgren JU (1987) Effects of antiestrogens on bone in castrated and intact female rats. Breast Cancer Res Treat 10:31–35

21. Gottardis MM, Jordan VC (1987) The antitumor actions of keoxifene (raloxifene) and tamoxifen in the N-nitrosomethylurea-induced rat mammary carcinoma model. Cancer Res 47:4020–4024

22. Love RR, Mazess RB, Barden HS, Epstein S, Newcomb PA, Jordan VC, Carbone PP, Demets DL (1992) Effects of tamoxifen on bone mineral density in postmenopausal women with breast cancer. N Eng J Med 326:852–856

23. Cummings SR, Eckert S, Krueger KA, Grady D, Powles TJ, Cauley JA, Norton L, Nickelsen T, Bjarnason NH, Morrow M, Lippman ME, Black D, Glusman JE, Costa A, Jordan VC (1999) The effect of raloxifene on risk of breast cancer in postmenopausal women: results from the MORE randomized trial. JAMA 281:2189–2197

24. Cummings SR, Ensrud K, Delmas PD, Reid DM, Goldstein S, Sriram U, Lee A, Thompson J, Armstrong RA, Thompson DD, Powles T, Zanchetta J, Kendler D, Neven P, Eastell R (2010) Lasofoxifene in postmenopausal women with osteoporosis. N Engl J Med 362:686–696

25. Jordan VC (1995) What if tamoxifen (ICI46,474) had been found to produce liver tumors in rats in 1973? Ann Oncol 6:29–43

26. Gottardis MM, Jordan VC (1988) Development of tamoxifen-stimulated growth of MCF-7 tumors in athymic mice after long-term antiestrogen administration. Cancer Res 48:5183–5187

27. Early Breast Cancer Trialists' Collaborative Group (EBCTCG) (2011) Relevance of breast cancer hormone receptors and other factors to the efficacy of adjuvant tamoxifen: patient-level meta-analysis of randomised trials. Lancet 378:771–784

28. Wolf DM, Jordan VC (1993) A laboratory model to explain the survival advantage observed in patients taking adjuvant tamoxifen therapy. Recent Results Cancer Res 127:23–33

29. Haddow A, David A (1970) Karnofsky memorial lecture. Thoughts on chemical therapy. Cancer 26:737–754

30. Yao K, Lee ES, Bentrem DJ, England G, Schafer JIM, O'Regan R, Jordan VC (2000) Antitumor action of physiologic estradiol on tamoxifen-stimulated breast tumors grown in athymic mice. Clin Cancer Res 6:2028–2036

31. Lewis JS, Meeke K, Osipo C, Ross EA, Kidawi N, Li Y, Bell E, Chandel NS, Jordan VC (2005) Intrinsic mechanism of estradiol-induced apoptosis in breast cancer cells resistant to estrogen deprivation. J Natl Cancer Inst 97:1746–1759

32. Anderson GL, Chlebowski RT, Aragaki AK et al (2012) Conjugated equine oestrogen and breast cancer incidence and mortality in postmenopausal women with hysterectomy: extended follow-up of the Women's Health Initiative randomised placebo-controlled trial. Lancet Oncol 13(5):476–486

33. Jordan VC, Ford LS (2011) Paradoxical clinical effect of estrogen on breast cancer risk: A "new" biology of estrogen-induced apoptosis. Cancer Prev Res 4:633–637

34. Ariazi EA, Cunliffe HE, Lewis-Wambi JS, Slifker MJ, Willis AL, Ramos P, Tapia C, Kim HR, Yerrum S, Sharma CGN, Nicolas E, Balagurunathan Y, Ross EA, Jordan VC (2011) Estrogen induces apoptosis in estrogen deprivation-resistant breast cancer via stress responses as identified by global gene expression across time. Proc Natl Acad Sci U S A 108 (47):18879–18886

35. Jordan VC, Collins MM, Rowsby L, Prestwich G (1977) A monohydroxylated metabolite of tamoxifen with potent antiestrogenic activity. J Endocrinol 75:305–316

36. Vogel VG, Costantino JP, Wickerham DL, Cronin WM, Cecchini RS, Atkins JN, Bevers TB, Fehrenbacher L, Pajon ER, Wade JL, Robidoux A, Margolese RG, James J, Lippman SM, Runowicz CD, Ganz PA, Reis SE, McCaskill-Stevens W, Ford LG, Jordan VC, Wolmark N (2006) The Study of Tamoxifen and Raloxifene (STAR): report of the National Surgical Adjuvant Breast and Bowel Project P-2 Trial. JAMA 295:2727–2741

37. Vogel VG, Costantino JP, Wickerham DL, Cronin WM, Cecchini RS, Atkins JN, Bevers TB, Fehrenbacher L, Pajon ER, Wade JL, Robidoux A, Margolese RG, James J, Runowicz CD, Ganz PA, Reis SE, McCaskill-Stevens W, Ford LG, Jordan VC, Wolmark N (2010) Update of the NSABP Study of Tamoxifen and Raloxifene (STAR) P-2 Trial: preventing breast cancer. Cancer Prev Res 3:696–706

38. Jordan VC (2008) The 38th David A. Karnofsky lecture: the paradoxical actions of estrogen in breast cancer–survival or death? J Clin Oncol 26:3073–3082

39. Jordan VC (1984) Biochemical pharmacology of antiestrogen action. Pharm Rev 36:245–276

40. Jordan VC (2006) 75th Anniversary Edition British Journal of Pharmacology Special Issue. Tamoxifen (ICI46,474) as a targeted therapy to treat and prevent breast cancer. Br J Pharmacol 147:S269–S276

41. Jordan VC (2009) A century of deciphering the control mechanisms of sex steroid action in breast and prostate cancer: the origins of targeted therapy and chemoprevention. Cancer Res 69:1243–1254

Appendix B: Selected Awards That Recognize the Contribution of Tamoxifen and Raloxifene to Medicine

2013	Fellow of the AACR Academy
2013	Fellow of the City and Guilds (London)
2012	ASPET Goodman and Gilman Award
2011	St. Gallen International Breast Cancer Award
2009	Elected to National Academy of Sciences (USA) (Fig. A.6)
2009	Fellow of the Academy of Medical Sciences (UK)
2008	Honorary Fellowship of the Royal Society of Medicine (Fig. A.7)
2008	American Society of Clinical Oncology 38th David A. Karnofsky Award
2007	Gregory G. Pincus Award and Medal. Worcester Foundation for Biomedical Research
2006	American Society Award for Chemoprevention, American Society of Clinical Oncology
2005–2009	Endowed Chair: Alfred G Knudson Chair in Basic Science, Fox Chase Comprehensive Cancer Center
2005	Honorary Doctor of Science Degree. University of Bradford, England
2003	The Charles F. Kettering Prize of the General Motors Cancer Research Foundation.
2002	Officer of the Most Excellent Order of the British Empire (OBE)
2002	American Cancer Society Medal of Honor (Basic Research Award).
2002	Inaugural Dorothy P. Landon American Association for Cancer Research (AACR) Prize in Translational Research.
2001	Bristol Myers Squibb Award and Medal for Distinguished Achievement in Cancer Research
2001	Honorary Doctor of Medicine Degree. University of Leeds, England
2001	Honorary Doctor of Science Degree. University of Massachusetts
2000	Strang Award. Cornell Medical School
2000	Honorary Fellowship Award and Medal. Faculty of Medicine of University Colllege, Dublin
1999–2004	Endowed Chair: Diana, Princess of Wales Professor of Cancer Research, Robert H. Lurie Cancer Center, Northwestern University Feinberg School of Medicine
1994	William L. McGuire Memorial Award. San Antonio Breast Cancer Symposium
1993	Cameron Prize Award. University of Edinburgh
1993	American Society for Pharmacology and Experimental Therapeutics Award for Experimental Therapeutics. Contributions to research on human disease

(continued)

1993	Gaddum Memorial Award for research contributions to pharmacology, British Pharmacological Society
1992	Inaugural Brinker International Breast Cancer Award for Basic Science. Susan G. Komen Foundation
1989	Eighth Bruce F. Cain Memorial Award American Association for Cancer Research

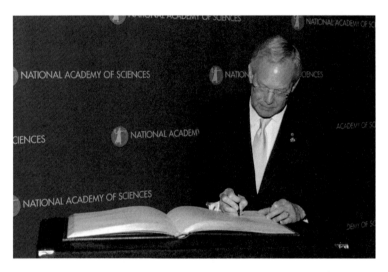

Fig. A.6 Signing the "Great Book" of Members of the National Academy of the Sciences USA during the Induction Ceremony on April 24, 2010

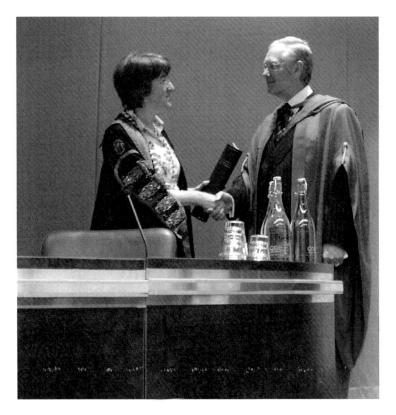

Fig. A.7 Honorary Fellowship of the Royal Society of Medicine awarded by Professor Ilora Finlay, Baroness Finlay of Llandaff, president of the Royal Society of Medicine (2008). This honor is awarded to individuals of international standing who have eminently distinguished themselves in the service of medicine and the fields which influence it. The Society permits, at most, 100 people into this elite group at any one time. In 2008, there were only 89 Honorary Fellows worldwide. In 2009, I received the Jephcott Medal from the Royal Society of Medicine, and in 2010, I was elected as the president of the Royal Society of Medicine Foundation in North America

Printed by Publishers' Graphics LLC
LMO130809.15.16.22